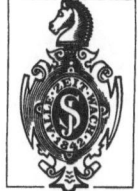

H. K. Seitz U. A. Simanowski N. A. Wright (Eds.)

Colorectal Cancer:
From Pathogenesis to Prevention?

Foreword by B. C. Morson

With 34 Figures

Springer-Verlag Berlin Heidelberg New York
London Paris Tokyo 1989

Priv.-Doz. Dr. med. Helmut Karl Seitz
Medizinische Universitätsklinik
Innere Medizin IV (Gastroenterologie)
Bergheimer Straße 58
D-6900 Heidelberg 1

Dr. med. Ulrich A. Simanowski
Medizinische Universitätsklinik
Innere Medizin IV (Gastroenterologie)
Bergheimer Straße 58
D-6900 Heidelberg 1

Professor Dr. med. Nicholas A. Wright
Department of Histopathology
Royal Postgraduate Medical School
Hammersmith Hospital
Du Cane Road
London W12 0HS, UK

ISBN 978-3-642-85932-8   ISBN 978-3-642-85930-4 (eBook)
DOI 10.1007/978-3-642-85930-4

Library of Congress Cataloging-in-Publication Data
Colorectal cancer. Includes index.
1. Colon (Anatomy)–Cancer–Etiology. 2. Colon (Anatomy)–Cancer–Prevention. 3. Rectum–Cancer–
Etiology. 4. Rectum–Cancer–Prevention. I. Seitz, H. K. (Helmut Karl), 1950–. II. Simanowski,
U. A. (Ulrich Arno), 1949–. III. Wright, Nicholas A. [DNLM: 1. Carcinoma. 2. Colorectal Neoplasms.
WI 520 C719364] RC280.C6C666 1989 616.99′4347 89-5871
ISBN 978-3-642-85932-8

© Springer-Verlag Berlin Heidelberg 1989
Softcover reprint of the hardcover 1st edition 1989

Typesetting: Konrad Triltsch, Würzburg.

2123/3020-543210 – Printed on acid-free paper

To Gisela and Steffi

Foreword

The past 20 years have seen a surge of research into colorectal cancer, which is a reflection of the need to improve our methods of treating patients suffering from this increasingly common form of cancer. Greater knowledge of the basic mechanisms involved in colorectal carcinogenesis is an essential prerequisite to improvements in cancer prevention.

In this volume the editors have brought together an impressive list of experts to cover the epidemiology, pathophysiology, morphology and basis for new diagnostic and therapeutic approaches to early detection and prevention. This broad scientific approach provides the reader with up-to-date review of our current state of knowledge of colorectal carcinogenesis and indicates how this information can be used to generate more research and create new opportunities for diagnosis and treatment.

This is a book of knowledge and ideas, some of them still at the stage of theoretical interest, but others with practical potential for the care of patients. I recommend it to those who have a research interest in colorectal carcinogenesis, as well as to readers who wish to know just how far medical scientists have progressed in their efforts to achieve the ideal of cancer prevention.

London, Spring 1989

Basil C. Morson, C.B.E., V.R.D., F.R.C.P., F.R.C.S., F.R.C.P.ath.

Preface

Colorectal carcinoma represents one of the most common cancers and therefore one of the leading causes of death in the highly industrialized countries. Migration studies have shown that exogenous factors, especially diet, play an important role in its aetiology. Abundance (e.g., fat) and deficiency (e.g., fiber) characterize the Western diet, and both seem to play significant roles in the pathogenesis of colorectal cancer.

During the last three decades major approaches have been directed at finding therapeutic measures against tumors already present, neglecting the preventive approach. In spite of innumerable efforts, the results to date have been disappointing.

In 1986 Bailar and Smith (New England Journal of Medicine 314: 1226–1232) published a large retrospective survey concerning the development of cancer mortality patterns in the United States from 1950 to 1982. The National Cancer Institute have announced that their goal is to achieve a 50% reduction in cancer-related mortality by the year 2000 (see Fig.). However, since 1950, the overall cancer mortality has risen continuously instead of falling. It seems unrealistic to expect that, in spite of all the tremendous but futile financial and scientific effort, we will soon find a major breakthrough in cancer treatment which will increase cure rates in the near future and reduce current cancer mortality by 50%. Bailar and Smith have therefore concluded

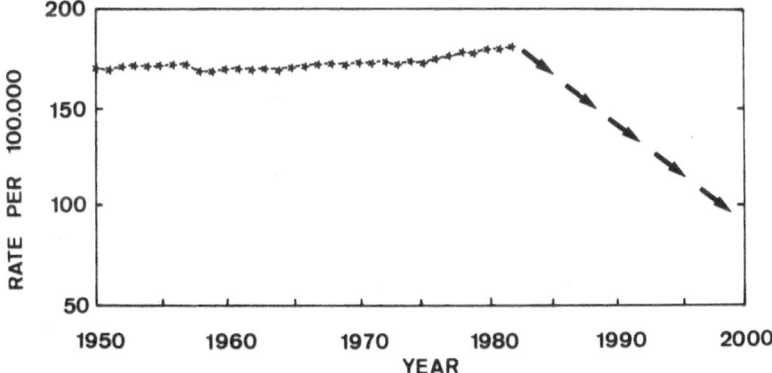

Fig. 1. Mortality from cancer of all sites, 1950 through 1982, in the United States population. Age was adjusted to the United States population of 1980. Extension to the year 2000 is shown to reflect the stated goal of the National Cancer Institute. (Reprinted, by permission of the New England Journal of Medicine 314: 1226, 1986)

"that some 35 years of intense effort focused largely on improving treatment must be judged as a qualified failure. ... On the basis of past medical experience with infectious and other nonmalignant diseases, however, we suspect that the most promising areas are in cancer prevention rather than treatment. ... Such a shift in research emphasis seems necessary if substantial progress against cancer is to be forthcoming." We believe that this statement is especially true for colorectal cancer.

This book compiles the current knowledge and concepts concerning the epidemiology and aetiology of colorectal cancer from the viewpoint of different scientific methodologies, which we hope will prepare the ground for a preventative approach to this problem of deep political, scientific and, not least importantly, humane concern.

Heidelberg and London, April 1989   Helmut K. Seitz
                                                                     Ulrich A. Simanowski
                                                                     Nicholas A. Wright

Table of Contents

Epidemiology

Geographic Epidemiology of Colorectal Cancer: The Role of Dietary Fat

G. N. Stemmermann

Japan-Hawaii Cancer Study, Kuakini Medical Center, 347 N. Kuakini Street, Honolulu, Hawaii 96817, USA

Contents

> It is well documented that Western style nutrition with a fat intake of approximately 40% of calories is associated with a higher risk of cancer of the breast, ovary and endometrium ... and quite definitely with left sided colon cancer
>
> Weisburger (1986).

> Our findings stress even more strongly that the effects of migration on cancer occurring are complex and that the Westernization of diet is a gross oversimplification; and by itself it provides an inadequate explanation for the gradients of cancer incidence in migrant populations
>
> Shimizu et al. (1987).

Introduction

The divergent views expressed by these two statements reflect the general lack of agreement as to the importance of dietary fat upon the induction and promotion of large bowel cancer. This chapter will summarize information in respect of the geographic distribution of large bowel cancer and will attempt to explain the basis of the controversial views concerning the impact of fat upon colorectal cancer risk. Special emphasis will be given to studies of indigenous and migrant Japanese because they are frequently cited as evidence that fat intake is a major risk factor for large bowel cancer.

Geographic Variation in Cancer of the Large Bowel

The first precise documentation of the great geographic variation in the frequency of cancer of the colon and rectum appeared in Segi's now classic tabulations of cancer mortality (1960) and mortality from other diseases (Segi et al. 1966) in 30 countries. His tables indicated that in the years 1952–1953, Japanese men had the lowest colon cancer age-adjusted mortality rates −2.2; while highest rates were found in men in Scotland −20.1. Subsequent editions of these tabulations were expanded to include mortality data from an additional 22 countries (Segi 1984). The international variation of colon cancer mortality rates from these expanded tables is shown in Fig. 1. The ten populations with the highest colon cancer mortality rates live in the prosperous countries of western Europe, North America, Australia, and New Zealand. The ten populations with the lowest rates live in the developing countries of Latin America, Africa, and Southeast Asia. The international differences in rectal cancer mortality are not as great as in colon cancer.

There are significant geographic variations in the mortality rates for large bowel cancer within specific countries. Thus, mortality rates for colorectal cancer are highest in the northeastern region of the United States (Blot et al. 1976) and, in all regions, they are highest in urban areas with high income. The highest death rates in China are found along the Yangtse River and in the central provinces on the eastern coast (Li 1982). The Chinese pattern may be related to the distribution of schistosomiasis japonica rather than variations in life style or diet.

Colon cancer in Japan shows distinct regional gradients that are not apparent with rectal cancer (Tajima et al. 1985). Male death rates from colon cancer are highest in Niigata prefecture and in the major metropolitan centers (e.g., Tokyo, Kanagawa, Nagoya, Osaka, Kyoto, Fukuoka), while female death rates are highest in northern Japan, Tokyo, and Kanagawa. The tendency for the highest rates to occur in an urban setting is consistent with registry data from other populations (see below).

Similar geographic variations in large bowel cancer incidence rates have been recorded in tumor registries from the five continents (Waterhouse et al. 1982). This tabulation also documents steep urban-rural and intraregistry racial gradients in the incidence rates of these tumors, with urban rates generally higher than rural rates. Thus the Warsaw, Poland registry lists urban, male colon cancer rates to be 11.6, while the rural rates are 5.2. A rural to urban gradient probably explains the observations in Austria that found higher incidence of colorectal cancer in Vienna than in Tyrol (Hanusch et al. 1985).

Wide racial variations in colon cancer incidence rates have been recorded in the United States, New Zealand, and Singapore (Waterhouse et al. 1982). United States Whites have much higher rates than Amerindians or Hispanics. Polynesians in New Zealand and Hawaii display much lower rates than the Caucasian populations of these registries, while the Malay and Indian populations show much lower rates than

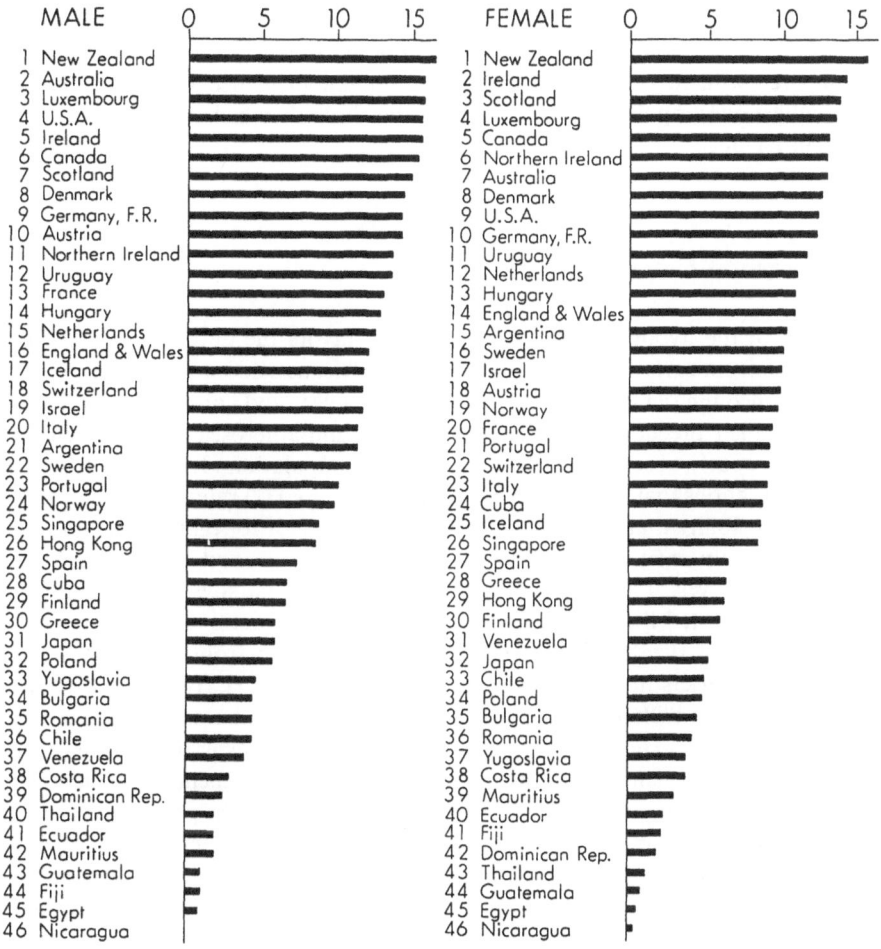

Fig. 1. The age-adjusted death rates for malignant neoplasms of the the intestine except rectum, 1978, from 46 different countries. (Adapted from Segi 1984)

do Chinese in Singapore. As in international studies, these subsets of populations show smaller urban-rural and racial contrasts when rectal cancer is the targeted tumor.

The concept that environmental differences account for these variations in colon cancer incidence and mortality is based on the observation that migrants from low-risk countries acquire the risk of the host countries. This observation has been made among Polish migrants to the United States (Staszewski and Haenszel 1965) and Australia (Staszewski et al. 1971), and Japanese migrants to Hawaii (Haenszel and Kurihara 1968). The post-World War II prosperity of Japan has been marked by a gradual evolution toward a Western life style. This represents migration in time rather than space and has also resulted in a rising incidence of colon cancer (Aoki et al. 1987).

The Japanese migrants to Hawaii have been considered ideal subjects for assessing the impact of different epidemiologic variables upon disease trends because they can be compared with two populations that yield reliable incidence and mortality data – the indigenous population of Japan and the discrete racial populations of the Hawaiian Islands.

Fat-Colorectal Cancer Hypothesis

The origin of the hypothesis that a high-fat diet favors the development of colon cancer dates from early observations that black Africans seldom developed diseases commonly encountered in Western society. Colon cancer and coronary heart disease (CHD) and their precursors, adenomatous polyps and atherosclerosis, respectively, were conspicuously absent from the black African population (Trowell and Burkitt 1981). Observations that Japanese experienced very low CHD rates (Keys et al. 1967) raised the possibility that fat intake was a major risk factor for that disease since the Japanese diet contained very little fat by Western standards, and Japanese had very low blood lipid levels. The observation that Japanese also had low colon cancer rates (Segi 1960) suggested that fat intake might influence this tumor as well.

Almost 90% of the Japanese migrants to Hawaii came from economically depressed rural districts in the following prefectures: Hiroshima, Yamaguchi, Kumamoto, Fukuoka, and Okinawa. They were hired as contract laborers in the sugar and pineapple industries. Those who remained in Hawaii at the expiration of their contracts gained employment as artisans, small merchants, and independent farmers. The second generation continued in these trades, and many entered the professions as well. The long-term result has been increasing affluence and employment in less physically demanding occupations. It is apparent that epidemiologic studies of the impact of the environment upon the shift in the frequency of any disease in this population should take more than diet into account.

Table 1 lists the macronutrient consumption of 2183 Japanese men living in Hiroshima, Japan, and 8006 Japanese men living in Honolulu, Hawaii, during the years 1965–1968. The data were derived from a 24-h recall examination of the two cohorts (Kagan et al. 1974). The migrants consumed more energy, protein, fat, cholesterol, and sucrose than their Hiroshima contemporaries, and smaller quantities of complex carbohydrate.

Dietary, social, and economic changes have resulted in major differences in the physical and biochemical characteristics of the two populations, as shown in Table 2. Hawaiian men are taller and heavier than those in Hiroshima. Their increased weight is due to subcutaneous fat rather than muscle mass. They also have higher hematocrit, serum cholesterol, and uric acid levels. In the case of body weight, back skinfold, and serum cholesterol, the differences are wider among the youngest men. This probably reflects the experience of first generation migrants who are concentrated among the oldest men and show the least Western acculturation.

It is unlikely that fat intake alone accounts for all of these changes, but it has been anticipated that the increased frequency of CHD and colon cancer among Hawaiian Japanese would be characterized by increased consumption of fat and a reduced

Table 1. Mean diet values of Japanese men in Japan and Hawaii from 24-h recall

Nutrient	Japan	Hawaii
Calories	2132	2274
Total protein (g)	76	94
(%)[a]	14.3	16.7
Animan protein	40	71
Vegetable protein	37	24
Total fat (g)	36	85
(%)[a]	14.1	33.2
Total carbohydrate (g)	339	260
(%)	63.2	46.4
Alcohol (g)	28	13
(%)[a]	8.7	3.7
Cholesterol (mg)	457	545

[a] Percentage of total calories.

Table 2. Mean values for selected variables by age and site

Variable	Site	Age				
		45–59	50–54	55–59	60–64	65–69
Men (n)	J	322	436	454	519	452
	H	1832	2792	1593	1338	451
Height (cm)	J	162.1	161.6	161.0	159.6	158.9
	H	164.3	163.6	162.6	160.5	159.8
Weight (kg)	J	55.3	56.1	55.5	53.7	51.7
	H	65.9	64.3	62.8	60.3	59.3
Arm skinfold (mm)	J	7.7	8.0	8.4	8.2	7.5
	H	8.0	8.0	8.0	7.8	8.1
Back skinfold (mm)	J	9.9	10.5	10.7	10.4	9.3
	H	17.4	16.7	16.3	15.5	14.9
Hematocrit (%)	J	43.6	43.1	42.7	41.8	41.9
	H	45.1	44.8	44.6	44.2	44.0
Cholesterol (mg/100 ml)	J	176.3	176.4	174.9	178.1	176.6
	H	219.4	219.4	218.7	216.7	211.1
Uric acid (mg/100 ml)	J	5.3	5.4	5.3	5.3	5.5
	H	6.1	6.0	5.9	5.9	6.0

J, Japan; H, Hawaii

intake of complex carbohydrate among those who subsequently developed both diseases.

This was not an unreasonable hypothesis. With few exceptions, the two diseases tend to be most common in the same countries (Fig. 2) and both occur more frequently in Hawaiian Japanese than those in Japan. Correlational studies have shown a close association between national per capita fat intake and colon cancer (Armstrong and Doll 1975), and several experimental studies have supported these results. High fat

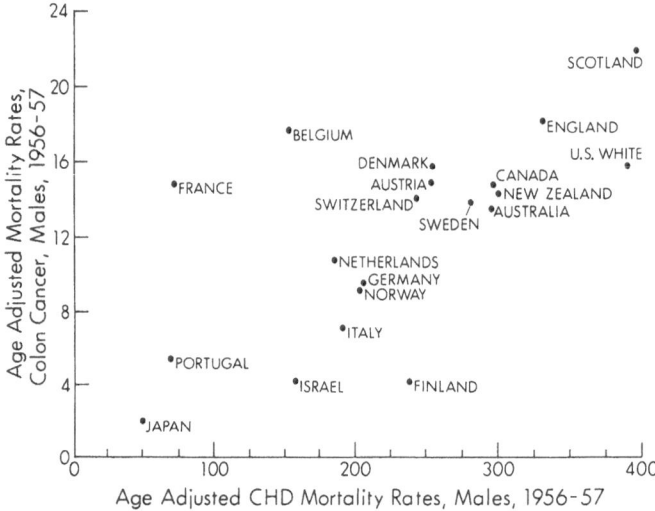

Fig. 2. Comparison between age-adjusted death rates from colon cancer and CHD, 20 countries. (Adapted from Segi 1960; Segi et al. 1966)

intake increases the frequency of large bowel cancer in rats exposed to a variety of carcinogens (Reddy et al. 1974, 1977) as does an atherogenic diet (Broitman et al. 1977). The replacement of complex carbohydrate by fat in the diet raises the level of serum cholesterol, an established risk factor for CHD (Keys et al. 1967).

Although Hawaiian Japanese show increased mortality and incidence rates for both CHD and colon cancer, the match is not perfect. Their colon cancer rates exceed those of their Caucasian neighbors (Waterhouse et al. 1982), but their CHD rates are intermediate between those of Japan and United States Whites (Haenszel and Kurihara 1968). Colon cancer rates are rising steeply among Hawaiian Japanese (Stemmermann et al. 1987), but their CHD rates are stable (Reed and Feinlieb 1983).

These inconsistencies are reproduced in other populations. Thus CHD rates are high in Finland, but colon cancer rates are low (Fig. 2). Native Hawaiians experience high rates of CHD (Reed and Feinlieb 1983), but low rates of colon cancer (Waterhouse et al. 1982). A similar pattern is found among Maoris in New Zealand. Specifically, Maori CHD rates equal those of non-Maoris and are rising (Prior and Tasman-Jones 1981), while their colon rates are only one-half of those of non-Maoris and are falling (Smith et al. 1985). France, where CHD mortality rates are low and colon cancer rates are high (Fig. 2), represents a contrasting pattern. It is apparent, therefore, that if increased fat intake does favor the development of either CHD or colon cancer, it probably does not act alone, nor does it have an equal influence on the two diseases.

An indirect relation between fat intake and colon cancer has been proposed through its influence upon the degradation of bile salts (Hill et al. 1977) and upon the level of fecal neutral steroids (Hill and Aries 1971; Wynder and Reddy 1974). Each of these is the subject of a separate chapter in this volume and will only be discussed briefly here in respect of the Hawaiian Japanese experience.

Hawaiian Japanese have higher fecal concentrations of deoxycholic acid (a degraded bile acid) than Japanese in Akita prefecture (Mower et al. 1979). The findings for other bile acids were unremarkable or inconsistent with the hypothesis that high levels of degraded bile acids increase colon cancer risk. Fecal bile acid production was not associated with Western foods, but two Japanese foods (pickled turnip and pickled plum) were negatively associated with modified fecal bile acids (Mower et al. 1978). These results suggest, but do not strongly support, a relation between bile salts and colon cancer risk.

Hawaiian Japanese have higher fecal concentrations of cholesterol and animal steroids than Japanese in Akita prefecture. There are no statistically significant differences in the concentrations of degraded coprostanol and coprostanone. The degraded fractions are actually greater in Akita than Hawaii (Nomura et al. 1983). These findings do not support a relation between fecal neutral steroid patterns and colon cancer risk.

Fat Intake and Colon Cancer: Other Correlational Studies

There were major changes in patterns of food consumption in Japan in the 20 years from 1959 to 1979 (Kuratsune et al. 1986), as shown in Table 3. Fat intake more than doubled, and animal protein consumption rose 1.2 times. Carbohydrate intake dropped, but energy intake was stable over time. This shift in dietary practice was greatest in the major metropolitan centers and least in rural communities (Tajima et al. 1985). It was matched by an increased mortality from left-sided colon cancer that was most conspicuous in urban centers. This has been attributed to a greater degree of westernization of the diet of urban Japanese.

Other correlational studies have failed to show an association between fat intake and colon cancer risk. These include Mormons and non-Mormons in Utah (Lyon and Sorenson 1978), Hawaiians and other races in Hawaii as show in Fig. 3 (Kolonel et al. 1981), and Maoris in New Zealand (Smith et al. 1985). The Maori experience is especially noteworthy. Maori males derive 46% of their calories from fat (F), with 39% from carbohydrate (C) (F : C = 1.18) (Prior and Tasman-Jones 1981). This compares with Hawaiian Japanese men who derive 33.5% of their calories from fat, with 46.4% derived from carbohydrate (F : C = 0.72) (Stemmermann et al. 1984), but who have colon cancer rates three-fold higher than those of Maoris (Waterhouse et al. 1982).

Table 3. Energy and nutrient intake per head by Japanese in 1959, 1970, and 1979. (From Kuratsune et al. 1986)

Year	Calories	Protein			Fat	Carbo-hydrate
		Total	Animal	Vegetable		
	(kcal)	(g)	(g)	(g)	(g)	(g)
1959	2148	70.1	24.3	45.8	24.0	413
1970	2210	77.6	34.2	43.4	46.5	368
1979	2113	78.4	39.4	39.0	54.8	315

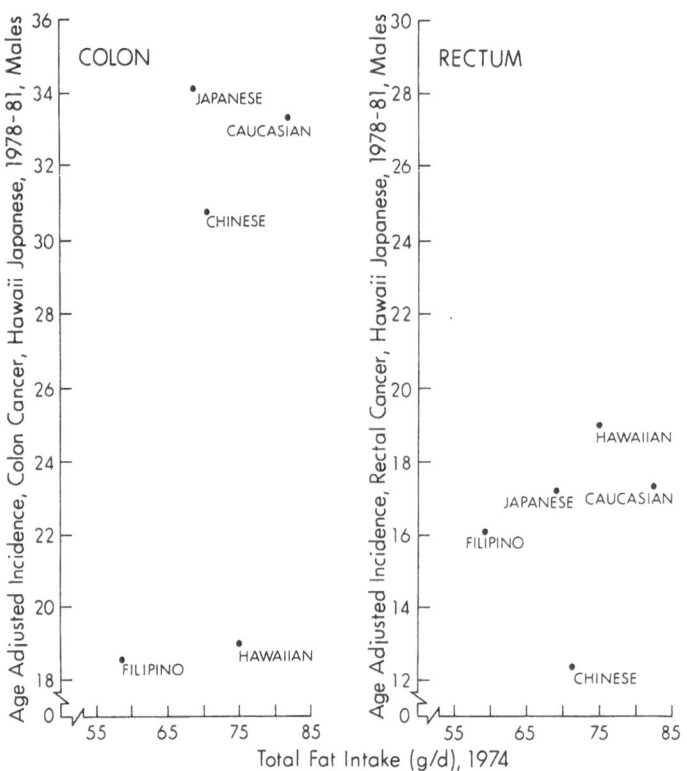

Fig. 3. The relation of fat intake to the age-adjusted incidence rates of colon and rectal cancer among men of different races in Hawaii. (Adapted from Hawaii Tumor Registry, unpublished data; Kolonel et al. 1981)

The inconsistencies that have emerged from these correlational studies have been attributed in part to the inability of identifying the dietary practices of those members of any population who actually acquire colon cancer. Moreover, information is not available concerning other factors that might influence cancer risk in large populations (e.g., obesity, occupation, alcohol consumption).

Measurements of the impact of different variables upon cancer risk of specific individuals can be performed directly, using one of two methods: the case-control study and the prospective cohort study. Although each method compares the experience of cancer patients with control subjects, they are not without their own problems. Dietary data collected for prospective studies might not hold true for the future, and dietary measurements taken at the time of cancer diagnosis might not reflect past experience.

Fat Intake and Colon Cancer: Case-Control Studies

A recent review (Kolonel 1987) lists 11 case-control studies that assess the impact of fat intake upon colon cancer risk, and at least six more have appeared since then

(Berry et al. 1986; Berta et al. 1985; Kune et al. 1987; MacQuart-Moulin et al. 1986; Potter and McMichael 1986; Tuyns 1986). Of these 17 reports, seven show an association between dietary fat and colon cancer, and ten do not. In some of these studies, the level of fat intake was inferred from the data on meat consumption. Two of these involve Japanese subjects: Hawaiian Japanese showed a direct association between meat intake and colorectal cancer (Haenszel et al. 1973), while the Japanese in Miyagi did not (Haenszel et al. 1980). It is apparent that the case-control approach has not resolved the inconsistencies that have emerged from correlational studies.

Fat Intake and Colon Cancer: Prospective Studies

None of the five prospective studies cited by Kolonel (1987) shows a direct association between fat and colon cancer. In addition, a study of parallel cohorts in Norway and Minnesota failed to show an association between meat and colon cancer (Bjelke 1978). Two cohort studies involve Japanese subjects. Hirayama (1981) found an inverse relation between meat intake and colon cancer in Japan, as did a study of the Japan-Hawaii cohort study of Hawaiian Japanese men (Stemmermann et al. 1984b). The updated data from the Hawaiian study are reproduced in Table 4 and include the results of a parallel study of CHD in this population. Fat intake is inversely related to colon cancer risk whether stated as grams per day or as a percentage of total calories. Rectal cancer is not associated with fat intake by either measurement, while CHD is directly and significantly related to protein and fat intake as a percentage of total calories, and inversely related to carbohydrate intake (McGee et al. 1984). These data support the hypothesis that CHD and colon cancer affect different subsets of the westernized Japanese population.

It should not be inferred that an inverse relation between dietary fat and colon cancer indicates that a high fat intake is protective against the tumor. It is possible

Table 4. Macronutrient consumptions, males, Japan-Hawaii Cancer Study

	Calories	Protein		Fat		Carbohydrates		Cholesterol
	per day	(g per day)	(% Cal)	(g per day)	(% Cal)	(g per day)	(% Cal)	(mg per day)
Controls n = 6025	2295	95.0	16.7	86.4	33.5	263.7	46.5	550.5
Colon cancer n = 155	2222	92.2	16.6	79.7[b]	31.6[c]	258.2	47.0	507.4
Rectal cancer n = 77	2380	96.0	16.6	88	33.3	263.7	44.3	571.8
Other cancer n = 767	2326	94.6	16.5	85.2	32.6[c]	265.9	46.3	566.6
CHD[a] n = 456	2229[b]	94.7	17.2[c]	86.4	34.7[c]	249.8	45.0[c]	561.8

[a] From McGee et al. (1984); [b] $P \leqq 0.05$; [c] $P \leqq 0.01$.

that the interrelationships of dietary fat with other factors can explain this association. However, it may be remarked that the National Science Foundation set a goal of 30% calories from fat in order to reduce cancer risk (Grobstein 1982). The men in the cohort who most closely approach this level are those who have experienced the highest rates of colon cancer.

Fat Intake and Cancer of Subsites Within the Large Bowel

It is generally recognized that colon cancer and rectal cancer differ in respect of geographic distribution and in respect of their relation to different epidemiologic variables and in their recent trends. Rectal cancer predominates in populations which are at low risk for colon cancer and is more likely to involve the distal 6 cm of that bowel segment (Haenszel 1982). It is less widely understood that subsites within the colon also differ in these respects. The bowel subsite most commonly affected in high-risk westernized populations is the sigmoid colon.

Connecticut, an affluent American state, has shown increased frequency of cancer of the sigmoid colon and ascending colon over a 34-year period (Snyder et al. 1977), a change that is greatest among persons older than 65 years of age. Japan has experienced a steep rise in cancer of the left colon between 1969 and 1981 (Tajima et al. 1985). This trend affects both sexes. There has also been a smaller rise in the death rates in cancer of the right colon over the same period. This pattern parallels a rise in fat consumption relative to carbohydrate intake.

The Hawaiian Japanese experience is shown in Fig. 4. Although rectal cancer rates are fairly stable for both sexes, cancer of the left colon (descending and sigmoid segments) and of the right colon (cecum, ascending, transverse segments) have shown increases in men and women, with the steepest rise being recorded in the left colon – 2.3 times over a period of 25 years. The ratio of cancer of the left colon to the rectum has risen from 0.98 to 2.1 over the same time period for Hawaiian Japanese men, and similar shifts in subsite distribution have occurred among Hawaiian Japanese women.

By 1987, the men in the Japan-Hawaii cohort of 8006 Hawaiian Japanese men had acquired 77 rectal cancers and 155 colon cancers since they were examined in the years 1965–1968. The fat intake of men who developed cancers at specific subsites in the large bowel is shown in Table 5. Tumors of the ascending colon and cecum were significantly and inversely related to total fat intake when stated as a percentage of total calories, as was cancer of the sigmoid colon when stated as grams per day. Sigmoid cancer was also inversely related to cholesterol intake and total calories.

These findings suggest that, if dietary fat promotes large bowel cancer, its influence is weakest in the cecum and ascending colon, and that a high fat intake has played little part in the steep rise in frequency of cancer of the sigmoid and ascending segments of the colon in this population.

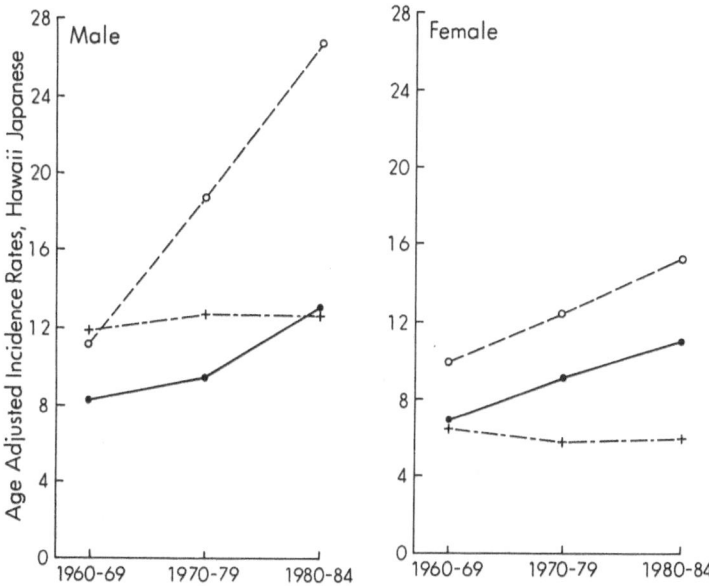

Fig. 4. Recent trends in cancer of the rectum and colonic subsites among Hawaiian Japanese. *Solid circles,* right colon cancer (cecum, ascending, transverse); *open circles,* left colon cancer (descending, sigmoid); *crosses,* rectal cancer (rectosigmoid, rectum)

Table 5. Adjusted mean daily intake of fat and cholesterol, and energy adjustment for age at the time of examination and ethanol intake was done by analysis of covariance

	Fat intake						Dietary Cholesterol	Calories
	Total		Saturated		Unsaturated			
	(g per day)	(% Cal)	(g per day)	(% Cal)	(g per day)	(% Cal)	(mg per day)	
Cecum, ascending colon (n = 35)	76.1[a]	28.2[c]	52.2	18.6[d]	23.9	9.7	489	2345
Transverse, descending colon (n = 15)	97.2	32.8	71.3[a]	24.4	25.9	8.4	620	2533[a]
Sigmoid colon (n = 95)	78.0[b]	33.0[b]	53.3[b]	22.6	24.7	10.4	484[b]	2098[d]
Rectosigmoid colon (n = 33)	93.7	36.2[a]	67.5	26.0[a]	26.2	10.1	582	2367
Rectum (n = 44)	85.1	32.8	62.9	24.1	22.1	8.7	557	2297
Control (n = 6025)	86.9	33.6	60.3	23.3	26.5	10.3	552	2305

[a] $P < 0.1$; [b] $P \leq 0.05$; [c] $P \leq 0.001$; [d] $P \leq 0.01$.
Mean is significantly different from control mean.

Dietary Fat: A Source of Energy

Colon cancer is most common among prosperous persons who "enjoy" a sedentary occupation (Blot et al. 1976; Garabrant et al. 1984; Gerhardsson et al. 1986; Haenszel et al. 1975; Lynch et al. 1975). The steep rise in Hawaiian Japanese colon cancer rates is synchronous with a rise in family income. In 1977 the mean Hawaiian Japanese family income was $ 19 431, compared to Hawaiian Whites whose mean family income was $ 19 005 (Annual Report, Hawaii Department of Health Annual Statistical Report). In contrast, the races with the lowest family incomes – Hawaiians ($ 13 615) and Filipinos ($ 12 683) – have comparably low incidence rates of colon cancer, in spite of great differences in fat consumption (Fig. 3). Lastly, the Hawaiian Japanese men who have shown the greatest weight gain between the ages of 25 and 55 are at highest risk of acquiring colon cancer (Nomura et al. 1985a). These findings suggest that higher energy input than expenditure is in some way related to colon cancer. Energy balance depends upon the level of energy intake, the efficiency of absorption, the level of basal metabolism, and the level of physical activity. Because it is difficult to measure some of these factors, body weight or body mass index provides a surrogate measure of energy balance.

Energy intake is highly correlated with all macronutrients, but the strongest correlation is with fat (Lyon et al. 1987). It is therefore possible that studies showing a direct association of colon cancer with fat intake actually reflect the energy intake of sedentary populations.

Influence of Fat Absorption on Colon Cancer Risk: The Postgastrectomy State

Dietary intake is not synonymous with nutrition, as is clearly demonstrated by patients who have had a subtotal gastrectomy. Among the 8006 Hawaiian Japanese men who were examined in the years 1965–1968, there were 407 who had previously undergone subtotal gastrectomy. Although their macronutrient intake was neither qualitatively nor quantitatively different from men with an intact stomach, their physical and biochemical attributes differed significantly from those of other men (Table 6). Their lower body weight, lower hematocrit and lower serum lipid levels all suggest less efficient absorption of nutrients among gastrectomy subjects (Stemmermann et al. 1984a). They also show evidence of metabolic bone disease (Klein et al. 1987). This has been attributed to alterations on vitamin D metabolism.

In our study (unpublished work in progress) of gastrectomy and non-gastrectomy subjects, cancer surveillance yielded a higher than expected number of cancers in the colon, rectum, lung, and prostate among gastrectomy subjects. The 11 colon cancers and seven rectal cancers among them yield age-adjusted odds ratios of 1.42 for the colon and 1.78 for the rectum. The number of cancers developed by these men is still too small to establish a statistically significant increase in risk at these sites, but they do suggest that, in themselves, neither low body weight nor diminished fat absorption is protective against large bowel cancer. An increase in frequency of colorectal cancer following gastrectomy has been reported by Ross et al. (1982) and

Table 6. Age-adjusted means, selected epidemiologic variables versus operation status

	No gastrectomy ($n = 7599$)	Gastrectomy ($n = 407$)
Age at first examination (unadjusted)	54.4	55.6
Weight at first examination (kg)	63.6	58.6[a]
Weight at age 25 (kg)	58.9	59.7[b]
Systolic BP (mmHg)	134	128[a]
Diastolic BP (mmHg)	82	77[c]
Hematocrit (%)	44.7	44.0[a]
Serum cholesterol (mg/dl)	219	204[a]
Serum triglyceride (mg/dl)	233	190[a]
Alcohol (oz per month)	13.6	16.2[c]
Cigarettes per day	10.1	14.1[a]

[a] $P \leq 0.001$; [b] $P \leq 0.05$; [c] $P \leq 0.01$.
All P values result from comparing the mean for a given surgical group to the mean for the 7599 nongastrectomy men.

by Bundred et al. (1985), suggesting that this early observation among the Hawaiian Japanese is not unique.

If gastrectomy does increase the risk of large bowel cancer, dietary fat might play a role in this effect in one of two ways: (a) diminished fat absorption carries with it diminished absorption of fat soluble vitamins; thus, it has been established that blood vitamin E level is reduced after this operation (Leonard et al. 1966); (b) impaired fat absorption will result in an increased fecal concentration of unabsorbed free fatty acids and bile salts.

Interaction of Dietary Fat and Calcium

It has been suggested that the collective action of fat, phosphorus, and calcium in the diet might influence large bowel cancer risk (Newmark et al. 1984). Specifically, it has been proposed that increased fat intake leads to increased levels of free, ionized fatty acids and bile salts in the feces. The toxic and potentially promoting effect of fatty acids and bile acids might be inhibited if they were converted into insoluble calcium soaps.

A case-control study of Hawaiian Japanese men with colon cancer could find no association between dietary calcium intake and colon cancer risk (Heilbrun et al. 1986). This was true whether phosphorus intake was high or low, or whether fat intake was high or low (Table 7). Adult Japanese consume less calcium than Caucasians because lactose intolerance discourages their use of milk products. It has been suggested that this accounts for their high colon cancer rates (Garland and Garland 1986), and that vitamin D deficiency accounts for the high colon cancer rates in northern countries, as shown in Table 8. Hawaiian Japanese, however, fail to demonstrate an association between vitamin D and large bowel cancer (Heilbrun et al. 1985). If, as has been suggested, calcium exerts its protective effect in conjunction with a high fat intake, the Hawaiian Japanese may not be an appropriate population for testing

Table 7. Age-adjusted odds ratios of colon cancer by level of dietary intake of fat, calcium, and phosphorus

		Low phosphorus (< 1032 mg per day)		High phosphorus (≧ 1032 mg per day)	
Calcium (mg per day)	≧ 445	1.00[a] (6)	1.09 (4)	1.39 (11)	0.70 (28)
	< 445	1.33 (30)	1.03 (9)	1.02 (3)	1.05 (8)
Fat (g per day)		< 61	≧ 61	< 61	≧ 61

[a] Referent group. Table entries are the age-adjusted odds ratio, with the number of colon cancer cases in parentheses.

Table 8. Adjusted odds ratios[a] of colon cancer and of rectal cancer by quartile of dietary variables

	Quartile of dietary variable				Linear trend P value[c]
	1 (low)	2	3	4 (high)	
Colon cancer					
Vitamin D (IU/1000 cal)	0.81	1.13	1.12	1.00	0.524
Calcium (mg/1000 cal)	1.32	1.05	0.72	1.00	0.274
Vitamin D + calcium	1.45	1.02	1.53	1.00	0.467
Rectal cancer					
Vitamin D (IU/1000 cal)	1.25	0.66	2.34[b]	1.00	0.965
Calcium (mg/1000 cal)	0.88	0.86	1.59	1.00	0.480
Vitamin D + calcium	1.00	0.73	1.54	1.00	0.580

[a] From logistic regression models, adjusting colon cancer risk for age at examination, and rectal cancer risk for age at examination and alcohol intake (oz per month).
[b] Odds ratio is significantly different from unity ($P < 0.05$).
[c] From separate logistic models, with a coded version of the diet variable used to denote quartiles.

this hypothesis since their fat intake does not reach the levels of United States Whites. The early results of the postgastrectomy subset, however, could be explained on the basis of high levels of fecal fatty acids combined with low calcium and vitamin D intake. A definitive conclusion must await analyses from other populations.

Role of Dietary Fat in Vitamin Transport

It has been suggested that the antioxidant properties of some fat-soluble vitamins may inhibit cancer induction (Peto et al. 1981; Tannenbaum 1983). The availability of such a vitamin at the tissue level depends upon its concentration in food, the efficiency of fat absorption from the gut, and its transport in the blood stream.

Table 9. Median values of fasting serum triglycerides, serum vitamin E levels, and vitamin E: serum triglycerides

Cancer	Patients n	Serum triglycerides (mEq/liter)	Serum vitamin E (μg/dl)	Vitamin E: triglycerides
Colon	27	6.0[a]	12.53	2.07[b]
Rectum	13	5.0	11.60	2.03
Stomach	30	4.6	12.80	2.69
Lung	40	5.8	12.55	2.31
Bladder	13	3.8	13.60	2.71
Controls	102	4.2	12.80	2.95

[a] $P < 0.05$; [b] $P < 0.005$ (determined by the nonparametric multiple comparisons procedure of Dunn).

There is a good correlation between carotene intake and its blood level, but the blood α-tocopherol level must be adjusted to the blood lipid level if it is to be used as a surrogate for vitamin E intake (Willett et al. 1983). The tissue level of tocopherol in normal, obese, and hyperlipemic rats is related to the serum tocopherol : total lipid ratio (Catignani and Fuller 1982), and it is now considered essential to state the tocopherol concentration in the terms of its relation to total blood lipid (Horwitt et al. 1972).

A case-control study of Hawaiian Japanese cohort men has not indicated a relation between bowel cancer and the serum levels of retinol, β-carotene, or α-tocopherol (Nomura et al. 1985b). The α-tocopherol : triglyceride ratio, however, was significantly and inversely related to colon cancer, as shown in Table 9 (Stemmermann et al. 1985). The blood triglyceride level in this population is directly associated with alcohol intake (Yano et al. 1984) and large bowel cancer (Stemmermann et al. 1985). There may be an interaction between alcohol intake, fat intake, and fat-soluble vitamin intake in respect to cancer risk, supporting the suggestion of D'Antonio et al. (1986). These findings suggest the possibility that circulating triglyceride and body fat might constitute a biologic sink that sequestrates vitamin E at the expense of mucosal cells. This might explain the high rates of colon cancer in Hawaiian Japanese and is a hypothesis that should be tested.

Role of Fat upon the Formation of Adenomatous Polyps of the Large Bowel

It is generally accepted that colorectal cancers arise from adenomatous polyps, and that the two conditions have a similar geographic distribution. These polyps are seldom found among sub-Saharan Blacks (Bremner and Ackerman 1970; Templeton 1973), but are common in high-risk populations (Clark et al. 1985; Helwig 1947). The great difference in colon cancer frequency among indigenous and migrant Japanese is matched by comparable differences in the frequency of adenomatous polyps. Among 202 Hawaiian Japanese autopsy subjects, 125 (62%) had adenomatous polyps (Stemmermann and Yatani 1973), while 179 of 669 (27%) indigenous Japanese autopsy subjects had polyps when examined by the same technique (Sato et al. 1976).

Table 10. Age-adjusted mean number of adenomatous polyps per subject by quartile of non-dietary variables

Variable	Quartile of variable				Test for linear trend	
	Q1 (low)	Q2	Q3	Q4 (high)	$\hat{\beta}$[a]	P value[c]
Body habitus						
Boda mass index	1.72	1.14	1.46	0.76	−0.261	0.141
Weight gain since age 25	1.21	2.17	0.93	0.79	−0.208	0.284
Physical activity index	1.37	1.26	1.34	1.19	−0.039	0.826
Laboratory variables						
Serum cholesterol	1.25	1.39	1.48	1.12	−0.022	0.898
Uric acid	1.05	1.36	1.31	0.98	+0.016	0.927
Glucose	1.08	1.41	0.87	1.78	+0.175	0.318
Hematocrit	1.19	1.05	1.13	1.73	+0.170	0.356
Social variables						
Age at examination	1.05	1.28	0.93	1.98	+0.247[b]	0.220[d]
Alcohol intake	1.04	0.87	1.61	2.34	+0.407	0.020
Current smoking	1.32	0.57	1.86	1.10	+0.026	0.870
Past or current smoking	1.20	1.02	1.84	1.09	+0.048	0.795

[a] Bivariate regression model coefficient for exposure variable quartiles.
[b] Univariate regression model coefficient for age quartiles.
[c] For testing whether $\hat{\beta}$ is significantly different from zero.
[d] From analysis of variance, for comparing the four means.

Table 11. Age-adjusted means of 24-h nutrient intake for men with and without adenomatous polyps

Nutrient	Subjects with adenomatous polyps ($n = 73$)	Subjects without adenomatous polyps ($n = 76$)	P value[a]
Calories	2037.6	2178.0	0.253
Protein (g)	83.2	89.4	0.281
Animal protein (g)	62.6	65.9	0.526
Vegetable protein (g)	20.6	23.5	0.072
Fat (g)	75.9	77.4	0.793
Saturated fat (g)	51.9	53.6	0.736
Unsaturated fat (g)	24.0	23.8	0.966
Cholesterol (mg)	535.2	542.8	0.886
Carbohydrate (g)	230.2	259.4	0.104
Simple carbohydrate (g)	74.3	86.7	0.170
Complex carbohydrate (g)	155.8	172.7	0.225

[a] For comparison of age-adjusted means, by analysis of covariance methods.

Atherosclerosis is a precursor to CHD, in much the same sense as adenomatous polyps precede colorectal cancer. The degree of aortic and coronary artery atherosclerosis is significantly and directly related to the presence and multiplicity of adenomatous polyps in the Hawaiian Japanese autopsy subjects (Stemmermann et al. 1986). This suggests that they develop in response to shared environmental events. The subsequent development of CHD and colon cancer in subsets of these Hawaiian Japanese men must result from the superimposition of other risk factors upon the initiators of the precursor lesions.

A review of epidemiologic risk factors among cohort men with and without adenomatous polyps at autopsy (Stemmermann et al. 1988) is summarized in Table 10. Men with polyps were no more obese than controls at the time of their examination in the years 1965–1968, nor had they experienced excessive weight gain after age 25. The data from their dietary examination indicated a similar energy intake, and lesser amounts of all macronutrients than controls (Table 11). None of these variations were statistically significant. Alcohol intake, however, was insignificantly related to the multiplicity of polyps (Table 10). Alcohol is an enzyme inducer and may interact with the intake of fat-soluble vitamins and serum lipids to favor cancer induction while inhibiting the development of end stage CHD (D'Antonio et al. 1986).

Conclusion

Changes in the dietary practices of Japanese in Japan and Hawaii are characterized by increased consumption of fat and protein, but decreased intake of complex carbohydrate. There is a trend toward increasing colon cancer risk in both populations. The dietary changes have been greater among Hawaiian Japanese and they have been operating over a longer period of time. The increase in colon cancer is also far greater among Hawaiian Japanese. These correlational findings are consistent with the hypothesis that a high fat intake favors the development of colon cancer in parallel with the risk of acquiring other Western diseases that have been related to dietary fat (e.g., CHD). Correlational studies of other groups, however, do not support this cause and effect relationship. This is especially true of Polynesians in New Zealand and Hawaii who experience low colon cancer rates in the face of a fat intake that is greater than that of most Western populations.

The relation of fat intake to colon cancer in case-control studies of Japanese and other populations have also been inconsistent, and prospective cohort studies of Japanese have shown a stronger relation of fat to CHD to colon cancer.

The effects of fat intake cannot be easily separated from those of dietary factors with which it is closely correlated (e.g., protein, fat-soluble vitamins) or from those with which it bears a reciprocal relation (complex carbohydrate); or from the synchronous effects of the profound social changes that continue to affect Hawaiian Japanese.

Future studies of large bowel cancer may be more fruitful if they focus upon obesity, alcohol consumption, fat-soluble vitamin transport and metabolism, and upon the effects of non-dietary variables: methods of food preparation, physical activity, economic status, and the mechanisms by which urbanization might influence large bowel function or disease.

References

Aoki K, Sasaki R, Mizuno S (1987) Changes in mortality of all forms of malignant neoplasms among Japanese for the last decades. Gann Monogr 33:33–43

Armstrong B, Doll R (1975) Environmental factors and cancer incidence and mortality in different countries, with special reference to dietary practices. Int J Cancer 15:617–631

Berry EM, Zimmermann J, Peser M, Ligumsky M (1986) Dietary fat, adipose tissue composition, and the development of cancer of the colon. JNCI 77:93–97

Berta JL, Coste T, Ravtureau J, Guilloud-Bataille M, Pequignot G (1985) Diet and rectocolonic cancers. Results of a case control study. Gastroenterol Clin Biol 9:348–353

Bjelke E (1978) Dietary factors and the epidemiology of cancer of the stomach and large bowel. Aktuel Ernaehrungsmed Klin Prax (Suppl) 2:10–17

Blot WJ, Fraumeni JF, Stone BJ, McKay FW (1976) Geographic patterns of large bowel cancer in the United States. J Natl Cancer Inst 57:1225–1231

Bremner CG, Ackerman LV (1970) Polyps and carcinoma of the large bowel. Cancer 26:991–999

Broitman SA, Vitale JJ, Vavrousek-Jakuba E, Gottlieb LS (1977) Polyunsaturated fat, cholesterol and large bowel tumorignesis. Cancer 40:2455–2463

Bundred NJ, Whitfield BCS, Stanton E, Prescott GC, Kingsworth AN (1985) Gastric surgery and the risk of subsequent colorectal cancer. Br J Surg 72:618–619

Catignani GL, Fuller PA (1982) Tissue tocopherol levels in normal, obese and hyperlipemic rats. Ann NY Acad Sci 393:167–168

Clark JC, Collan Y, Eide TJ, Esteve J, Ewen S, Gibbs NM, Jensen OM, Koskela E, Maclennan R, Simpson JG, Stalsberg H, Zaridge DG (1985) Prevalence of polyps in an autopsy series from areas with varying incidence of large bowel cancer. Int J Cancer 36:179–186

D'Antonio JA, LaPorte RE, Dai W, Hom DL, Wozniczak M, Kuller LH (1986) Lipoprotein cholesterol, vitamin A and vitamin B in an alcoholic population. Cancer 57:1798–1802

Garabrant DH, Peters JM, Mack TM, Bernstein L (1984) Job activity and colon cancer risk. Am J Epidemiol 119:1005–1014

Garland CF, Garland FC (1986) Calcium and colon cancer. Hum Nutr Clin Nutr 5:161–166

Gerhardsson M, Norell SE, Kiviranta H, Pedersen NL, Ahlbom A (1986) Sedentary jobs and colon cancer. Am J Epidemiol 123:775–780

Grobstein C (1982) Diet, nutrition and cancer. National Academy Press, Washington

Haenszel W (1982) Contribution of migrant population to study of cancer risk. In: Aoki K, Tominaga S, Hirayama T, Hirota Y (eds) Cancer prevention in developing countries. University of Nagoya Press, Nagoya, Japan, pp 351–362

Haenszel W, Kurihara M (1968) Studies of Japanese migrants. I. Mortality from cancer and other diseases among Japanese in the United States. J Natl Cancer Inst 40:43–68

Haenszel W, Berg JW, Segi M, Kurihara M, Locke FB (1973) Large bowel cancer in Hawaii Japanese. J Natl Cancer Inst 51:1765–1779

Haenszel W, Correa P, Cuello C (1975) Social class differences among patients with large bowel cancer in Colombia. J Natl Cancer Inst 54:1031–1035

Haenszel W, Locke FB, Segi M (1980) A case control study of large bowel cancer in Japan. J Natl Cancer Inst 64:17–22

Hanusch J, Friedl HP, Schemper M, Schiessel R (1985) Incidence and regional distribution of colorectal cancers in Austria. Wien Klin Wochenschr 97:456–460

Heilbrun LK, Nomura AMY, Hankin JH, Stemmermann GN (1985) Dietary vitamin D and calcium and risk of colorectal cancer. Lancet 1:925

Heilbrun LK, Hankin JH, Nomura AMY, Stemmermann GN (1986) Colon cancer and dietary fat, phosphorus, and calcium in Hawaiian-Japanese men. Am J Clin Nutr 43:306–309

Helwig E (1947) The evaluation of adenomas of the large bowel and their relation to carcinoma. Surg Gynecol Obstet 84:36–49

Hill MJ, Aries VC (1971) Faecal steroid composition and its relationship to cancer of the large bowel. J Pathol 104:129–139

Hill MJ, Drasar BS, Williams RE (1977) Faecal bile acids and clostridia in patients with cancer of the large bowel. Lancet 1:535–539

Hirayama T (1981) A large-scale cohort study on the relationship between diet and selected cancers of digestive organs. In: Bruce WR, Correa P, Lipkin M et al. (eds) Gastrointestinal cancer: endogenous factors. Banbury report vol 7. Cold Spring Harbor, NY, pp 409–429

Horwitt MK, Harvey CC, Dahm CH, Searcy MT (1972) Relationship between tocopherol and serum lipid levels for determination of nutritional adequacy. Am J Acad Sci 203:223–236

Kagan A, Harris B, Winkelstein W, Johnson KG, Kato H, Syme SL, Rhoads GG, Gay ML, Nichaman MZ, Hamilton HR (1974) Epidemiologic studies of coronary heart disease and stroke in Japanese men living in Japan, Hawaii and California: demographic, physical, dietary and biochemical characteristics. J Chronic Dis 27:345–364

Keys A, Aravanis C, Blackburn HW et al. (1967) Epidemiologic studies related to coronary heart disease: characteristics of men aged 40–59 in seven countries. Acta Med Scand [Suppl]: 460:1–392

Klein KB, Orwoll ES, Lieberman DA, Meier DE, McClung MR, Parfitt AM (1987) Metabolic bone disease in asymptomatic men after partial gastrectomy with Billroth II anastomosis. Gastroenterology 92:608–616

Kolonel LN (1987) Fat and colon cancer: how firm is the epidemiologic evidence? Am J Clin Nutr 45:336–341

Kolonel LN, Hankin JH, Nomura AMY, Chu SY (1981) Dietary fat intake and cancer incidence among five ethnic groups in Hawaii. Cancer Res 41:3727–3728

Kune S, Kune GA, Watson LF (1987) Case control study of dietary etiological factors: the Melbourne colorectal cancer study. Nutr Cancer 9:21–42

Kuratsune M, Honda T, Englyst HN, Cummings JH (1986) Dietary fibre in the Japanese diet. In: Hayashi Y, Nagao M, Sugimura T et al. (eds) Diet, nutrition and cancer. Japan Sci Soc Press, Tokyo/VNU, Utrecht, pp 247–253

Leonard PJ, Losowsky MS, Pulvertaft CN (1966) Vitamin E levels after gastric surgery. Gut 7:578–580

Li JY (1982) Investigation of geographic patterns of cancer mortality in China. NCI Monogr 62:17–42

Lynch HT, Guigis H, Lynch J, Brodkey FD, Magee H (1975) Cancer of the colon: socio-economic variables in a community. Am J Epidemiol 102:119–127

Lyon JL, Mahoney AW, West DW, Gardner JW, Smith KR, Sorenson AW, Stanish W (1987) Energy intake: its relationship to colon cancer risk. JNCI 78:853–861

Lyon JL, Sorenson AW (1978) Colon cancer in a low risk population. Am J Clin Nutr 31:5227–5230

Macquart-Moulin G, Ribol E, Corner J, Charnay B. Berthezene P, Day N (1986) Case control study on colorectal cancer and diet in Marseilles. Int J Cancer 38:183–191

McGee D, Reed D, Yano K, Kagan A, Tillotson J (1984) Ten year incidence of coronary heart disease in the Honolulu heart program: relation to nutrient intake. Am J Epidemiol 119:667–676

Mower HF, Ray RM, Stemmermann GN, Nomura AMY, Glober G (1978) Analysis of fecal bile acids among Japanese in Hawaii. J Nutr 108:1289–1296

Mower HF, Ray RM, Shoff R, Stemmermann GN, Nomura AMY, Glober G, Kamiyama S, Shimada A, Yamakawa H (1979) Fecal bile acids in two Japanese populations with different colon cancer risks. Cancer Res 39:328–331

Newmark HL, Wargovich MJ, Bruce WR (1984) Colon cancer and dietary fat, phosphate and calcium: a hypothesis. JNCI 72:1323–1325

Nomura AMY, Wilkins TD, Kamiyama S, Heilbrun LK, Shimada A, Stemmermann GN, Mower HF (1983) Fecal neutral steroids in two Japanese populations with different colon cancer risks. Cancer Res 43:1910–1913

Nomura AMY, Heilbrun LK, Stemmermann GN (1985a) Body mass index as a predictor of cancer in men. JNCI 74:319–323

Nomura AMY, Stemmermann GN, Heilbrun LK, Salkeld RM, Vuilleumier JP (1985b) Serum vitamin levels and the risk of cancer of specific sites in men of Japanese ancestry in Hawaii. Cancer Res 45:2369–2372

Peto R, Doll R, Buckley JD, Sporn MB (1981) Can dietary beta carotene materially reduce human cancer rates? Nature 290:201–208

Potter JD, McMichael AJ (1986) Diet and cancer of the colon: a case control study. JNCI 76:557–569

Prior I, Tasman-Jones C (1981) New Zealand and Pacific Polynesians. In: Trowell HC, Burkitt D (eds) Western diseases: their emergence and prevention. Arnold, London, pp 227–267

Reddy BS, Weisburger JH, Wynder EL (1974) Effects of dietary fat level and dimethylhydrazine on fecal acid and neutral sterol excretion and colon carcinogenesis in rats. J Natl Cancer Inst 52:507–511

Reddy BS, Watanabe K, Weisburger JH (1977) Effect of high fat diet on colon carcinogenesis in F344 rats treated with 1,2-dimethylhydrazine, methylazoxymethanol acetate, or methyl-nitrosourea. Cancer Res 37:4156–4159

Reed DM, Feinlieb M (1983) Changing patterns of cardiovascular disease in the Pacific Basin: report of an international workshop. J Community Health 8:182–205

Ross AHM, Smith MA, Anderson JR, Small WP (1982) Late mortality after surgery for peptic ulcer. New Engl J Med 30:519–522

Sato E, Ouchi A, Sasano N, Ishidate T (1976) Polyps and diverticulosis of large bowel in autopsy population of Akita prefecture, compared to Miyagi. Cancer 37:1316–1321

Segi M (1960) Cancer mortality for selected sites in 24 countries (1950–1957). Department of Public Health, Tohoku University School of Medicine, Sendai, Japan, pp 206–211

Segi M (1984) Age adjusted death rates for cancer for selected sites in 46 countries. Segi Institute of Cancer Epidemiology, Nagoya, Japan

Segi M, Kurihara M, Tsukahara Y (1966) Mortality for selected causes in 30 countries (1950–1961). Kosei, Tokyo, pp 118–125

Shimizu H, Mack TH, Ross RK, Henderson BE (1987) Cancer of the gastrointestinal tract among Japanese and white immigrants to Los Angeles County. JNCI 78:223–228

Smith AH, Pearce NE, Joseph JG (1985) Major colorectal cancer aetiological hypotheses do not explain mortality trends among Maoris and non Maoris in New Zealand. Int J Epidemiol 14:79–85

Synder DN, Heston JF, Meigs JW, Flannery JT (1977) Changes in site distribution of colorectal carcinoma in Connecticut, 1940–1973. Dig Dis 22:791–797

Staszewski J, Haenszel W (1965) Cancer mortality among the Polish-born in the United States. J Natl Cancer Inst 35:291–297

Staszewski J, McCall MG, Stenhouse NS (1971) Cancer mortality in 1962–1966 among Polish migrants to Australia. Br J Cancer 25:599–610

Stemmermann GN, Yatani R (1973) Diverticulosis and polyps of the large intestine. Cancer 31:1260–1270

Stemmermann GN, Heilbrun LK, Nomura AMY, Rhoads GG, Glober GA (1984a) Late mortality after partial gastrectomy. Int J Epidemiol 13:299–303

Stemmermann GN, Nomura AMY, Heilbrun LK (1984b) Dietary fat and the risk of colorectal cancer. Cancer Res 44:4633–4637

Stemmermann GN, Nomura AMY, Heilbrun LK, Mower H, Hayashi T (1985) Colorectal cancer in Hawaiian Japanese men: a progress report. NCI Monogr 69:125–131

Stemmermann GN, Heilbrun LK, Nomura AMY, Yano K, Hayashi T (1986) Adenomatous polyps and atherosclerosis: an autopsy study of Japanese men in Hawaii. Int J Cancer 38:789–794

Stemmermann GN, Nomura AMY, Kolonel LN (1987) Cancer among Japanese-Americans in Hawaii. Gann Monogr 33:99–108

Stemmermann GN, Heilbrun LK, Nomura AMY (1988) The association of diet and other factors with adenomatous polyps of the large bowel: a prospective autopsy study. Am J Clin Nutr 47:312–317

Tajima K, Hirose K, Nakagawa N, Kuroishi T, Tominaga S (1985) Urban-rural difference in the trend of colorectal cancer mortality with special reference to the subsites of colon cancer in Japan. Jap J Cancer Res (Gann) 76:717–728

Tannenbaum SR (1983) *N*-nitroso compounds: a perspective on human exposure. Lancet 1:629–632

Templeton AC (1973) Tumours in a tropical country. Heinemann, London, pp 52–70

Trowell H, Burkitt D (1981) Western diseases: their emergence and prevention (Preface). Arnold, London, pp XIII–XVI

Tuyns AJ (1986) A case control study on colorectal cancer in Belgium. Preliminary results. Soz Praventivmed 31:81–82

Waterhouse J, Muir C, Shanmugaratnam K, Powell J (1982) Cancer in five continents, vol IV. International Agency for Research on Cancer, Lyon, France

Weisburger JH (1986) Application of the mechanisms of nutritional carcinogenesis to the prevention of cancer. In: Hayashi Y, Nagao M, Sugimura T et al. (eds) Diet, nutrition and cancer. Japan Sci Soc Press, Tokyo/VNU, Utrecht

Willett WC, Stampfer MJ, Underwood BA, Taylor JO, Hennekens CH (1983) Vitamin A, E and carotene: effects of supplementation on their plasma levels. Am J Clin Nutr 38:559–566

Wynder E, Reddy BS (1974) Metabolic epidemiology of colorectal cancer. Cancer 34:801–806

Yano K, Reed DM, McGee D (1984) Ten year incidence of coronary heart disease in the Honolulu heart program. Am J Epidemiol 119:653–666

Genetic Predisposition to Colorectal Cancer

D. G. Harnden

Cancer Research Campaign, Paterson Institute for Cancer Research,
Christie Hospital and Holt Radium Institute, Manchester, M2O 9BX, UK

Contents

Introduction

Genetic factors in cancer have been recognised for many years but have been widely regarded as of only minor interest. There has been a growing appreciation recently of the part played by heredity in many cancers including colorectal cancer. The present brief review touches on the main topics but for an in-depth coverage of the field the reader is referred to the recent monograph edited by P. M. Lynch and H. T. Lynch (1985)

Relative Importance of the Genetic Element in Colorectal Cancer

Any mention of genetic predisposition to colorectal cancer instantly brings to mind the diseases associated with multiple colonic polyps where there is usually a strong familial incidence. It is important, however, to get these diseases into perspective, no matter how dramatic and interesting they may be. In the United Kingdom there are about 27 000 new cases of colorectal cancer each year, and of these only about 0.6% (150 or so) can be attributed to familial adenomatous polyposis (FAP) (Bussey 1982). This is roughly in accord with an estimated gene frequency of 1 in 10 000. Further, the presence of colonic polyps is only one of a number of well-established conditions, some genetic, some not, associated with an increased predisposition to colorectal cancer. Amongst these are previous colonic cancer, previous polyps, hereditary non-polyposis colorectal cancer (HNPCC), inflammatory bowel disease, family history of colonic cancer, previous cancer of the bladder or breast. Thompson and Pearlman (1982) conclude that only 12% – 15% of all colonic cancers show one or more of these predisposing factors. In other words, more than 85% of all colorectal cancers occur in patients for whom there is no apparent risk factor.

Does this then mean that for the majority of cases of colorectal cancer, genetic factors are unimportant? On the contrary, there are very good reasons to suspect that genetic factors may play a part in many cases of colorectal carcinoma. In those cases where a genetic element has been recognised (FAP, HNPCC or family history of colorectal cancer) the notion that the disease is hereditary, at least to some degree, depends upon the recognition of the familial incidence of the disease. It is, however, quite possible for there to be an important genetic component in the disease without overt familial clustering (Bodmer 1986). Let us suppose that the carrier of a dominant gene is at a 100-fold increased risk of developing carcinoma and that the disease has a normal population incidence of 1 in 1000; then there is still only a 1 in 10 chance of a gene carrier developing the disease, and the probability of familial clustering is low. The contribution that such a genetic factor will make to the overall incidence of the disease will depend on the gene frequency in the population. For example, if the gene frequency is relatively low, say 1 in 1000, then roughly 10% of cancers of this type will be directly attributable to this gene. It will be seen, therefore, that a substantial proportion of cancer may be attributable to a genetic susceptibility without that being immediately obvious from the disease pattern in the population. For purely practical reasons, most studies concentrate on the minority of familial cases, but it should always be borne in mind that, if a genetic component can be identified in the non-familial majority of cases, this would have a much greater potential for prevention and early diagnosis.

Interaction of Genetic and Environmental Factors

It is probably better, however, to avoid a rigid demarcation into "genetic" cases and "non-genetic" cases. It is clear that environmental factors are vitally important in the aetiology of carcinoma of the colon, and the detailed evidence is considered elsewhere in this volume. Briefly, the geographical variations are so large and the immigrant population effects are so striking that one is forced to the conclusion that environmental factors, possibly dietary factors, are the major causal agents in determining the occurrence of colorectal cancer. Some workers go further and suggest that 80% (or some other high percentage) of cases are "caused by the environment". In the context of prevention, this is both unhelpful and misleading. A more realistic and positive approach is to accept it as likely that environmental factors are important in *all* cases of carcinoma of the colon. Equally genetic factors play a part in all cases. In some instances, genetic factors will be more important; in others environmental factors will be more important – it is all a matter of degree. For example, in FAP we are studying one end of a spectrum where the genetic component is very stong, but even here it is reasonable to suppose that the development of carcinoma in patients with polyps is affected, to some extent, by environmental factors. Situations where the genetic component is strong relative to the environmental component are likely to be rare, and for the majority of cancers of the colorectum, the environmental component will be the most important influence. However, the significant environmental factors will be operating on a very varied human population. If we are to understand these environmental factors, it is critical that we also examine the variability of the population.

Inherited versus Acquired Genetic Changes

Genetic Change in the Cancer Cell

In any discussion of genetics and cancer it is important to distinguish between (a) constitutional genetic variation which affects all the cells of the body and which is associated with inherited susceptibility, and (b) genetic changes confined to the cancer cells themselves which will occur in both hereditary and sporadic cases. While many different hypotheses have been put forward to explain the nature of the change from the normal cell to the cancer cell, there is now a wide measure of agreement that an alteration in the genome of the cell, either structural or regulatory, must be involved. In some cases there are easily recognised structural changes in the chromosomes or in the DNA. Since we know that many carcinogenic agents (radiation, carcinogenic chemicals, oncogenic viruses) can cause such genetic damage, it is reasonable to postulate that this genetic change is an important part of the neoplastic process. In other cases, no structural change in the DNA has been demonstrated, but there is clear evidence of misregulation of the expression of the genome.

Interaction Between Inherited and Acquired Genetic Change in Cancer

Recent studies have shown that, for several diseases, constitutional genetic change and genetic abnormality in the tumour cells are related. For instance, constitutional genetic lesions (usually deletions) which are present in all the cells of some cancer-prone individuals are also present in the cancer cells of patients who do not have a predisposition. The prototype of this kind of association is found in retinoblastoma. Patients with deletions of chromsome 13 involving band 13q14 have a characteristic malformation syndrome, the severity of which depends on the extent of the lesion but often includes retinoblastoma (Harnden and Herbert 1982). Patients with constitutional deletions involving chromosome 13 but not including band 13q14 do not get retinoblastoma. It was shown by Cavanee et al. (1983) that the cells of a proportion of retinoblastoma tumours in patients who have no constitutional genetic abnormality also show chromosome deletions or other rearrangements involving the band 13q14. The conclusion is that there is, at this locus, a gene whose function is in some way associated with the development of retinoblastoma and that the disease may arise as a consequence of either inherited or acquired lesions at this locus, or a combination of the two. While DNA sequences at or close to this locus have been isolated (Friend et al. 1986), the gene itself has not yet been isolated, nor is its function known. It has, however, been speculated (Knudson 1985) that the gene may be important in the development of the retina and also that it may be an "anti-oncogene", i.e. that it in some way antagonises the activity of one of the now numerous proto-oncogenes whose malfunction has been firmly associated with the development of neoplasia. Similar associations have now been recognised between chromosome lesions at 11p13 and Wilms' tumour (Koufos et al. 1984, 1985).

Genetic Change in FAP

The two relatively rare tumours mentioned above could have been special cases, but recent studies have shown that similar considerations apply to carcinoma of the colon. In 1985 Herrera et al. reported on a 42-year-old patient with a deletion of the long arm of chromosome 5 who had mental retardation, multiple developmental abnormalities and FAP of the Gardner's syndrome type. Following up on this due Bodmer et al. (1987) have located the FAP gene at chromosome 5q21–q22. Even more interesting, in an accompanying paper Solomon et al. (1987) have shown, using a highly polymorphic minisatellite DNA probe, that in 20% of 45 cases of non-familial colorectal carcinoma, there has been loss of one allele of genes located on the long arm of chromosome 5 as compared with normal tissue from the same subject. The most likely mechanism is loss of the whole chromosome.

This observation is in accord with the concept, developed particularly from retinoblastoma and Wilms' tumour, that a proportion of tumours are associated with loss of one allele at a critical locus thus leaving in a hemizygous condition an abnormal gene located on the other chromosome. These genes are therefore recessive at the cellular level in spite of the dominant inheritance pattern in the families. The majority of the cells of the retina or the colonic mucosa are not abnormal in patients who carry the mutant gene. Therefore, one normal copy is sufficient for normal function. If, however, that normal copy is lost, the abnormal gene is expressed, by either partial or complete loss of function, leading to a focal clonal expansion. Subsequent changes lead on to full malignancy. In the case of retinoblastoma, the probability of further change is high so that almost all the focal lesions become malignant. In polyposis the probability is less for a single lesion, but, because of the very large number of lesions, the probability of one or more becoming malignant is very high. Thus in either case a carrier of the gene has a high probability of malignancy, and hence, even though the gene is recessive, the inheritance pattern in the family will appear to be that of a dominant gene, and the family must be counselled appropriately.

The "Two Mutation" Hypothesis

The above description applies particularly to familial cases, but Knudson (1971) has proposed that such a "two mutation" hypothesis could explain both hereditary and non-hereditary cases of certain cancers. In the hereditary cases, the first "mutation" is inherited and the second one is acquired in a somatic cell, while in the sporadic cases both mutations are somatic (and sequential in the same cell) and the lesions are therefore rare. This concept was derived from the epidemiology of the diseases; however, it fits well with the observations which have been made in recent years on the chromosomes and DNA of cancer-susceptible patients.

Other Chromosomal Abnormalities in Colorectal Tumours

There were several earlier reports of other chromosome abnormalities in polyps and in carcinoma of the colon and rectum. For example, Mark et al. (1973) reported on seven polyps from a patient with Gardner's syndrome. In six out of seven polyps, an extra chromosome of the D (13–15) group was present. Mitelman et al. (1974) examined five polyps from a patient with polyposis and no stigmata of Gardner's syndrome. Very few adequately banded cells were examined, but trisomy for chromosome 14 was observed in several cells and also in two cells from two other patients with sporadic polyps.

In a series of papers, Reichman and her colleagues describe the chromosome banding of human large bowel cancers. They report a variety of abnormalities but eventually focus on chromosome 1, (Reichman et al. 1984). However, in an earlier paper (Reichman et al. 1981), a deletion of the long arm of chromosome 5 (5q–) is reported in eight out of 31 cases. Four of these cases were in the near diploid range, and 5q– was singled out as the most common rearrangement. It is not too surprising that no special attention was paid to this since the 5q– chromosomes appear in a background of many other varied abnormalities, both structural and numerical.

A report of a constitutional chromosome polymorphism at band 2q21.3 in patients with FAP (Gardner et al. 1985) has not been confirmed.

Association of Carcinoma of the Colon and Rectum with Normal Traits

While the most obvious instances of a genetic effect in cancers of the colon and rectum are those where familial clustering occurs, there are a small number of reports of an association between normal (inherited) traits and these cancers.

Histocompatibility Type

There are extensive studies on the association of particular diseases, including malignant diseases, with HLA type. In some these are very clear and probably meaningful relationships, as in Hodgkin's disease (Dausset et al. 1982). There are relatively few studies on colon cancer. Dausset et al. (1982) refer to two population studies on colon and one study on rectal cancer from the International HLA and Disease Registry which were negative for HLA association. Lynch et al. (1975) have shown a strong association between the occurence of carcinoma in members of a large pedigree and the histocompatibility haplotype A2 B12. However, in this family there were a variety of different neoplasms, and only a small number had carcinoma of the colon. Another interesting family is reported by Sivak et al. (1981) who found an association between haplotypes A3 B18 and A2 B17 with colonic carcinoma. Similarly, Katano et al. (1980) and Dupré et al. (1975) report association between colorectal cancer and haplotypes A9 B35 and A2 B12, respectively, the latter being in a polyposis family. More recent reports (Illeni et al. 1986; Alcalay et al. 1982) also show an association between HLA type and colorectal cancer. Kune and Serjeantson (1984), on the other hand, in a carefully controlled study, showed no significant differences between cases and controls for any of the large number of HLA antigens studied. Thus, no consistency of pattern has emerged, so the results are difficult to interpret.

Blood Groups

Similarly, there are reported associations between blood groups and malignancy. The best known is that between carcinoma of the stomach and blood group A (McConnell 1966). Once again, there are few studies on blood groups and carcinoma of the colon. McConnell lists several studies prior to 1966 which show no significant correlation. More recently, Halvorsen (1986), in a retrospective study of 747 cases, found an AB0 and Rh blood group distribution similar to that of healthy blood donors. There was a slight distortion in the stage distribution of carcinoma of the colon, with Rh− patients having a more favourable distribution than Rh+ cases. In a brief communication, Mousseron-Canet (1984) reported a distorted sex ratio of blood group distribution among patients with colorectal carcinoma. They suggest that certain AB0 incompatabilities between mother and foetus, especially a group 0 mother sensitised against an A foetus, may have a lower than usual risk of certain cancers.

The evidence, therefore, for association of either blood group or histocompatibility type with carcinoma of the colorectum is not strong.

Ethnic Groups

There are very substantial differences in the incidence of colorectal cancer in different parts of the world. The overwhelming body of evidence suggests that these differences are due to environmental factors rather than genetic factors. However, Wellington et al. (1979), in a very complex multivariate analysis, conclude that even when all other variables are taken into consideration, there is a residual ethnic effect for carcinoma of the colon which relates particularly to a high incidence in groups in the United States of particular European origin. Similarly Culter and Young (1979) conclude that some of the differences they observe between ethnic groups in the United States, including a statistically significant excess of cancers of the colon and rectum in white males, may be real.

Syndromes Associated with Colorectal Cancer

A few years ago it would have been relatively simple to describe the various syndromes which appear to confer a susceptibility to carcinoma of the colon and rectum. An excellent summary of the older literature is given by McConnell (1966). McKusick (1983) is able to list three principal forms of intestinal polyposis associated with increased susceptibility to carcinoma of the colon which he terms "intestinal polyposis type 1" (familial polyposis of the colon, FPC); "intestinal polyposis type II" (Peutz-Jeghers syndrome, PJS) and "intestinal polyposis type III" (Gardner's syndrome, GRS). McKusick notes that there are demarcation problems, especially between types I and III but concludes that "the intrafamilial consistency of phenotype is too great for FPC and GRS to be due to precisely the same mutation". He does agree, however, that they may be due to different mutant alleles of the same gene.

In view of recent studies which seem to blur the distinction between types I and III, these will be considered together under the general name of FAP.

Familial Adenomatous Polyposis

Classically "polyposis coli" [FPC, adenomatosis of the colon and rectum (ACR) or familial intestinal polyposis type I (FIP I)] is described as a dominantly inherited syndrome in which multiple adenomatous polyps occur in, and are confined to, the colon and rectum and where the probability of malignant change is very high. The penetrance of the gene is very high so that virtually all gene carriers develop polyps and a high proportion get carcinoma of the colon; indeed, most develop the disease at an early age. Gardner's syndrome (FIP III) is classically defined as a dominantly inherited syndrome in which multiple adenomatous polyps occur throughout the gastrointestinal tract, frequently associated with extraintestinal symptoms (Gardner 1962). Again there is a high probability of malignant change in the polyps. Gardner noted an association with a number of benign neoplasms such as osteomata and fibromata as well as epidermal cysts. Osteomata and overlying fibromas characteristically occur on the mandible and forehead, while sebaceous and epidermal cysts may occur in the back. Mesentric fibromatosis may occur following surgery.

Extracolonic Polyps

The particular difficulty that has arisen with the neat classification (FPC and Gardner's syndrome) is that it is now clear that virtually all patients with polyposis have polyps throughout the gastrointestinal tract. In 1977 Yao et al. drew attention to duodenal lesions in patients with familial polyposis of the colon. Tonelli et al. (1981, 1985) have reported their own findings and reviewed the literature on extracolonic polyps in polyposis. In their 1985 study they carried out detailed examinations of 24 patients from 20 unrelated families, all of whom had a colectomy for multiple polyposis. They found fundic gland polyps in three patients (12.5%), antral adenomas in three (12.5%), duodenal adenomas in 14 (58.3%); ileal polyps in five (20.8%) and ileal lymphoid polyps in five (20.8%). Only two patients had polyps at all sites. The ages of those with and without polyps were similar. Of the 24 patients, 13 had "Gardner's stigmata" and 11 did not; extracolonic polyps were present in both groups though duodenal adenomas were more common in those patients with Gardner's features. They suggest that the terms "familial gastrointestinal polyposis" or "adenomatous polyposis of the gastrointestinal tract" would be appropriate names for all cases. Utsonomiya et al. (1981) also consider the two syndromes together under the name "adenomatosis coli". Extraintestinal stigmata of Gardner's syndrome were found in only 42.8% of the cases, while 70% had polypoid lesions of the stomach, 100% had polyps of the duodenum, and 70% had polpys of the jejunum. Adenomatous polyps of the entire gastrointestinal tract are found in some members of almost all families regardless of whether or not Gardner's features are present.

More recently Jarvinen and Sipponen (1986), in a comparison of FAP with juvenile polyposis using endoscopy, found that 90% (45 of 50) of patients with FAP had upper gastrointestinal polyps. Shemesch et al. (1985) found adenomas in one or more upper gastrointestinal tract sites in all of 17 patients with Gardner's syndrome. There is thus wide agreement that polyps are not confined to the colon even in families regarded as having classical polyposis coli.

Penetrance and Expressivity

It is of considerable interest that a series of patients from widely different locations should give reasonably comparable results with respect to extracolonic polyps. Similarly, a consideration of several different series shows that virtually all the gene carriers develop polyps, i.e. the pentrance of the gene is high. However, the severity and extent of the disease (expressivity) appears to be variable both within and between families. Some patients have enormous numbers of polyps, 10 000 or more, which may cover the entire surface of the colon and rectum. The average number of adenomas in colectomy specimens is about 1000, and the tumours are fairly evenly distributed around the colon and rectum (Bussey 1982). Bussey also suggests that a figure of 100 adenomas may be a practical dividing line between polyposis cases and "non-polyposis cases" since the polyposis cases may have counts down to 150 and non-polyposis cases, though usually having fewer than 20 polyps, may have polyp counts up to 80 or so. On the other hand, individual patients within families where the gene is clearly expressed may have only small numbers of polyps. This makes the distinction between the various forms of this disease even more difficult. It also raises the whole question of the role of the progression of adenomatous polyps to carcinoma in both familial and non-familial cases of carcinoma of the colon. It can, however, be a firm conclusion that any adenomatous polyp carries a risk of undergoing malignant change, and so the more polyps, the higher the risk of carcinoma.

As might be expected, therefore, there is a wide variation in the age of diagnosis of both polyps and of carcinomas. There is good agreement between the London series

(Bussey 1975) and the Japanese series (Utsonomiya et al. 1981). About 50% of gene carriers have polyps by late adolescence, and 90% have polyps by 25 years. These patients may be symptom free until around the age of 30 years. Large bowel cancer is found in 50% of gene carriers by the late 20s and in 90% by the age of 40 years. If anything, the progression is slightly slower in the Japanese cases.

Peutz-Jeghers Syndrome

PJS is almost certainly a different entity. It is inherited in an autosomal dominant manner. The main feature is polyps of the gastrointestinal tract which are most often hamartomatous (McAllister and Richards 1977). The second feature which character-ises this syndrome is the presence of melanised spots on the lips, buccal areas and digits. Females in these families are prone to develop granulosa cell tumours of the ovaries.

The polyps tend to be concentrated in the upper gastrointestinal tract, but in some patients polyps are also found in the large bowel (Bumbic et al. 1986). Peutz-Jeghers polyps rarely undergo malignant transformation, and, in view of the distribution of the polyps, this rare syndrome contributes little to the incidence of colorectal cancer. However, rare cases are reported. For example Narita et al. (1987) report a case where 52 colonic polyps were removed endoscopically. The majority were hamartomatous, but in three polyps adenomatous change and foci of adenocarcinoma were found.

Rarely isolated hamartomatous polyps of the Peutz-Jeghers type occur in patients with no other features of the Peutz-Jeghers or other polyposis syndromes (Bott et al. 1986).

Juvenile Polyposis

In this rare, dominant condition the polyps are normally hamartomatous; they may be few in number but may also be very numerous (Veale et al. 1966). They have a very low probability of undergoing malignant change, but there are several reports of relatives of patients developing gastrointestinal cancer. There are also occasional reports of colonic cancer in the patients themselves. Rozen and Baratz (1982) describe a mother and son with multiple juvenile colonic polyps. The mother developed an adenocarcinoma of the colon, but there was no evidence of the occurrence of adeno-matous polyps. However, "adenomatous features" were noted both in the original polyps of the mother and in a number of the polyps of the son.

The findings of Jarvinen and Sipponen (1986), while broadly in agreement, lead to slightly different conclusions. Gastroduodenal polyps were found in 11 of 12 patients with juvenile polyposis. Most of the polyps in these patients were hyperplastic. One focal adenomatous lesion in an antral hypoplastic polyp and one duodenal adenoma were found. These cases are contrasted with polyps in familial adenomatosis patients where the majority of the gastroduodenal polyps were either hamartomatous or adenomatous. It is concluded that, while both groups of diseases show upper gastro-intestinal polyps, each has its own characteristic pattern.

A rare variant associated with hereditary haemorrhagic telangiectasia and pulmonary arteriovenous malformations (Cox et al. 1980) may be associated with a higher risk of malignancy.

Turcot Syndrome

Turcot syndrome is an association between polyposis of the colon and malignant tumours of the central nervous system. The polyps are adenomatous, and though relatively few in number compared with classical colonic polyposis, there tends to be a greater proportion of large polpys. Itoh et al. (1979), on the basis of their own cases and a review of the literature, concluded that this is a recessive form of polyposis, and this is the general view. However, it has been suggested that Turcot syndrome is simply an unusual presentation of Gardner's syndrome (Yaffee 1964). More recently Costa et al. (1987) have reported on a family in which there are three members affected with colonic adenomatosis, one of whom has a brain tumour and is considered to be a case of Turcot syndrome. They conclude that the disease is determined by an autosomal gene with "pleiotropic effect and variable expressivity".

Familial Incidence of Non-polyposis Carcinoma of the Colon and Rectum

Increased Incidence in Relatives

For many cancers there is some evidence that cancer of the specific type is more common in close relatives of cases with that cancer. This is also true for carcinoma of the colon and rectum. One very careful study by Lovett (1976) records the cancer incidence in the families of 209 patients admitted to St. Mark's Hospital, London for treatment of carcinoma of the colon and rectum. Particular care was taken to avoid selection of cases and any case referred to St. Mark's because of a strong family history was excluded from the study as were any cases with evidence of polyposis. A total of 47 deaths due to large bowel cancer were recorded among 430 deaths of first degree relatives. This was considerably in excess of expectation based on the Registrar General's mortality statistics for the appropriate period, and the author concludes that first degree relatives of patients with bowel cancer have a three-fold increase in risk of developing the same cancer.

Almost every surgeon is able to quote, from his own experience, unusual familial aggregations of cancer of the colon and rectum. Further, there are many reports in the literature of multiple cases of cancer of the colorectum occurring in the same family. For example, Purtillo et al. (1987) report the remarkable occurrence of many cases of mucinous carcinoma of the colon in a black family. Similarly, Dunstone and Knaggs (1972) report on a very large family in which 22 of 50 recorded deaths were due to carcinoma of the colon or rectum. A further five living members of the family had been treated for carcinoma of the large bowel. The cases spanned three generations, and there was no evidence of polyposis.

It is important, but sometimes difficult, to distinguish between a familial incidence which may have a genetic basis and those situations where there are several cases of these relatively common cancers in near relatives purely by chance. Indeed, for some time many cancer epidemiologists were not impressed by these familial clusters on the grounds that they were felt to be part of a random distribution of cancers to which attention had been drawn simply because of the grouping together of several cases. Now, however, largely as a result of the work of Lynch and his associates (Lynch and Lynch 1985, 1986; Lynch et al. 1975, 1976, 1981), it is widely agreed that there are some exceptional families where it is highly likely that a susceptibility to colonic cancer is inherited in an autosomal dominant manner and that it is possible to lay down criteria for the recognition of such families. As stressed earlier, this does not mean that genetic factors are not important in families which do not meet these criteria.

Hereditary Non-polyposis Colorectal Cancer

The clearly familial cases have come to be known as the "cancer family syndrome" (Lynch et al. 1981), but this is something of a misnomer since there is no syndrome associated with the disease in individual patients. What is meant by this term is a familial aggregation of cancer which can be defined in a particular way. Alternative names that have been used are "Lynch syndrome I" for familes where there is familial, site-specific, non-polyposis colon cancer and "Lynch syndrome II" (cancer family syndrome) where non-polyposis colon cancer occurs in association with other forms of cancer. These are also inappropriate terms of same reason. However, Lynch and Lynch (1987) have now proposed that familial aggregations of these diseases be known as HNPCC types a and b, and this seems a very satisfactory terminology.

The prototype cancer family was described by Warthin (1913, 1925) who reported a very large pedigree in which there were many cases of carcinoma of the uterus, stomach and, in the later generations, intestine including colon. Warthin draws particular attention to the early age of onset (average less than 40 years). It was, however, Lynch and his associates who, in a series of papers, drew attention to the fact that the high cancer incidence often held up in extended pedigrees thus removing the criticism that these were chance findings and he also went a long way to defining and formalising the criteria for the recognition of these families (e.g. Lynch et al. 1976, 1981; Lynch and Lynch 1985). It is hard to summarise the features better than Lynch et al. have done themselves so I will quote them directly from their 1981 paper.

> The following criteria for the syndrome can be established:
> 1) A high frequency of adenocarcinoma of the colon endometrium and ovary (breast, stomach, other adenocarcinomas, and possibly lymphomas, may be additional components of the tumour spectrum).
> 2) In the case of colonic cancer a significant excess of proximal colonic involvement.
> 3) Significantly early age of cancer onset (mean of approximately 45 years) when compared to sporadically occurring counterparts in the general population (mean onset, approximately 65 years).

4) An excess of multiple primary cancer in affected patients.
5) Pedgree expression consistent with an autosomal dominant mode of genetic transmission.
6) Occasional occurrence of sebaceous adenomous epitheliomas and carcinomas in patients with the syndrome cancers (Torre's syndrome).
7) An increased frequency of prolonged survival in cancer affected patients.

This description of course predates the new nomenclature and encompasses both types of HNPCC. Other authors have confirmed and extended this definition. For example, Mecklin et al. (1986) have proposed that the finding of a high proportion of mucinous carcinomas should be a further indication of HNPCC. In a study of 100 separate tumours in 75 patients with colorectal carcinoma they found 35% – 39% of mucinous carcinomas in familial patients as compared to 20% in controls – patients with carcinoma of the colon and no hereditary background. There was also a higher proportion of poorly differentiated tumours in the hereditary cases, and, while the incidence of additional adenomas was similar in both groups, the adenomas in the HNPCC cases more often had dysplastic or villous features. This would also bring the family described by Purtillo et al. (1987) mentioned earlier within the definition of HNPCC. In spite of the setting of these criteria there is still considerable difficulty in deciding whether or not an individual patient belongs to such a family.

A recent study from Finland (Mecklin and Jarvinen 1986) pinpoints the problem very nicely. They suggest that 5% or more of colorectal cancer patients may have HNPCC and pose the questions of how to recognise these patients and should their assignment to this category affect their treatment. In a study of 22 HNPCC families they identified 200 cancer patients of whom 122 had colorectal carcinoma. They confirmed the principal features identified by Lynch: an early age of onset (mean 41 years), a proximal location of the colonic tumour (54% in the right colon) and a high frequency of multiplicity. However, only 40% had a clear family history of cancer at the time of diagnosis. Thus for an individual patient the decision as to whether or not the case is one of HNPCC remains difficult and may only be made after extensive family studies over a period of several years. Where a patient is clearly identified as belonging to a HNPCC family, however, lifelong follow-up examinations of the remaining colon and rectum are advised.

Colonic Cancer in Twins

One of the classic methods for determining genetic origin of a disease is to compare concordance rates in monozygotic and dizygotic twins. Few formal studies have been carried out on cancer in twins but these tend to show no increased concordance. For example, in a large study by the Danish Twin Registry and the Danish Cancer Registry (Holm et al. 1982) there was no excess concordance in monozygotic twins for colorectal cancer occurring in a population where neither twin had died before 15 years of age. There are, however, isolated positive reports. Johnson and Thompson (1986) report a remarkable instance where a pair of monozygotic male twins aged 73 presenting within 5 months of each other. Each had three moderately differentiated adenocarcinomas of the colon. There is no history of bowel disease in the immediate family, though their father had died of carcinoma of the bladder. Both twins also had multiple subcutaneous lipomas but no other abnormality. Reference is made in this report to two other instances of concordance for colonic cancer in monozygotic twins, in one case simultaneous and in the other pair at a time interval of 2 years. Clearly this is a rare occurrence and does little to support the idea of a general strong genetic aetiology for colon cancer. However, where a disease is not inherited directly, but rather a susceptibility is inherited (dependent perhaps on further environmental influences) the absence of a twin effect is not too surprising.

Types of Inherited Susceptibility

Many diseases and indeed many clinical syndromes are found to be heterogeneous in their aetiology. This is also true of genetic disease where the same condition may arise as the result of different types of genetic lesion. It is clear that cases of cancer of the colon and rectum will have a variety of different causes, and even amongst those cases with a significant genetic background, the precise genetic mechanisms may be different. One can recognise at least three different types of inherited susceptibility.

Inherited Lesion as Part of Genetic Change in Cancer Cell

In some cancers, we have already noted that a lesion is inherited which is similar if not identical to that found in the cancer cells of sporadic cases. If we assume that a series of genetic changes lead to cancer, inheritance of one of these changes will increase the probability that full malignancy will be reached. The recognition of a lesion on the long arms of chromosome 5 in colonic cancers could suggest that this mechanism may operate in some cases of inherited colorectal cancer.

Inherited Genetic Instability

In diseases such as xeroderma pigmentosa (XP), it seems clear that an unusual sensitivity to a specific environmental agent (ultraviolet light) is associated with the development of cancer. In XP the mechanism is a DNA repair defect suggesting that the inherited genetic lesion is not itself part of the genetic change in the cancer cell but may lead to such change secondarily, in the cells of affected individuals. Evidence that this occurs in colorectal cancer has not been forthcoming but can not be ruled out at this stage, though clearly any effect cannot be as dramatic as that in XP.

Effects on Progression and Surveillance

Most often it is considered that genetic susceptibility operates at the initiation of carcinogenesis. Thus it appears that by some means cellular transformation to malignancy is more probable. It is quite possible, however, that even if the transformation frequency is unaltered, the probability of development of full malignancy may be modified by genetic factors which either enhance the probability of progression or decrease the probability that a potentially malignant cell is recognised and eliminated. Increased sensitivity to promoting agents could be one such mechanism.

It is well documented that hormone balance can affect the probability of malignant progression in experimental systems, and the hormone dependence of certain breast cancers is well documented. There is, however, little or no evidence that colorectal cancer is influenced by endocrine factors. There is a slight excess of both colon and rectal cancer in males as measured by age-specific incidence rates (Fraser and Adelstein 1982). Similarly, immunological factors, which again may be under genetic control, can influence tumour progression. However, the Immunodeficiency Cancer Registry, which records cases of cancer occurring in patients with primary immunodeficiency diseases, shows no association between immunodeficiency and colorectal cancer (Filipovich et al. 1980).

Mechanisms of Inherited Susceptibility

Initiation and Promotion

Current models of carcinogenesis are all based on the concept of a multistage process, evidence for which comes both from mathematical models of age incidence and from experimental evidence. One such scheme is the initiation and promotion model which arises from studies on mouse skin chemical carcinogenesis but fits well with other situations including the human cancers where specific stimuli are known. The precise nature of these steps is not known for certain, but much evidence points to the first step, initiation, being an irreversible genetic change while the subsequent promotional steps may involve either further genetic changes, or alterations in either the cellular environment or the capacity of the cell to respond to environmental stimuli. Initiating agents, such as benzo[a]pyrene, may act as complete carcinogens if given in adequate dose. If, however, the dose is low, they may cause changes which are inapparent unless a further promoting stimulus is applied. Promoting agents, such as the phorbol esters, will not cause cancers even when administered in large doses. However, repeated small doses given after (even a long time after) a low dose of an initiating agent will lead to malignancy. In colon cancer it has been suggested that bile acids and specific dietary constituents might act as promoting agents (McMichael and Potter 1985).

It has been argued by several authors that the inherited genetic abnormality in diseases such as FAP is akin to initiation, and that the colonic mucosa in these patients simply requires the application of one or more promoting influences for neoplasia to occur. A number of attempts have been made to show that cells from patients with FAP are abnormal in their response to promoting agents, with conflicting results. Kopelovich et al. (1979) report that fibroblasts from FAP patients treated with tetradecanoyl-phorbol-13-acetate (TPA) produce moderately differentiated fibrosarcomas on inoculation into the anterior chamber of the eye of nude mice. Antecol and Mukherjee (1982) were, however, unable to reproduce this result.

Biochemical and Kinetic Changes

There are a number of reports of biological or biochemical differences between the cells of the colonic mucosa in patients with familial colonic cancers as opposed to controls. For example, Chesa et al. (1986) describe an immunohistochemical study in which they show that reactivity to monoclonal antibodies against two particular groups of cytokeratins differs in normal mucosa as compared to mucosa from polyposis patients. Cytokeratins reacting with antibodies AE1 and AE3 are expressed in the more mature areas of the normal mucosa (surface and upper crypts) but throughout the glands and surface mucosa in patients with polyposis. Similarly, solitary tubular polyps and hypoplastic polyps are composed largely of non-expressing cells, while polyps of high malignant potential and colonic carcinomas show a preponderance of AE1- and AE3-positive cells. The cytokeratins recognised by these antibodies thus appear to be markers for tissues at high risk of malignancy.

A similar alteration in the distribution of cellular activities has been described in a series of papers by Lipkin and his colleagues (Lipkin and Deschner 1977; Lipkin 1978). In the normal colon, proliferation of epithelial cells is largely confined to the basal and middle regions of the crypts. This pattern is disordered not only in polyps, but also in the apparently normal mucosal cells of FAP patients and in some symptom-free members of FAP families. In FAP patients the cells of the surface mucosa frequently show continuing DNA synthesis as measured by incorporation of tritiated thymidine in short-term culture. This disruption of normal behaviour is sometimes seen in the mucosa of patients with isolated polyps.

A further indication that differentiation patterns are disturbed in this disease comes from Davies et al. (1983) who reported that in polyps and carcinomas of patients with polyposis coli various isoenzyme patterns resembled those of the foetus or liver rather than those of normal colon.

Chromosomal Abnormality and Instability

There are many reports of chromosomal abnormalities in both cultured skin cells, mucosal cells and lymphocytes from patients with FAP. Danes (1978) reported increased levels of polyploidy in epithelial cell containing cultures from FAP patients and also in cultured colonic mucosa. Danes and Alm (1979) observed these changes in both patients with and those without Gardner's stigmata but not in all and they suggest that it reflects a degree of genetic heterogeneity. Delhanty et al. (1980, 1983) also observed increased tetraploidy in a low proportion of cultured cell lines from skin biopsies of patients with FAP, and also chromosome instability in lymphocytes, fibroblasts and colon cells from an FAP patient.

Pero et al. (1986) report an increased level of spontaneous chromosome aberrations in fibroblasts from FAP cases. Similarly, Heim et al. (1985) report an increased frequency of spontaneous structural chromosome abnormalities in fibroblasts cultured from FAP patients. In a large study covering 57 cell strains they found an increase of a variety of chromosome and chromatid aberrations in strains from patients as compared with those from controls. Moreover, an excess of chromosome aberrations was also noted in the patients' cells following treatment with N-methyl-N'-

nitro-*N*-nitrosoguanidine (MNNG). While the differences between mean values were highly significant, there was considerable overlap between individual observations from patients and controls. However, in a study using lymphocytes Kasukawa et al. (1985) found no difference between FAP patients and controls with respect to spontaneous numerical chromosome abnormalities and only a slight excess of structural aberrations in the patients.

The overall impression, therefore, is that there is some evidence of chromosome instability in cells from patients with FAP. It is, however, somewhat inconsistent from patient to patient and is not at present useful in distinguishing individual affected members in a family though it may be a helpful in combination with other parameters.

Sensitivity to Environmental Agents

There is no clinical evidence to suggest that patients with FAP or other familial susceptibility to colon cancer are unusually sensitive to drugs, radiation or other environmental agents. However, a large number of studies have been carried out on cultured cells from these patients. In a review of these reports Harnden et al. (1984) conclude that while individual studies show a marked sensitivity to killing or to cellular transformation by radiation, viruses or chemicals, there is a lack of consistency about these reports which makes it very difficult to say that FAP cells are unusually sensitive to any particular agent, e.g. some studies show FAP cells to be sensitive to cell killing by MNNG while others fail to find such a sensitivity. None of the positive reports have been followed up by convincing confirmation of an effect that would be useful in a diagnostic situation. Furthermore, there are no real clues from these studies which suggest which particular environmental agents might be interacting with the abnormal inherited gene to produce the clinical problem.

Activation of Oncogenes

There are a number of reports of the activation of specific oncogenes in colorectal cancer. Most often, c-Ki-*ras* is activated (Cunningham and Weinberg 1984). One report describes the activation of the c-Ha-*ras* (Greenhalgh and Kinsella 1985) in cell lines from a carcinoma of the colon. Of particular interest in the present context, Yuasa et al. (1986) report the recognition of an activated c-K-*ras* 2- gene in a cell line derived from a metastatic deposit in a lymph node of a patient with FAP. The topic of oncogenes is dealt with in detail by James and Sikora (this volume).

The Relevance of Heredity in Cancer Prevention

Knowledge of genetic causes of carcinoma of the colon and rectum has already provided important information for the management of some patients with this disease. An increasing understanding should make further contributions in the future. There are three ways in which genetic knowledge can makes contribution.

Antenatal Diagnosis

With the recognition of a DNA probe tightly linked to the FAP gene (Bodmer et al. 1987) it should be possible, at least in some families, to identify affected individuals antenatally using chorionic villus sampling by 7–9 weeks' gestation, thus giving the possibility of selective termination of pregnancy.

Identification of Individuals at Risk

Similar, the availability of this probe and others will certainly now identify individuals at risk in a family. This has the double advantage of early reassurance to those not at risk and the concentration of screening procedures on those known to be at risk.

While the probe so far identified has been linked to FAP, it may also be useful in other non-polyposis families. Even if not, similar probes for the other familial cases will be found.

Family Histories and Screening

Even without DNA probes or other sophisticated laboratory techniques, much can be and is already done to help members of these "at risk" families. The importance of taking a simple family history from those cases where there is a high index of suspicion must be stressed. In those instances where there is reason to believe that the condition is familial appropriate examination of all individuals at risk is indicated, with a view to possible surgical intervention. It is important to stress that adequate genetic counselling of these families is essential. The level of anxiety is often very high and with the new techniques being made available, it will now be possible to offer most family members some practical advice and help. Cases that are identified early have a greatly improved probability of survival though lifelong surveillance may be necessary.

References

Alcalay M, Bontoux D, Maire P, Matuchansky C, Alcalay D, Tanzer J (1982) HLA B27 and colorectal cancer. N Engl J Med 307:443–444

Antecol MH, Mukherjee BB (1982) Effects of 12-O-tetradecanoylphorbol-13-acetate on fibroblasts from individuals genetically predisposed to cancer. Cancer Res 42:3870–3879

Bodmer WF (1986) Inherited susceptibility to cancer. In: Franks LM, Tiech NM (eds) Introduction to the cellular and molecular biology of cancer. Oxford University Press, Oxford, pp 93–110

Bodmer WF, Bailey CJ, Bodmer J, Bussey HJR, Ellis A, Groman P, Lucibello FC, Murday VA, Rider SH, Scambler P, Sheer D, Solomon E, Spurr NK (1987) Localisation of the gene for familial adenomatous polyposis on chromosme 5. Nature 328:614–616

Bott SJ, Hanks JB, Stone DD (1986) Solitary hamartomatous polyp of the duodenum in the absence of familial polyposis coli. Am J Gastroenterol 81:993–994

Bumbic S, Stepanovic R, Nestrovic B (1986) Peutz-Jeghers syndrome – juvenile instestinal polyposis – review of 5 cases. Z Kinderchir 41:178–180

Bussey JH (ed) (1975) Familial polyposis coli. The John Hopkins University Press, Baltimore

Bussey HJR (1982) Genetic factors. In: Duncan W (ed) Colorectal cancer. Springer, Berlin Heidelberg New York, pp 45–58 (Recent results in cancer research, vol 83)

Cavenee WK, Dryja TP, Philips RA, Benedict WF, Godebout R, Gallie BL, Murphree AL, Strong LC, White RL (1983) Expression of recessive alleles by chromosomal mechanisms in retinoblastoma. Nature 305:779–784

Chesa PG, Rettig WJ, Melamed MR (1986) Expression of cytokeratins in normal and neoplastic colonic epithelial cells. Implications for cellular differentiation and carcinogenesis. Am J Surg Pathol 10:829–835

Costa OL, Silva DM, Colnago FA, Vieira MS, Musso C (1987) Turcot syndrome: autosomal dominant or recessive transmission. Dis Colon Rectum 30:391–394

Cox KL, Frates RC, Wong A, Gandhi G (1980) Hereditary generalised juvenile polyposis associated with pulmonary ateriovenous malfunction. Gastroenterology 78:1566–1570

Cunningham JM, Weinberg RA (1984) Detection and analysis of oncogenese in colon carcinoma. Prog Cancer Res Ther 29:403–411

Cutler SJ, Young JL (1979) Demographic patterns of cancer, incidence in the United States. In: Fraumeni JF (ed) Persons at high risk of cancer. Academic, New York, pp 307–342

Danes BS (1978) Increased in vitro tetraploidy: tissue specific within the heritable colorectal cancer syndromes with polyposis coli. Cancer 41:2330–2334

Danes BS, Alm T (1979) In vitro studies on adenomatosis of the colon and rectum. J Med Genet 16:417–422

Dausset J, Colombani J, Hors J (1982) Major histocompatibility complex and cancer with special reference to human familial tumours (Hodgkin's disease and other malignancies). Cancer Surv 1:119–149

Davis MB, Swallow DM, Delhanty JDA (1983) Isozyme analyses of the large intestine with special reference to carcinoma of the colon and familial polyposis coli. Disease Markers 1:283–297

Delhanty JDA, Davis MB, Wood J (1983) Chromosome instability in lymphocytes, fibroblasts and colon-epithelial-like cells from patients with FPC. Cancer Genet Cytogenet 8:27–50

Delhanty JDA, Pritchard MB, Bussey HJR, Morson BC (1980) Tetraploid fibroblasts and familial polyposis coli. Lancet i:1365

Dunstone GH, Knaggs TWL (1972) Familial cancer of the colon and rectum. J Med Genet 9:451–456

Dupre N, Nouza E, Raffoux C, Morvan JC, Gras JP (1975) Polypose rectocolique familiale et systeme HLA à propos d'une observation. Bordeaux Med 30:2125–2130

Filipovich AH, Spector BD, Kersey JH (1980) Immunodeficiency in humans as a risk factor in the development of malignancy. Prev Med 9:252–259

Fraser P, Adelstein AM (1982) Recent trends in colorectal cancer. In: Duncan W (ed) Springer, Berlin Heidelberg New York, pp 1–10 (Recent results in cancer research, vol 83)

Friend SH, Bernard SR, Rogel JS, Weinberg RA, Rappaport JM, Albert DM, Dryja TP (1986) A human DNA segment with properties of the gene which predisposes to retinoblatoma. Nature 323:643–646

Gardner EJ (1962) Follow up study of a family group exhibiting dominant inheritance for a syndrome including intestinal polyps, osteomas, fibromas and epidermal cysts. Am J Hum Genet 14:376–390

Gardner EJ, Woodward SR, Hughes JP (1985) Evolution of chromosomal diagnosis for hereditary adenomatosis of the colorectum. Cancer Genet Cytogenet 15:321–334

Greenhalgh DA, Kinsella AR (1985) c-Ha-*ras* not c-Ki-*ras* activation in three colon tumour cell lines. Carcinogenesis 6:1533–1535

Halvorsen TB (1986) ABO blood groups, rhesus types and colorectal adenocarcinoma. A retrospective study of 747 cases. Scand J Gastroenterol 21:979–983

Harnden DG, Herbert A (1982) Association of constitutional chromosome rearrangements with neoplasia. Cancer Surv 1:149–173

Harnden DG, Morten JEN, Featherstone T (1984) Dominant susceptibility to cancer in man. In: Klein G, Weinhouse S (eds) Recent Advances in cancer research, vol 41. Academic, London, pp 185–255

Heim S, Johansen SG, Kolnig AM, Strombeck B (1985) Increased levels of spontaneous and mutagen induced chromosome aberrations in skin fibroblasts from patients with adenomatosis of the colon and rectum. Cancer Genet Cytogenet 17:333–346

Herrera L, Kakati S, Gibas L, Pietrzak E, Sandberg AA (1986) Gardner's syndrome in a man with an interstitial deletion of 5q. Am J Med Genet 25:473–476

Holm NV, Hauge M, Jensen OM (1982) Studies of cancer aetiology in a complete twin population: breast cancer, colorectal cancer and leukaemia. Cancer Surv 1:17–32

Illeni MT, Agazzi C, Doci R, Lombardo C, Maschereti E, Audisio RA (1986) Human leukocyte antigens and sister chromatid exchanges in families with multiple adenomatosis coli. Cancer Detect Prev 9:459–468

Itoh H, Ohsato K, Yao T, Iida M, Watanabe H (1979) Turcot's syndrome and its mode of inheritance. Gut 20:414–419

Jarvinen HJ, Sipponen P (1986) Gastrointestinal polyps in familial and adenomatous and juvenile polyposis. Endoscopy 18:230–234

Johnson CD, Thomson H (1986) Six synchronous colonic cancers in a pair of monozygotic twins. Dis Colon Rectum 29:745–746

Kasukawa T, Watanabe T, Endo A (1985) Cytogenetic and cytokinetic analysis of lymphocytes from patients with hereditary adenomatosis of the colon and rectum. Cancer Genet Cytogenet 16:73–79

Katano M, Fujiwara H, Toyoda K, Torisu M (1980) Immunogenetic studies of familial large bowel cancer. Gann 71:583–588

Knudson AG (1971) Mutation and cancer: statistical study of retinoblasma. Proc Natl Acad Sci USA 68:820–823

Knudson AG (1985) Hereditary cancer, oncogenes and anti oncogenes. Cancer Res 45:1437–1443

Kopelovich L, Bias NE, Helson L (1979) Tumour promotor alone induces neoplastic transformation of fibroblasts from humans genetically predisposed to cancer. Nature 282:619–621

Koufos A, Hansen MF, Lampkin BC, Workman ML, Copeland NG, Jenkins NA, Cavenee WK (1984) Loss of alleles at loci on human chromosome 11 during genesis of Wilm's tumour. Nature 309:170–172

Koufos A, Hansen MF, Copeland NG, Jenkins NA, Lampkin BC, Cavenee WK (1985) Loss of heterozygozity in three embryonal tumours suggests a common pathogenetic mechanism. Nature 316:330–334

Kune GA, Serjeantson S (1984) HLA and colorectal cancer. Med J Aust 141:199

Lipkin M (1978) Susceptibility of human population groups to colon cancer. Adv Cancer Res 27:281–304

Lipkin M, Deschner EE (1977) Gastointestinal neoplasia: an investigate approach. In: Mulvihill JJ, Miller RW, Fraumeni JF (eds) Genetics of human cancer. Raven, New York, pp 369–375

Lovett E (1976) Family studies in cancer of the colon and rectum. Br J Surg 63:13–18

Lynch HT, Lynch J (1987) Genetic predictability and minimal cancer clues in Lynch syndrome II. Dis Colon Rectum 30:243–246

Lynch HT, Thomas RJ, Terasaki PI, Ting A, Guirgis HA, Kaplan AR, Magee H, Lynch J, Craft C, Chaperon E (1975) HLA in cancer family "N". Cancer 36:1315–1320

Lynch HT, Krush AJ, Thomas RJ, Lynch J (1976) Cancer family syndrome. In: Lynch HT (ed) Cancer genetics. Thomas, Springfield, pp 355–388

Lynch HT, Lynch PM, Albano WA, Lynch JF (1981) The cancer syndrome: a status report. Dis Colon Rectum 24:311–322

Lynch PM, Lynch HT (eds) (1985) Colon cancer genetics. Van Nostrand Reinhold, New York

Mark J, Mitelman F, Dencker H, Norryd C, Tranberg KG (1973) The specificity of the chromosomal abnormalities in human colonic polyps. A cytogenetic study of multiple polyps in a case of Gardner's syndrome. Acta Pathol Microbiol Scan 81 A:85–90

McAllister AJ, Richards KF (1977) Peutz-Jeghers syndrome: experience with twenty patients in five generations. Am J Surg 134:717–720

McConnell RB (ed) (1966) The genetics of gastrointestinal disorders. Oxford University Press, London

McKusick VA (ed) (1983) Mendlian inheritance in man, 6th edn. The Johns Hopkins University Press, Baltimore

McMichael AJ, Potter JD (1985) Host factors in carcinogenesis: certain bile acid metabolic profiles that selectively increase the risk of proximal colon cancer. J Natl Cancer Inst 75:185–191

Mecklin JP, Jarvinen HJ (1986) Clinical features of colorectal carcinoma in cancer family syndrome. Dis Colon Rectum 29:160–164

Mecklin JP, Sipponen P, Jarvinen HJ (1986) Histopathology of colorectal carcinoma and adenocarcinoma in cancer family syndrome. Dis Colon Rectum 29:849–853

Mitelman F, Mark J, Nilsson PG, Dencker H, Norryd C, Transberg KG (1974) Chromosome banding pattern in human colonic polyps. Hereditas 78:61–68

Mousseron-Canet MM (1984) Blood groups, sex and frequency of colorectal carcinoma. Lancet ii:926–927

Narita T, Eto T, Ito T (1987) Peutz-Jeghers syndrome with adenomas and adenocarcinomas in colonic polyps. Ann J Surg Pathol 11:76–81

Pero RW, Heim S, Bryngelsson C (1986) Lower rates of thymidine incorporation with DNA of skin fibroblasts from patients with adenomatosis of the colon and rectum. Carcinogenesis 7:541–545

Purtillo DT, Geelhoed GW, Li FP, Yang JP, Thurber WA, Darrah J, Cassel C (1987) Mucinous carcinoma in a black family. Cancer Genet Cytogenet 24:11–15

Reichman A, Martin P, Levin B (1981) Chromosome banding patterns in human large bowel cancer. Int J Cancer 28:431–440

Reichman A, Martin P, Levin B (1984) Chromosome in human large bowel tumours: a study of chromosome 1. Cancer Genet Cytogenet 12:295–301

Rozen P, Baratz P (1982) Familial juvenile colonic polyposis with associated colon cancer. Cancer 49:1500–1503

Shemesh E, Pines A, Bat L (1985) Spectrum of extracolonic gastrointestinal involvement in Gardner's syndrome. Int J Med Sci 21:973–976

Sivak MV, Schleutermann-Sivak D, Braun WA, Sullivan BH (1981) A linkage study of HLA and inherited adenocarcinoma of the colon. Cancer 48, 76–81

Solomon E, Voss R, Hall V, Bodmer WF, Jass JR, Jeffreys AJ, Lucibello FC, Patel L, Rider SH (1987) Chromosome 5 allele loss in human colorectal carcinomas. Nature 328: 617–619

Thompson JS, Pearlman N (1982) Cancer of the colon and rectum in high risk patients. Dis Colon Rectum 25:461–463

Tonelli F, De Masi E, Astarita L, Nardi F (1981) Gastric and duodenal polyps associated with familial polyposis coli: personal experience and review of the literature. Ital J Gastoenterol 13:32–39

Tonelli F, Nardi F, Bechi P, Taddei G, Gozzo P, Romagnoli P (1985) Extracolonic polyps in familial polyposis coli and Gardner' syndrome? 28: 664–668

Utsonomiya J, Iwama T, Hirayama R (1981) Familial large bowel cancer. In: Decosse JJ (ed) Clinical surgery international, vol 1. Churchill Livingstone, Edinburgh, pp 16–33

Veale AM, McColl I, Bussey HJR, Morson BC (1966) Juvenile polyposis coli. J Med Genet 3:5–6

Warthin AS (1913) Heredity with reference to carcinoma: as shown by the study of cases examined in the pathological laboratory of the University of Michigan. Arch Intern Med 12:546–555

Warthin AS (1925) The further study of a cancer family. J Cancer Res 9:279–286

Wellington DG, MacDonald EJ, Wolf PF (1979) Cancer mortality: environmental and ethnic factors. Academic Press, New York

Yafee HS (1964) Gastric polyposis and soft tissue tumours. Arch Dermatol 89:806–808

Yao T, Iida M, Ohsato K, Watanabe H, Omae T (1977) Duodenal lesions in familial polyposis of the colon. Gastroenterology 73:1086–1092

Yuasa Y, Oto M, Sato C, Miyaki M, Iwama T, Tonomura A, Namba M (1986) Colon carcinoma K-ras 2 oncogene of a familial polyposis coli patient. Jpn J Cancer Res 77:901–907

Acquired Conditions of Increased Risk of Colorectal Cancer

R. R. Frentzel-Beyme

Institute of Epidemiology and Biometry, Deutsches Krebsforschungszentrum,
D-6900 Heidelberg, FRG

Contents

Introduction

The fact that colorectal cancer is a major cause of morbidity and mortality and that it has become a major prematurely killing disease in almost every Western population makes this neoplastic entity a central target for preventive efforts. Some previously suggested associations between increased risk and dietary factors have recently turned out to be inconsistent in adequately conducted studies which have to be considered to be of importance, thus leaving doubts regarding the value of certain recommendations. This absence of factors which increase risk consistently makes it mandatory to focus on other more likely indicators for elevated risks and also on more manageable factors in prevention.

Assuming that the unresolved controversy regarding dietary factors may impede the formulation of recommendations for primary prevention, and in view of the failure to recognize relevant risk factors for colon cancer, some other lines of research may be of interest, among them the concept of looking at high-risk groups (Smith et al. 1985). The acquired conditions which increase the risk for colon and rectal cancer will consequently have to be considered more closely.

While prominent researchers maintain that Western-style nutrition with a fat intake of approximately 40% of calories is associated with a higher risk of cancer of the breast, ovary, endometrium, colon, and with the left-sided colon in particular (Weisburger and Wynder 1987), the evidence recently published by other groups at the National Cancer Institute in the United States (Jones et al. 1987) and in Japan (Shimizu et al. 1987) have challenged the contention that breast cancer is related so strongly with fat intake and have proposed that for colon cancer the Westernization of diet might be a gross oversimplification, especially as an explanation for the gradients of cancer incidence in migrant populations such as Japanese immigrants in Hawaii and the United States (Shimizu et al. 1987).

Rural to urban ratios are more likely explained by general life style, i.e., the impact of the environment should take more than dietary aspects into account (Stemmermann, this volume). In his review, Stemmermann shows that if increased fat intake does favor the development of either cardiovascular heart disease or colon cancer, it probably does not act alone, nor does it have an equal influence on the two diseases. The obvious weakness of most studies referred to again and again, especially correlation ones, is that it was impossible to identify the dietary practices and actual fat intake of those persons who actually acquired colon cancer. Various risk factors, such as those having a reputation as "multiple risk factors" (obesity, smoking, alcohol consumption, occupation) were not simultaneously assessed, let alone considered in the analyses (Stemmermann et al. 1984a).

Therefore, only prospective, historical-prospective, or certain controlled studies include personal information from the patients and compare any frequencies of prevalent factors with information identically collected from comparable population samples as controls are able to provide reliable, valid information for adequate comparisons. Such an approach was used by the International Agency for Research on Cancer (IARC) collaborative studies on radiation risk for incident cancer secondary to radiotherapy given for treatment of cervical cancer and will serve as an exemplary case for the study of risk associations (Day and Boice 1983). The cohort study part of this study resulted in one important finding, viz. the clarification of an assumed relationship of second primary cancers at the rectum or colon with radiation treatment of cancer of the cervix.

Although most patients in whom colorectal cancer develops are "standard-risk" patients who are mostly above 50 years of age, with incidence peaks at 75–80 years, incidence is increased at a lower age in special populations of persons with a family history of polyposis syndromes, nonpolyposis inherited colon cancer syndrome, familial cancer syndrome, and ulcerative colitis. In women, groups with an elevated risk include patients who have had genital or breast cancer. This chapter reviews other more anecdotal reports of associations without sufficient evidence to be causal, but of importance for prevention and relevant for the population at large.

Requirements for Etiological Associations in Cancer

The first observations of etiologically important factors are often made by physicians who quantify their observations of unusual frequencies of certain "factors" in a group of patients. Such observations can appear to be mini-epidemics, even outbreaks. Even if these epidemics are not necessarily causal in nature, the coincidence of findings already has a chance of becoming a "syndrome." A whole array of possible risk associations or increases of the probability of developing colorectal cancer has been compiled in the literature. A typical case of this type of report is the increased occurrence of overt diabetes mellitus found among patients with colon or rectal carcinoma which was even statistically significantly different from a chance coincidence (Williams et al. 1984). The reported clusters of cancer in patients with acromegaly may also fall into this category (Ituarte et al. 1984).

Reports on the coincident occurrences of cancer and diabetes and speculation concerning the relationship between the two diseases have been found in the medical literature for about 100 years. Theoretical concepts (the effect of diabetes on the incidence of cancer, the effect of diabetes on the clinical course of cancer, and vice versa) were published in 1888 by Tuffier (cited by Kessler 1971). In a large cohort study including 21 447 diabetic patients of the Boston Joslin Clinic who were followed up for 30 years, a 25% sample of the 10 066 deaths was analyzed for the distribution of cancer deaths. Compared with the expected deaths, a statistically insignificant increase of intestinal (colon) cancer deaths was found is women, and a borderline significant decrease of rectal cancer was found in men; the observed and expected numbers for colon cancer in men and for rectal cancer in women were similar (Kessler 1970 a, b). The nature of the coincidences found repeatedly is not yet clear, although even a negative association of cancer and diabetes in males of certain populations has been discussed as being genetically related to glucose-6-phosphate-dehydrogenase variants (Kessler 1971). The obvious importance of sex-specific analyses shows that, apart from a review of the existing literature, epidemiological approaches are required to clarify the clinical findings of increased occurrences of any kind before any conclusions are drawn.

The ultimate test of causality is practically impossible since experiments in humans are considered unethical. One scientific approach, however, is to reconstruct the experiment which occurred in nature, which is the essence of epidemiology and the so-called paradigm of nonexperimental epidemiological research (Rothman 1986). Epidemiology has developed the methods to distinguish between etiologically relevant associations and chance occurrences or coincidental observations. One of the aims of any research into such etiologically important factors is the use of this knowledge for prevention, either primary or secondary. Casuistic reports have a role in that they indicate possible etiological associations. A systematic search for scientific evidence beyond descriptive reports requires controlled studies; however, not only a statistical appraisal, but also the determination of a risk estimate gives information regarding the intensity of a putative risk association. The risk ratio (RR) is based on epidemiologically sound planning of a study, usually including all, and especially representative, cases of the population. This estimate can be given in terms of the dimension of the problem (e.g., as an etiological fraction) or in terms of prevention.

Therapeutic conditions

Radiation

One example of the importance of epidemiological study methods is the dual approach by the IARC in the study of radiation risk which resulted in identification of the radiation-induced risk for rectal cancer, whereas no significant association could be found for colon cancer (Day and Boice 1983). This exemplary case serves the purpose of demonstrating the risk concept and the approaches usually needed for the assessment of the character of a seemingly important hazard (which in this case could be the iatrogenic and thus man-made association between radiotherapy and cancer).

In an editorial, Schottenfeld (1983) referred to epidemiological studies of medically exposed populations in general and the complexity of both damage at the tissue and at the cell levels, as well as risk prediction by mathematical models. According to this review the linear nonthreshold model was considered useful in defining the upper limits of risk for the radiation levels usually applied in medical diagnosis and therapy.

A follow-up of 20–30 years is generally required to give a useful estimate of radiation risk. Given an age at first exposure of 40–50 years, this requirement of an adequate epidemiological study can only be fulfilled if the majority of a study population survive to a high age of at least 70 years on average. The conclusion of a study by Sandler and Sandler (1983) was that the large number and improved survival of women who are treated by radiation for gynecological malignancy makes the issue of radiation-induced cancers of the colon and rectum an important one. Whether or not the risk in these patients is due to their gynecological cancer or to the radiation was considered not to be as important as the magnitude of this risk. For the estimation on this risk large-scale follow-up studies would be needed.

The international radiation study of the IARC was planned to make such an evaluation on a large scale possible, in that many thousands of women were followed up in different countries with cancer registries for the incidence cancer of the colon or rectum. Over 180 000 women with clinical diagnosis and therapy of cervical cancer were appropriate targets for careful surveillance for incident colorectal cancer. Second primary tumours appeared after an interval of between 1.2 and 31 years after radiation for the first primary tumor. The finding of an increased risk for rectal cancer but no increased risk for colon cancer was almost as surprising as the paradox finding that the longer the follow-up, the lower the RR became. Another paradox was that no excess of cancer of the rectum was found in patients with in situ cancer obviously treated by radiotherapy (Day and Boice 1983).

The absence of an overall excess has to be seen as an important finding in view of the high dose received by the colon and the significant excess mortality from colon cancer observed in patients irradiated for ankylosing spondylitis, in women irradiated for metropathia hemorrhagica, and among atomic bomb survivors (cited in Day and Boice 1983). Since cervical cancer patients are often of low socioeconomic status and may, therefore, have a lower risk of colon cancer, it may have been inappropriate to use only general population rates for predicting second tumors of the colon. The existence of a nonirradiated "internal" control cohort helped, however, to identify this effect as only marginal, if it exists at all. After all, the absence of increasing risk since the time of irradiation is another sign of a lack of any radiation effect. Nevertheless, a case-control approach was considered as helpful in determining radiation doses in women both with and without second primary cancers at particular sites, such as colon or rectum, and is to be seen as another requirement for the establishment of an etiological association.

Ureterosigmoidostomy

The clinical problem of adenocarcinoma of the colonic mucosa as a recognized complication in ureterosigmoidostomy patients has been estimated to amount to an approximately 500 times higher risk of cancer (referred to in Crissey et al. 1980). In children operated on for congenital malformation, such as exstrophy of the bladder or incontinentia, the risk was still higher, with latency periods of 5–50 years.

The hypothesis that colonic epithelium is susceptible to urine-borne carcinogens was studied in an experimental rat model (Crissey et al. 1980). The variables studied were urinary stream, feces, and the two different epithelia. Exclusion of feces was achieved by aproximal colostomy leaving a urine-bathed rectal bladder. Adenocarcinoma of the colon appeared adjacent to the junction of the epithelia where the urine joined the fecal stream. Unless fecal matter was present, no adenocarcinoma appeared at the junction, thus disproving a susceptibility of colonic mucosa to urine-borne carcinogens.

The current model seems to include not only hydrolytic enzymes in the urine, (known from bladder carcinogenesis research using β-naphthylamine), but also conjugated carcinogens in the stool that are activated by the junction of the two streams (where both are at the greatest concentration). The model therefore suggests that children with colon conduits do not have an increased risk of developing adenocarcinoma of the colonic mucosa.

Lasser and Acosta (1975) recommend, however, based on their review of case reports, that patients who have undergone ureteroanastomosis should be followed up for the rest of their lives. Hammer (1982) recommends starting these regular examinations 5 years after the operation and repeating them every 2 years. Cases of adenomatous polyps at the ureterocolonic junction, which are considered as precancerous lesions, have also been described (Hanley and McGarity 1971).

Gastrectomy

Partial gastrectomy (GE) as a possible factor of acquired increased risk has been mentioned in connection with follow-up studies of patients after surgery for peptic ulcer (Ross et al. 1982). An observed number of 16 colorectal carcinomal deaths differed considerably from the expected figure of about nine resulting in an RR 1.8. Another seemingly related finding was an increased RR of 2.82 for carcinoma of the pancreas after GE. The real nature of such associations could be examined with an adequately designed follow-up survey, including the proper assessment of potentially suspect confounders such as smoking habits. Thus, another case of a "synergism" could be shown as the reason for an association. The findings of Ross et al. (1982) induced a replication of their study in Hawaii. The mortality pattern of 407 Japanese males with partial FE was compared with that of 7599 unoperated males. After age adjustment, an inverse risk for colorectal cancers was found, with a RR of 0.58, pointing in the direction of a decreased risk (Stemmermann et al. 1984 b). The findings of Ross et al. (1982) were considered as primarily caused by smoking habits, although no information was obtained on smoking status in their study. The authors simply commented: "Thus, we found that diseases known to be related to smoking contributed more towards mortality than diseases traditionally linked with the sequelae of gastric surgery.

Bundred et al. (1985) considered smoking and did not find an influence on the relative risk of subsequent colorectal carcinoma in patients with gastric surgery (RR 2.1, confidence limits 1.1–4.0), although they refer to alcohol consumption as being frequently associated with smoking, peptic ulceration (stomach), as well as with colorectal cancer.

Environmental Conditions

Occupational Exposure

The hazards connected with a specific occupational exposure are usually best investigated, from the point of view of epidemiological methods and completeness of follow-up, by the cohort approach based on total risk populations of exposed workers. The number of cancer deaths observed are compared with the numbers expected on the basis of a reference population not exposed to the occupational hazard, and the result is mostly presented as a standardized mortality ratio (SMR). An SMR above 100 indicates that more deaths were observed than would have been expected in an identical (age-adjusted) group of people. An RR indicates the increase of observed versus expected numbers as a simple ratio, confidence limits showing the statistical significance if the limits do not include 1.0 (or 100 in case of the SMR).

In colorectal carcinoma, which is rarely considered to be related to specific occupational exposures, few studies have linked an occupation with the occurrence of malignant neoplasia. A few risk factors in the working environment have been described and seem to have been analyzed using adequate methods. The 30% increase of the incidence of colorectal cancer over the last three to four decades would suggest an occupational hazard, but only if it had occurred in men exclusively (Berg and Howell 1975). It is, therefore, still uncertain whether occupational risks have contributed to a large extent to increasing rates in the Western populations.

The recent report of a finding of asbestos bodies in a carcinoma of the colon in an insulation worker with asbestosis (Ehrlich et al. 1985) stimulated discussion regarding the possibility of direct action of swallowed mucus or saliva containing asbestos fibers, as well as the action of cigarette smoke condensate on gastrointestinal tract mucosa (Davis 1986). In occupational risk studies among workers exposed to asbestos, chrysotile was found to be associated with an elevated risk for cancers of colon and rectum, increasing gradually with dust exposure accumulated for up to 9 years before death (McDonald et al. 1980). This confirmed earlier findings regarding shipyard workers in Italy and insulation workers in the United States (cited by

Goldsmith 1982), although there are also negative studies, thus making the evidence less convincing. In a review of the concept of asbestos as a systemic carcinogen, Goldsmith (1982) concluded from the data of 11 cohort studies that open questions concerning a specific carcinogenic risk of the gastrointestinal sites would require prospective studies of persons exposed to asbestos with the synchronous assessment of defence mechanisms or their depression (as a possible biological mechanism involving the immune system). The finding by Ehrlich et al. (1986) throws new light on the evidence necessary to fulfill one postulate in causal argumentation, namely that the putative etiological agent needs to have direct contact with the target tissue.

In his review of studies on the effect of asbestos in the water supply – hence an environmental exposure – Erdreich (1983) indicated that digestive tract cancers were found in one study to be associated with exposure to ingested asbestos; nevertheless, the risk should be considered, and measures to reduce exposures should be indicated.

The increased incidence of colon cancer and rectal tumors in pattern markers of the North American automobile industry was the topic of three mortality studies and two cross-sectional investigations with screening of pattern and model makers by sigmoidoscopy. The mortality studies by Schottenfeld et al. (1980) and Robinson et al. (1980) were not entirely convincing since the methodology was not totally adequate for the reliable identification of a risk. In these studies the proportion of cancer deaths among the occupational subgroup of pattern makers was compared with the proportion of the mortality from the same cancer type in the general population. The third study (Swanson and Belle 1982) could make use of the industry-based cancer registry, and it was possible to determine the consistently increased incidence of colorectal cancer in persons employed for 10–14 years (SMR 650), 15–19 years (SMR 492), 20–24 years (SMR 176), and more than 24 years (SMR 210). The pattern makers, who were mainly exposed to wood, had a greater incidence of cancer than would be expected to occur in groups of similarly aged white males in the metropolitan Detroit area if they were followed up for the same period of time. Another site of significant cancer excess was the salivary gland.

The subsequent screening of 14073 pattern makers by sigmoidoscopy using a flexible, 60-cm long instrument revealed 11 of 12 incident colorectal cancers. The sensitivity of this examination procedure was 92%, whereas the specificity was 85%. The high number (218) false positive results is explained by the large number of polyps found (15.5%), of which the majority proved to be benign upon pathological examination. One person with cancer had no detectable polyp but a strong hemoccult positive test (Bang et al. 1986).

To evaluate the effectivity of the hemoccult test in such screening programs, the information on its performance may be of interest. Of 2.6% positive test results (48 workers), three were found to be caused by malignant colon neoplasms, i.e., three of 12 cases were discovered using the test alone, yielding a sensitivity of only 25%. The rate of only 2.4% false positive results is fair, but given the weak sensitivity, more sensitive tests are needed for reliable screening programs of this kind.

The issue of an increased risk for cancer of the colon or rectum in the specific populations in the automobile industry, as mentioned above, is still under debate, and recently a mortality study of identical design to the North American one has been launched in the automobile industry of the Federal Republic of Germany, so far without any strong indication of an increased risk for this particular site.

Vobecky et al. (1978, 1983) reported an increased incidence of colorectal cancer mortality in Canadian synthetic textile factory workers producing acetate monofilaments for carpet fabrication. A cohort study revealed a ten-fold mortality risk and an RR of colorectal carcinoma morbidity of 11.4. In conjunction with this follow-up, these authors carried out a case-control study on those 43 workers who developed cancer in the years 1965–1979 and compared information concerning specific working conditions with three randomly selected control groups from the same company (Vobecky et al. 1984). The exposure of 44% of workers with cancer occurred in specific departments where extrusion of filaments took place, whereas only 21% of the controls had worked in this department. The RR of cancer for those working in these departments was 3.72 ($p < 0.005$). As a result of this study, prevention was effected, and data available after 1975 appeared to show that the risk might have disappeared. A confirmation of this circumstantial impression would require a thoroughly planned and conducted cohort study of the type previously described, based on those employed after 1975 and allowing for a latency period of observation, usually at least 10–15 years.

In the United States and the United Kingdom, industries with so-called white collar workers had comparably higher rates of colorectal cancers, thus suggesting a particular risk in primarily sedentary occupations. Several studies have since confirmed a much more vague but rather consistent, risk association for sedentary professions. Gerhardsson et al. (1986) studied the association between physical job activity and colon cancer by following 1.1 million Swedish men for 19 years. This epidemiological study on the basis of census information about occupation, age, social class, marital status, and residence had the advantage of evaluating cancer morbidity instead of mortality on the basis of a nationwide registry. The study determined the RR to be 1.3, with 90% confidence intervals of 1.2–1.5. The highest risk was found for the transverse colon (RR 1.6), the lowest for the sigmoid portion of the colon (RR 1.2). Rectal carcinoma risk was not increased above expectation. According to the authors, it was judged unlikely that confounding by food habits, leisure time activity, marital status, or geographical region could explain the association. The influence of residing time of dietary residues in the colon as an important factor for metabolic processes, already suggested by Burkitt (1971), is discussed as a very likely reason for the association found fairly consistently in several studies, mostly based on mortality alone. The authors point out that given the low physical activity in Western societies, any causal association would be of considerable importance for prevention. The average "sitting time" during working hours was used for the classification of sedentary occupations. Such jobs included clerks and company executives, bookkeepers and cashiers, (public) administrators, brokers and agents, bank officials and employees, post masters, accountants, railway engineers and assistants, as well as shoemakers, and 25 other occupations.

The influence of physical activity in occupation on mechanical grounds, perhaps by stimulated colon peristalsis, was studied by Garabrandt et al. (1984). Rectal cancer was not found to be associated with sedentary or light work, and limited physical activity was even related in a dose-response fashion to cancer, indicating etiologically important influences if other, essential risk factors could be identified more precisely at the same time. This finding was corroborated by another interesting study on life-time occupational exercise, showing a reduction of colon (but not rectal) cancer risk, depending on the degree of exercise or proportion of time in jobs including only sedentary or light work (Vena et al. 1985).

Many other occupational risk studies were either not confirmed by adequate studies carried out using the same approach and methodology, or they could not be confirmed upon reanalysis. This again shows the complexity of epidemiological research in differing populations without standardized methods and instruments of assessment of outcome variables such as cancer mortality or morbidity.

Schistosomiasis

Schistosomiasis is one acquired condition which was mentioned in an epidemiological context in connection with cancer fairly early. Up until now, however, pathogenetic mechanisms have not been entirely clear, especially in explaining certain inconsistencies such as absence of cancer in the severely infected patients. The environmental nature and geographical pathology become obvious when considering the saying from Napoleon's time that Egypt was the land of menstruating males, indicating that schistosomal cystitis because of infection early in youth coincided with puberty and caused hematuria, and was thus accepted as a normal token of maturity (Cheevers 1978). The high prevalence of bladder cancer in endemic schistosomiasis foci and the frequent association of *Schistosoma haematobium* infection with a distinctive type of bladder tumor made a causal association suspected as early as 1905 (Goebel 1905).

Because of its endemic nature *S. haematobium* seems to be, at least in Egypt, related to *S. mansoni*. Inflammatory polyps, the precursor lesion of colon cancer, also seem to be causally related not only to *S. mansoni* – the main predilection of *S. mansoni* being the large intestine – but also to *S. haematobium*. Cheevers (1978) points out that numerous case reports of coincidental schistosomiasis and colon cancer did not give sufficient evidence that cancer was more frequent in infected individuals. Whatever the past and present risk of schistosomal cancer, the risk will possibly increase if exposure to other carcinogens becomes more frequent.

Recent reports from the province in China where intestinal schistosomiasis is endemic, at least in studies conducted in the pathological departments of several hospitals, showed a causal relationship between schistosomiasis and colon cancer (En-Sheng 1981). Research into intervention efforts aimed at eradicating transmission by health measures, as recently reported from Tanzania where pockets of *S. haematobium* and *S. mansoni* exist, may indicate the part played by this helminthic infection in the etiology of colon cancer (Tanner and Degremont 1986).

Host Factors

Familial Predisposition and Parity

Breast Cancer Associated with Colon Cancer

Lynch et al. (1985) described epidemiological similarities between colorectal and breast cancer in terms of geographical, dietary, socioeconomic and migration-associated patterns, which do not apply, however, to rectal cancer, suggesting differing etiologies for colon and rectal cancers.

Albano et al. (1982) claim a well-established type of cancer on a hereditary basis on the one hand, and a relationship between breast and colon cancer on the other. The former claim is based on indices such as younger age at onset (both types of cancer below the age of 50 on average), an excess of proximal, i.e., right-sided lesions of the colon, and more bilateral occurrences in the hereditary breast cancer (Mecklin and Jarvinen 1986). The latter claim of an association had already been described before (overview given by Schottenfeld and Winawer 1982). Anecdotal reports of this kind have repeatedly suggested that survival rates in hereditary cancer may be significantly higher, which, in part might be ascribed to early detection because of closer surveillance of cancer family members. A verified case of colorectal cancer in a member of a cancer family requires life-long follow-up examinations of remaining parts of the colon and rectum (Mecklin and Jarvinen 1986).

The Japanese epidemiological study on familial predisposition to colon cancer seems to have confirmed findings on proximity (right-sided colon) as well as the multiplicity of the intestinal tumor, and also of the other so-called double primary cancers in other organs of the same patient (primarily rectal neoplasms) (Murata and Takahashi 1984). According to Anderson (1980), the risk of colon cancer in the family of patients with colon cancer is about three times higher than that in the general population. It does not seem clear, however, what the risk is of a member of such a family experiencing a manifest neoplasm during his/her lifetime. Experience from Switzerland seems to indicate that the simple and harmless family history method can be employed by any practitioner in the field for the identification of healthy persons at high risk for colorectal carcinoma (Weber et al. 1985).

The number of children as a variable, although not mentioned in previous work, has recently been considered in several studies. The question is pertinent in that an increased risk for breast cancer is found to be related to nulliparity or late pregnancy with only few children. Weiss et al. (1981) reported an excess of female colon cancer in relation to reproductive factors such as low parity. Women with colon cancer had fewer children than randomly allocated population-based control persons. Compared with the incidence in nulliparous women as reference, the rates in women with one or two and three or more children were reduced by 30% and 50%, respectively. No association was found between parity and rectal cancer. Hormonal factors such as contraceptive or noncontraceptive estrogen use were not related to colon cancer incidence. No information could be given about the roles of fertility or pregnancy, or the inability to undergo the physiological changes during child-bearing as possible factors. Because of the consistently found effect, also in relationship to breast cancer risk, the suggestion of a role of events in the reproductive life is made in order to stimulate further research into this line of thinking.

In a recent case-control study on 388 incident colon cancer cases and 787 control persons (Cragle 1984), of whom 71% and 67%, respectively, were interviewed [but due to other exclusion criteria (race, residence) only data from 200 cases and 407 controls were analyzed], a significantly negative risk association was found with the number of pregnancies. This feature could add to the similarities described between cancers of such different localizations as breast and colon. The very striking similarity, however, is the increase in incidence with age for both types of cancer (Lynch et al. 1985).

Another study including cases from a population-based cancer registry (Liff 1986) was designed to study information on parity. The study was based on 342 women with cancers of the colon and rectum and could clarify some of the reasons for the previously reported association of number of children and cancer (a relationship which was never considered for study in male cases). When parity information from all cases was evaluated, no association with cancer was observed, but within the subgroup of cases interviewed (only 61% of eligible cases in the registry could be included in the study, main reason for omission being death) there was a "possible" association. The author of this study thinks that methodological inadequacies could be responsible for differential reporting of parity information in the previous studies.

Mormon females had much lower rates of colon cancer in a large-scale study in Utah (Lyon et al. 1976), and the overall incidence of cancer of the colon and rectum in Utah is below that reported for the population of the United States as a whole and even for Californian Seventh Day Adventists. The birth rate of Mormons is referred to as being 60% higher than that of the United States as a whole (cited by Lyon et al. 1985).

Barrett's Esophagus and Colonic Tumors

Sonntag et al. (1985) reported on a previously unrecognized coincidence of the so-called Barrett's Esophagus and colonic tumors. This syndrome is considered to be one manifestation of the columnar cell replacement process of the distal esophagus in patients with peptic esophagitis. This pathological phenomenon is already under scrutiny in connection with adenocarcinogenesis of Barrett's esophagus. The incidence of esophageal adenocarcinoma is 30–40 fold higher in patients with a symptomatic columnar-lined esophagus compared with expected figures based on the general population or Veterans Administration populations (cited by Cameron et al. 1985), also it does not occur in the majority of such patients. Longevity was apparently unimpaired by a diagnosis of Barrett's esophagus. The association with cancer could be caused by the accidental detection because an unknown proportion of the general population probably has Barrett's esophagus but it remains undetected unless carcinoma develops. The clinical gastroesophageal reflux syndrome is often associated with Barrett's esophagus, even in children (Dahms and Rothstein 1984), and surgery to prevent reflux seems not to be effective in preventing the later development of carcinoma (if it does not even provoke such an occurrence). Similarly, the detection of colon cancer could be in part due to more intensive diagnostic procedures in gastroenterological patients with a risk of Barrett's esophagus. Criteria to diagnose Barrett's esophagus necessarily require biopsy for confirmation.

Sonntag et al. (1985), in a prospective study using colonoscopy in 63 patients, uncovered three patients with colonic carcinoma and 16 with benign adenomas. Five additional patients had had colon cancer surgery and three had had colonoscopic polypectomies for benign lesions. This high frequency makes a chance finding rather unlikely. But some important questions remain on factors which may be at work in this association. Bremmer and Hamilton (1985) discussed controversial aspects of Barrett's esophagus as a precancerous syndrome and claimed that there was no doubt that a columnar-lined esophagus had a malignant potential, requiring vigilant annual follow-up with endoscopical studies. This recommendation was based on a review of the literature suggesting that 10% of patients with Barrett's esophagus developed an adenocarcinoma. The role of heredity was introduced by Pero et al. (1983) who suggested that individuals who were genetically disposed to colon cancer had increased sensitivity to acquired DNA damage (via defective DNA repair synthesis as measured by unscheduled DNA synthesis). Such a mechanism could account for the relationship between colonic tumors and esophageal metaplasia, and the association between Barrett's esophagus and colon cancer. Confirmation of such an association as nonspurious requires additional prospective controlled studies.

Behavioral Characteristics

Homosexuality

The hypothesis that a venereally transmissible agent (or its treatment) is responsible for some proportion of the squamous cell carcinomas of the rectum or anus has been tested using the descriptive epidemiological approach on the basis of cancer registration data (Austin 1982). A higher rate of squamous cell carcinoma of the rectum or anus is associated with single males as a sociodemographic variable in some areas of the west coast of the United States. The observation of a 20-fold higher rate of syphilis among men with anal cancer compared with other cancer sites (Dalin et al. 1982) was in line with a specific risk associated with anal intercourse. Other observations supporting this reasoning are:

- A total of 24.4% of men with anal cancer had never been married compared with 7.8% of men with cancer of the colon and rectum.
- A higher rate of this cancer was found in men in some areas of the west coast of the United States which are noted for their homosexual communities.

It is interesting to note that 20%–25% of the adult population of San Francisco is thought to be homosexual. People remaining unmarried may, however, also be under increased risk for totally different reasons, for example, they often postpone the development of their private, independent life in favor of a dedicated care of one or both parents, the loss of whom could be detrimental as a major adverse life event (Grossarth-Maticek et al. 1984). The particular localization of the cancer, however, indicates that also very specific mechanical causes or causal mechanisms may have to be considered.

Models for Combined Acquired Conditions

In his mathematical approach for the combination of etiologically important variables Veale (1985) has postulated that the genetic argument in no way conflicts with variations in the incidence of bowel cancer that have been shown to be associated with defined epidemiological variables. In the model, the observed frequency of cancer among parents of index cases is consistent with a simple genetic penetrance. The possibility that too great a frequency of cancer in siblings of index cases could conflict with simple genetic penetrance is used to introduce strong intrafamilial environmental factors that are not excluded by any genetic model but make interpretation of family data more difficult. This same argument could also be used for the concept of susceptibility, which will be discussed later.

Sutherland and Bailar (1984) take this argument to consider a "multihit" theory for colon carcinogenesis along the lines of an adenoma-carcinoma sequence but point out that a large proportion of the population may be at risk of "four-hit" colon tumors following a nonadenoma etiological sequence. Keeping this in mind, many possible mechanisms are relevant for those heterogeneous parts of the population not under genetically determined susceptibility.

The newly adopted view of identifying the susceptibility of persons and populations for more effective prevention has led to recommendations (Lipkin 1985) which are also discussed in several other chapters of this volume. In this context, however, one aspect ought to be mentioned without expanding too much on the subject: familial aggregates which have been cancer-free for two or more generations should also be studied to answer the question of whether all acquired conditions are equally absent in these groups, or whether susceptibility is more important than exposure to individual risk factors (Veale 1985). The development of risk factor profiles would be necessarily influenced by such considerations, as has been the case in discussions regarding rodent strains and their different susceptibilities. Not least the findings of the influence of diet alone on cancer incidence in the (rodent) animal model (Roe 1987) has put an immense importance on the responsibility of any future design of risk factor-oriented investigations as well as causal research. The increased efforts in recommendations for prevention have to be seen in a similar way if these prescriptions are only valid for a minor subgroup of the total population.

Evidence is accumulating from research into the contribution of psychosocial factors to disease risk that not only the emotionally dependent personality type, but also a rational person with a lack of autonomy is under increased risk of manifest cancer (Grossarth-Maticek et al. 1988). This again points to a predictive type of suceptibility which, however, is accessible to prevention by prophylaxis using psychotherapy, or by other means, if it is administered before disease becomes clinically manifest. Since the basis of behavioral patterns may be linked to family traditions in a similar fashion as genetic influences, the combination of concepts and research efforts should be directed into more interdisciplinary research, including neurotransmitters and their activation by the stimulation of central nervous functions, and into future studies of populations with increased (Lipkin 1985) and those with considerably lower risk.

Until this is accomplished and more experience has accrued, recommendations given so far are "at least harmless," as admitted by those groups having promoted primary prevention rather energetically (Weisburger and Wynder 1987). The finding that Seventh Day Adventists and other populations with vegetarian life style or a diet-conscious way of life belong to low-risk populations (Schottenfeld 1982; Frentzel-Beyme et al. 1988) points in the same direction. A large proportion of the low cancer rates among Adventists may be explained by their abstinence from tobacco and alcohol. In view of a comparatively high meat consumption by Mormons, another religious group abstaining from tobacco and alcohol consumption, it is difficult to assert that a vegetarian diet is important in the prevention of colon cancer (Tollefson 1986).

In one comparatively large case-control study designed to show effects of genetic and environmental interaction (Cragle 1984), one statistically significant finding was a negative association of colon cancer with smoking (and number of pregnancies, see above). Hirayama (1981) showed an increased risk of colon cancer from cigarette smoking for those who drank alcohol daily. These conflicting findings illustrate not only the need for models to study the interactions, but also the necessity to be aware of the lack of relevant information on behavioral and psychosocial factors which ought to be included in future research efforts.

Conclusions

The prevention of colon cancer as a consequence of other clinically symptomatic conditions would require careful surveillance, although there is a lack of an evaluation of measures for their effectiveness. The reduction of medically indicated radiation is less urgent for the prevention of colon cancer, although it appears that it should be recommended for the prevention of rectal cancer, the rectum being one of a few sites which have been associated with radiation. After all, the conditions mentioned here (and other acquired conditions) cannot explain the large numbers of cases in hospitals. Occupational risk applies only to a small fraction of the population, mostly male, whereas schistosomiasis has only regionally limited importance, if at all. The small fraction of people whose sexual behavior possibly increases their risk should, however, not cause inclusion of more information on behavior to be neglected. Behavior can be addressed by therapeutic means, whereas other acquired conditions may not be redressable, nor can previous carcinogenic exposure be totally neutralized.

References

Albano WA, Recabaren JA, Lynch HT, Campbell AS, Mailliard JA, Organ CH, Lynch JF, Kimberling WJ (1982) Natural history of hereditary cancer of the breast and colon. Cancer 50:360–363

Anderson DE (1980) Risk in families of patients with colon cancer. In: Winawer SJ, Schottenfeld, Sherlock P (eds) Colorectal cancer: prevention, epidemiology, and screening. Raven, New York, p 410 (Progress in cancer research and therapy, vol 13)

Austin D (1982) Etiological clues from descriptive epidemiology: squamous carcinoma of the rectum or anus. NCI Monogr 62:89–90

Bang KM, Tillett S, Hoar SK, Blair A, McDougall V (1986) Sensitivity of fecal hemoccult testing and flexible sigmoidoscopy for colorectal cancer screening. J Occup Med 28:709–713

Berg JW, Howell MA (1975) Occupation and bowel cancer. J Toxicol Environ Health 1:74–89

Bremmer CG, Hamilton DG (1985) Barrett's esophagus: controversial aspects. In: De Meester TR, Skinner DB (eds) Esophageal disorders: pathophysiology and therapy. Raven Press, New York, pp 233–239

Bundred NJ, Whitfield BCS, Stanton E, Prescott RJ, Davies GC, Kingsnorth AN (1985) Gastric surgery and the risk of subsequent colorectal cancer. Br J Surg 72:618–619

Burkitt DP (1971) Epidemiology of cancer of the colon and rectum. Cancer 28:3–13

Cameron AJ, Ott BJ, Payne WS (1985) The incidence of adenocarcinoma in columnar lined (Barrett's) esophagus. N Engl J Med 313:857–859

Cheevers AW (1978) Schistosomiasis and neoplasia. J Natl Cancer Inst 61:13–18

Cragle DL (1984) The effects of genetic and environmental interaction in an epidemiologic investigation of colon cancer and water quality. Diss Abstr Int B Sci Eng 45:1739-B

Crissey MM, Steale GD, Gilles RF (1980) Rat model for carcinogenesis in ureterosigmoidostomy. Science 207:1079–1080

Dahms BB, Rothstein FC (1984) Barrett's esophagus in children: a consequence of chronic gastro-enterological reflux. Gastroenterology 86:318–323

Daling JR, Weiss NS, Klopfenstein LL, Cochran LE, Chow WH, Daifuku R (1982) Correlates of homosexual behaviour and the incidence of anal cancer. JAMA 247:1988–1990

Davis RM (1986) The prevalence and causes of colonic cancer (Letter to the editor). JAMA 255:2295

Day NE, Boice JD (1983) Second cancer in relation to radiation treatment for cervical cancer. From the International radiation study group on cervical cancer. IARC Lyon, pp 137–162 (IARC scientific publications, no 52)

Ehrlich A, Rohl AN, Holstein EC (1985) Asbestos bodies in carcinoma of the colon in an insulation worker with asbestosis. JAMA 254:2932–2933

En-Sheng Z (1981) Cancer of the colon and schistosomiasis. J R Soc Med 74:645

Erdreich L (1983) Comparing epidemiologic studies of ingested asbestos for use in risk assessment. Environ Health Perspect 53:99–104

Frentzel-Beyme R, Claude J, Eilber U (1988) Mortality among German vegetarians: first results after five years of follow-up. Nutr Cancer 11:117–126

Garabrandt DM, Peters JM, Mack TM, Bernstein L (1984) Job activity and colon cancer risk. Am J Epidemiol 119:1005–1014

Gerhardsson M, Norell SE, Kiviranta H, Pedersen NL, Ahlbom A (1986) Sedentary jobs and colon cancer. Am J Epidemiol 123:775–780

Goldsmith JR (1982) Asbestos as a systemic carcinogen: the evidence from eleven cohorts. Am J Ind Med 3:341–348

Goebel C (1905) Über die bei Bilharziakrankheit vorkommenden Blasentumoren mit besonderer Berücksichtigung des Carcinoms. Z Krebsforschung 3:369–513

Grossarth-Maticek R, Frentzel-Beyme R, Becker N (1984) Cancer risk associated with life events and conflict solution. Cancer Detect Prev 7:201–209

Grossarth-Maticek R, Eysenck HJ, Vetter H, Frentzel-Beyme R (1988) The Heidelberg prospective intervention study. In: Eylenbosch WJ, Van Larebeke N, Depoorter AM (eds) Primary prevention of cancer. Raven Press, New York, pp 199–212

Hammer B (1982) Hochrisikogruppen beim kolorektalen Karzinom. Schweiz Rundsch Med Prax 27:1130–1133

Hanley JM, McGarity WC (1971) Ureterosigmoidostomy and neoplasms of the colon. Arch Surg 103:69

Hirayama T (1981) A large-scale cohort study on the relationship between diet and selected cancers of digestive organs. In: Bruce WR, Correa P, Lipkin M, Tannenbaum SR, Wilkins TD (eds) Gastrointestinal cancer: endogenous factors. Banbury report, no 7. Cold Spring Harbor, New York, pp 409–429

Ituarte EA, Petrini J, Hershman JM (1984) Acromegaly and colon cancer. Am Inst Med 101:627–628

Jones Y, Schatzkin A, Green S, Block G, Brinton L, Ziegler R, Hoover R, Taylor PR (1987) Dietary fat and breast cancer in the NHANES I epidemiologic follow-up study. J Natl Cancer Inst 79:465–471

Kessler II (1970a) Cancer mortality among diabetics. J Natl Cancer Inst 44:673–686

Kessler II (1970b) A genetic relationship between diabetes and cancer. Lancet I:218–220

Kessler II (1971) Cancer and diabetes mellitus. A review of the literature. J Chronic Dis 23:579–600

Lasser A, Acosta AE (1975) Colonic neoplasms complicating ureterosigmoidostomy. Cancer 35:1218–1222

Liff JM (1986) The roles of parity and diet in the etiology of colon cancer in women. Diss Abstr. Int B Sci Eng 46:2276

Lipkin M (1985) Identification of populations with increased susceptibility to cancer of the large intestine. In: Lynch PM, Lynch HT (eds) Colon cancer genetics. Van Nostrand Reinhold, New York, pp 128–156

Lynch HT, Lynch PM, Keethley J (1985) Epidemiology of colon cancer. In: Lynch PM, Lynch HT (eds) Colon cancer genetics. Van Nostrand Reinhold, New York, pp 1–16

Lyon JL, Klauber MR, Gardner JW, Smart CR (1976) Cancer incidence in Mormons and non-Mormons in Utah, 1966–1970. N Engl J Med 294:129–133

McDonald JCM, Liddell FDK, Gibbs GW, Eyssen GE, McDonald AD (1980) Dust exposure and mortality in chrysotile mining 1910–1975. Brit J Ind Med 37: 11–24

Mecklin JP, Jarvinen HJ (1986) Clinical features of colorectal carcinoma in cancer family syndrome. Dis Colon Rectum 29:160–164

Murata M, Takahashi T (1984) An epidemiological study of familial predisposition to large bowel cancer. Gan No Rinsho 30:243–250

Pero RW, Miller GD, Lipkin M, Markowitz M, Gupta S, Winawer SJ, Enker W, Good R (1983) Reduced capacity for DNA repair synthesis in patients with or genetically predisposed to colorectal cancer. J Natl Cancer Inst 70:867–875

Robinson C, Waxweiler RJ, McCammon C (1980) Pattern and model makers, proportionate mortality 1972–1978. Am J Ind Med 1:159–165

Roe F (1987) The problem of pseudocarcinogenicity in rodent bioassays. In: Butterworth BE, Slaga TJ (eds) Nongenotoxic mechanisms in carcinogenesis. Banbury report no 25. Cold Spring Harbor, New York, pp 189–200

Ross AHM, Smith MA, Anderson JR, Small WP (1982) Late mortality after surgery for peptic ulcer. N Engl J Med 307:519–522

Rothman KJ (1986) Modern epidemiology. Little, Brown, Boston/Toronto

Sandler RS, Sandler DP (1983) Radiation induced cancers of the colon and rectum: assessing the risk. Gastroenterology 84:51–57

Schottenfeld D (1983) Radiation as a risk factor in the natural history of colon cancer (Editorial). Gastroenterology 84:186–190

Schottenfeld D, Warshauer ME, Zauber AG (1980) Study of cancer mortality and incidence in wood shop workers. Report to the General Motors Corporation, Detroit

Schottenfeld D, Winawer SJ (1982) Large intestine. In: Schottenfeld D, Fraumeni JF (eds) Cancer epidemiology and prevention. Saunders, Boston

Shimizu H, Mack TH, Ross RK, Henderson BE (1987) Cancer of the gastrointestinal tract among Japanese and white immigrants to Los Angeles County. J Natl Cancer Inst 78: 223–228

Smith AH, Pearce NE, Joseph IG (1985) Major colorectal cancer aetiological hypotheses do not explain mortality trends among Maoris and non-Maoris in New Zealand. Int J Epidemiol 14:79–85

Sonntag SJ, Schnell T, Cheijfec G, Chintam R, Wanner J (1985) Barrett's esophagus and colonic tumors. Lancet I:946–949

Stemmermann GN, Nomura AMY, Heilbrun LK (1984a) Dietary fat and the risk of colon cancer. Cancer Res 44:4463–4637

Stemmerman GN, Heilbrun L, Nomura A, Rhoads GG, Glober GA (1984b) Late mortality after partial gastrectomy. Int J Epidemiol 13:299–303

Sutherland JV, Bailar JC (1984) The multihit model of carcinogenesis: etiologic implications for colon cancer. J Chronic Dis 37:465–480

Swanson MG, Belle SH (1982) Cancer morbidity among woodmakers in the US automobile industry. J Occup Med 24:315–319

Tanner M, Degrenant A (1986) Monitoring and evaluation of schistosomiasis control with a primary health care program. Tropenmed Parasit 37:220–223

Tollefson L (1986) The use of epidemiology, scientific data and regulator authority to determine risk factors in cancer of some organs of the digestive system. 4. Colon cancer. Regul Toxicol Pharmacol. 6:24–54

Veale AM (1985) Colorectal cancer: investigation of a genetic model. In: Lynch PM, Lynch PM, Lynch HT (ed) Colon cancer genetics. Van Nostrand Reinhold, New York

Vena JE, Graham S, Zielezny M, Swanson MK, Barnes RE, Nolan J (1985) Lifetime occupational exercise and colon cancer. Am J Epidemiol 122:357–365

Vobecky J, Devroede G, Lacaille J, Watier A (1978) An occupational group with a high risk of large bowel cancer. Gastroenterology 75:221–223

Vobecky J, Caro J, Devroede G (1983) A case-control study of risk factors for large bowel carcinoma. Cancer 51:1958–1963

Vobecky J, Devroede G, Caro J (1984) Risk of large-bowel cancer in synthetic fiber manufacture. Cancer 54: 2547–2542

Weber W, Voegtli B, Buser M, Gencik A, Kayasseh L, Stalder GA, Torhorst J, Müller H (1985) Vergleich der Tumorinzidenz bei 251 Verwandten ersten Grades von 50 Patienten mit kolorektalen Karzinomen mit derjenigen der Baseler Bevölkerung. Schweiz Med Wochenschr 115: 1005–1006

Weisburger JH, Wynder EL (1987) Etiology of colorectal cancer with emphasis on mechanism of action and prevention. In: De Vita V, Hellman S, Rosenberg SA (eds) Important advances in oncology. Lippincott, Philadelphia, pp 197–220

Weiss NS, Daling JR, Chow WH (1981) Incidence of cancer of the large bowel in women in relation to reproductive and hormonal factors. J Natl Cancer Inst 67: 57–60

Williams JC, Walsh DA, Jackson JF (1984) Colon carcinoma and diabetes mellitus. Cancer 54: 3070–3071

Inflammatory Bowel Disease and Colorectal Cancer

A. J. Greenstein and D. B. Sachar

Departments of Surgery and Medicine (Division of Gastroenterology),
Mount Sinai School of Medicine of the City University of New York,
One Gustave L. Levy Place, New York, NY 10029-6574, USA

Contents

Introduction

One of the long-term risks of inflammatory bowel disease is the development of cancer. Patients with either non-specific or specific forms of disease are at increased risk for various types of intestinal (Greenstein et al. 1980, 1981; Gyde et al. 1980) or extraintestinal (Greenstein et al. 1985) cancers. The non-specific forms of chronic inflammatory bowel disease comprise ulcerative colitis and Crohn's disease, common in the British Isles, Scandinavia, Western Europe, and North America; a specific form with possible increased cancer risk is schistosomiasis, endemic in much of the Far East, China, the Philippines, Egypt, and the rest of Africa. The increased risk of colorectal cancer is unequivocal in ulcerative colitis, highly probable, albeit somewhat controversial, in Crohn's colitis, and still debatable in schistosomiasis. In each of these three forms of inflammatory bowel disease, there are cancers for which the risk is increased: reticuloendothelial tumors in ulcerative colitis and Crohn's disease (Greenstein et al. 1985; Hanauer et al. 1982), perineal cancers (Greenstein et al. 1985; Slater et al. 1984) and malignant melanoma (Greenstein et al. 1985) in Crohn's disease, and genitourinary (Alexis and Domingo 1986; Ghoneim et al. 1985) and hepatic (Kojiro et al. 1986) cancers in schistosomiasis, associated with *Schistosoma haematobium* and *Schistosoma japonicum*, respectively.

Table 1. Features of colorectal cancer in inflammatory bowel disease

	Ulcerative colitis	Crohn's disease	Schistosomiasis
Age at cancer (mean)	49	56	40
Cancer incidence 0/E[a]	7–29 X	4–20 X	0–8 X
Multicentral origin	Yes	Yes	Yes
Multiple cancers (%)	8–43	11	16
High-risk duration of disease (years)	8–10	15–20[c]	10[c]
High-risk extent of disease	Universal and left-sided	Relation to extent unknown	Universal and segmental
Occurrence at site of overt disease	Yes (95%)	Usually (66%)	Yes
Excluded bowel at risk	Yes[b]	Yes[b]	Not applicable
Pathology	Carcinoma	Carcinoma	Carcinoma
Stricture	Yes	Yes	Yes
Dysplasia-associated	Yes	Yes	Yes
Five-year survival (%)	45	35	46

[a] Observed/expected ratio.
[b] Excluded rectal stump in ulcerative colitis; excluded small or large bowel in Crohn's disease.
[c] Cases may also occur in first decade.

There are many similarities among these three forms of premalignant inflammatory bowel disease. In each of these diseases there is usually a long duration of inflammatory bowel disease preceding development of intestinal cancer. Premalignant change ("dysplasia") has been demonstrated in the epithelial cells of the intestinal tract in ulcerative colitis (Dobbins 1967; Lennard-Jones et al. 1977, 1983; Morson and Pang 1967) and Crohn's disease (Fleming and Pollock 1975; Warren and Barwick 1983), and in both the colon (Ming-Chai et al. 1980, 1981) and bladder in schistosomiasis (Ghonheim et al. 1985). Furthermore, the cancers associated with all three forms of disease tend to be multicentric in origin (Edwards and Truelove 1964; Clemmensen and Johansen 1972; Greenstein et al. 1980, 1986; Hamilton 1985; Hinton 1966; Ming-Chai et al. 1980, 1981). In both ulcerative colitis and schistosomiasis, the dysplasia and malignant changes almost invariably occur at sites of evident disease, whereas in Crohn's disease about one-third of cancers occur at sites remote from clinically obvious disease (Greenstein et al. 1980, 1987). Comparisons of the clinical and epidemiological features of the three forms of inflammatory bowel disease are shown in Table 1.

Historical Background

Although ulcerative colitis was first described as an entity by Sir Samuel Wilks in 1859 ("The morbid appearance of the intestine of Miss Banks." *The Medical Times and Gazette* 2:264, quoted by Goligher 1968) it was not until 1925 that Crohn and Rosenberg first described a patient with ulcerative colitis and colorectal carcinoma. Since then, many reports have confirmed the high incidence of large bowel cancer in ulcerative colitis (de Dombal et al. 1966; Devroede et al. 1971; Edwards and Truelove 1964; Greenstein et al. 1979 a; Slaney and Brooke 1959). There is now little doubt that the incidence is significantly increased.

The issue of an increased cancer incidence in Crohn's disease remains somewhat more controversial. For years after the early descriptions of this disease by Dalziel in 1913, and by Crohn et al. in 1932, and following the recognition of colonic involvement by Colp in 1934, and acceptance by Crohn in 1966, there were no reports of cancer associated with this form of inflammatory bowel disease. The firm belief thus developed that there was no relationship between Crohn's disease and cancer. In 1948, however, Warren and Sommers described the first case of carcinoma of the large bowel occurring in association with Crohn's disease (Warren and Sommers 1948). There are now at least 80 patients in whom cancer of the large bowel has been reported in association with Crohn's colitis, ileocolitis (Greenstein et al. 1980, 1981; Hamilton 1985), or regional enteritis (Greenstein et al. 1987).

Schistosomiasis has been recognized as an endemic disease for centuries in areas of the Far East and Africa. The first suggestion that cancer of the rectum may be related to *S. japonicum* was by Endo in 1908 (cited by Faust and Meleney 1924). Decades later, it was ultimately recognized that colorectal cancer was common in certain areas of the People's Republic of China where schistosomiasis was endemic. In Zhejiang and Jiangsu provinces, prevalence rates of up to 44 per 100 000 were nearly ten times the rates in other areas where schistosomiasis was uncommon (Chen et al. 1981; Ming-Chai et al. 1980, 1981). Indeed, Xu and Su have noted a significant correlation between colorectal cancer incidence and schistosomiasis prevalence (Xu and Su 1984). Moreover, certain clinical and histological similarities between schistosoma-related and ulcerative colitis-related colorectal cancers provide further evidence for a direct association (Chen et al. 1981; Ming-Chai et al. 1980, 1981).

Colorectal Cancer in Ulcerative Colitis

The risk of colorectal cancer is considerably increased for patients with ulcerative colitis, particularly for those with universal disease of long standing (deDombal et al. 1966; Devroede 1980; Greenstein et al. 1979 a; Prior et al. 1982). The relative risk is especially high in younger patients (Devroede et al. 1971). The mean age of occurrence of ulcerative colitis-related cancer is 49 years, versus 69 years for colorectal cancer in the general population (Greenstein et al. 1986).

Clinicopathological Features

Colorectal cancers in ulcerative colitis show characteristic clinico-pathological features. They are more diffuse, sometimes invisible to the naked eye, or may infiltrate the bowel wall causing stricture formation (V. Gumaste et al., in preparation). They are frequently multiple with an incidence of multiplicity of between 14% and 40%, compared with 4% for de novo colorectal cancer (Greenstein et al. 1986). Also, the proportion of right-sided cancers is greater (Greenstein et al. 1979b), largely due to the increased incidence of multiple synchronous cancers (Greenstein et al. 1986).

Ulcerative colitis-related cancers are often insidious in onset. Advanced cases are characterized by obstructive symptoms, rapid weight loss, and abdominal masses (Greenstein et al. 1979b). Strictures with or without obstruction are a particularly ominous sign and should be immediately evaluated by colonoscopy. Among 59 ulcerative colitis patients, ten of 52 non-obstructing strictures and all seven obstructing strictures proved to be malignant (V. Gumaste et al., in preparation).

Risk Factors

The principal risk for colorectal cancer in ulcerative colitis occurs after 10 years of disease, increasing with longer durations of disease, but probably independent of age at onset or severity of disease. The risk is greatest for pancolitis, although left-sided disease also carries an increased risk that seems to take 5–10 years longer to emerge. Actuarial calculations in some hospital series (deDombal et al. 1966; Devroede et al. 1971; Dobbins 1977; Greenstein et al. 1979) have shown cumulative cancer risks as high as 50% at 40 years, but the referral and ascertainment biases in such series are enormous (Sachar and Greenstein 1981). Other studies based on ambulatory populations (Katzka et al. 1983; Kewenter et al. 1978) show much lower risks, although still at levels considerably increased over age- and sex-matched populations, reaching up to 20% for all cases of colitis and 35% for universal colitis after 35 years of disease (Katzka et al. 1983). The risk is also increased in the remaining rectum of patients following ileorectal anastomosis (Baker et al. 1978; Grundfest et al. 1981; Lavery et al. 1982), reaching approximately 5% at 20 years, 13% at 25 years, and 25% at 30 years (Baker et al. 1978).

The only way to prevent colorectal cancer completely is the radical but generally impractical solution of prophylactic total proctocolectomy. Bonnevie et al. (1974) reported a zero cancer incidence at 30 years with a policy of early surgery. The challenge, however, is to design an acceptable and cost-effective surveillance program for the great mass of asymptomatic patients in whom purely prophylactic operation is inappropriate.

Early Detection and Prevention (Surveillance)

In high-risk ulcerative colitis patients, early cancer detection is of fundamental importance in preventing mortality. Older reports, with more advanced cancers, suggested a much higher cancer case-fatality rate for ulcerative colitis-related than for de novo colorectal cancer (Hinton 1966). Newer studies, however, have shown a cancer case-fatality rate in ulcerative colitis very similar to that for de novo colorectal cancer (Greenstein et al. 1976b; Hughes et al. 1978; Lavery et al. 1982; Ohman 1987; Ritchie et al. 1981; van Heerden and Beart 1983). The prognosis is dependent upon the Dukes stage of the tumor at the time of resection, with 5-year survival rates of 100% for stage A and 33% for stage C (Ohman 1982). Earlier diagnosis using endoscopy has improved the prognosis, not only by directly identifying earlier cancers, but also by finding premalignant changes associated with unsuspected early lesions elsewhere in the colon.

Precancerous epithelial dysplasia was described in 1967 by Morson and Pang. The detection of dysplasia by surveillance colonoscopy (Lennard-Jones et al. 1977, 1983) and the association between dysplasia and cancer (Dobbins 1977; Nugent and Haggitt 1984), especially in the presence of an elevated mass (Blackstone et al. 1981), mandate prophylactic colectomy when unequivocal dysplasia is documented in the absence of acute inflammation. The cost–benefit ratio has not been established for prophylactic colonoscopic surveillance. Most such programs commence after 10 years of disease, often on an annual or biannual schedule, but the effectiveness of such regimens in saving lives that would otherwise be lost is highly uncertain (Collins et al. 1987). Perhaps more sensitive indicators of premalignancy, such as DNA flow cytometry (Hammerberg et al. 1984), cell turnover kinetics (Deschner et al. 1977), mucin histochemistry, lectin binding, or monoclonal antibody identification of antigenic tumor markers (Itzkowitz et al. 1987) will ultimately prove to be more reliable "early warning" signs than routine histological examination for dysplasia.

Colorectal Cancer in Crohn's Disease

Incidence

There is some controversy regarding the increased incidence of colorectal carcinoma with Crohn's disease. Although many series omit mention of such cancers, high incidences in Crohn's disease were reported in two early publications from the United Kingdom (Atwell et al. 1965; Perrett et al. 1986), while two more recent series from the United States found 7–20 times the expected incidence in an age- and sex-matched population (Greenstein et al. 1981; Weedon et al. 1973). By now, there are quite a few studies suggesting an increased incidence of gastrointestinal cancer in Crohn's disease (Alexander-Williams 1976; Fielding et al. 1972; Greenstein et al. 1980, 1981; Gyde et al. 1980).

Clinicopathological Features

The clinical features of colorectal cancer occurring in Crohn's disease are difficult to differentiate from the original clinical features of the underlying inflammatory bowel disease. Diagnostic difficulties are further complicated by the occurrence of cancer in excluded distal bowel (Greenstein et al. 1978), or in association with enterovesical or colovesical fistulae (Greenstein et al. 1978; Lightdale et al. 1975), rectovaginal fistulae (Buchmann et al. 1980), colocutaneous fistulae (Church et al. 1985; Greenstein et al. 1978), or perianal fistulae (Greenstein et al. 1978; Slater et al. 1984; Zinkin and Brandwein 1980). Compared to de novo cases, colorectal cancers in Crohn's disease, as in ulcerative colitis, occur at an earlier age (48 years vs. 60 years), are more often located in the right colon (45%), and are more frequently diffusely infiltrating (Collins et al. 1987) or multiple (Keighley et al. 1975; Hamilton 1985; Korelitz 1983). Approximately one-third of cancers in our reported series occurred in areas of grossly normal bowel (Greenstein et al. 1980), including six cases of colorectal cancers in regional ileitis (Greenstein et al. 1987). These observations are consistent with the concept that Crohn's disease may affect the whole gastrointestinal tract, even in the absence of overt disease (Allan et al. 1975; Crucioli 1967; Ferguson et al. 1975; Goodman et al. 1976).

Surveillance of Crohn's Disease for Carcinoma

The issue of surveillance for cancer in patients with Crohn's disease remains controversial. Korelitz (Cooper et al. 1984; Korelitz 1983) and Shorter (1983) suggest the need for surveillance, while Butt (Butt et al. 1980; Butt and Morson 1981), Fielding (Fielding et al. 1972), and Warren (Warren and Barwick 1983; Warren and Sommers 1948) do not advise prophylactic measures, although they recommend "vigilance" in Crohn's disease. We agree with Hamilton (1985) that cost–benefit studies of surveillance protocols are thus needed in well-defined Crohn's disease populations.

Several factors make it difficult at this time to propose a rational surveillance program for Crohn's disease patients. These factors include the variety of cancers which occur in association with Crohn's disease: extraintestinal (Greenstein et al. 1985) and intestinal (Greenstein et al. 1980), small bowel (Frank and Shorey 1973; Fresco et al. 1982; Ginzburg et al. 1956), and large bowel (Greenstein et al. 1987; Hamilton 1985; Slater et al. 1984; Thompson et al. 1983). They also include several different modes of clinical presentation: cancers following long duration of disease (Greenstein et al. 1978), cancers coincident with onset of Crohn's disease (Darke et al. 1973; Hamilton 1985; Perrett et al. 1968; Thompson et al. 1983), cancers remote from overt disease (Frank and Shorey 1973; Greenstein et al. 1980; Hamilton 1985; Riddell et al. 1983), and cancers in excluded segments (Kim et al. 1976; Greenstein et al. 1978). Finally, they include features that make the diagnosis difficult to establish even when a lesion is suspected and sought: the inaccessibility of small bowel to endoscopic examination, the difficulty of evaluating segments of bowel that are either bypassed (Brown et al. 1970; Greenstein et al. 1978; Kim et al. 1976) or proximal to strictures (Greenstein et al. 1975), the "invisibility" (Fleming and Pollock 1975) or "occult" (Thompson et al. 1983) nature of the neoplasms, and the confounding of cancer symptoms with those of the underlying bowel disease.

Three distinctive microsopic features of intestinal cancer occurring with Crohn's disease were described by Fleming and Pollock: invisibility, mucosal dysplasia, and endometriosis-like invasion of the stroma. These characteristics complicate the issue of surveillance (1975). "Invisibility," which occurs occasionally, is defined as microscopic recognition when the cancer is difficult to perceive even on opening the operative specimen. Mucosal dysplasia, similar to that described in ulcerative colitis (Morson and Pang 1967), is found in 25% of cases (Fleming and Pollock 1975; Thompson et al. 1983; van Heerden and Beart 1980). An endometrial-like pattern occurs in almost 40% (Fleming and Pollock 1975).

Despite the difficulties of advising surveillance for Crohn's disease, several tentative proposals can still be offered. In regular clinical check-ups, an explanation should be sought for recurrence of old symptoms or for development of new symptoms, particularly intestinal obstruction, external fistula, intestinal bleeding, wiehgt loss, or perianal disease, especially if these symptoms develop after a long period of quiescent disease. Such symptoms warrant full work-up including endoscopy, radiological studies, and CT scan as appropriate. Excision of excluded segments should be included in any reoperation for recurrent disease.

On the other hand, no routine endoscopic surveillance program can be recommended at this time. It would require an elaborate and long-term controlled study to see whether earlier cancer diagnosis and better curative results could be achieved by regular colonoscopic surveillance. In view of the uncertainties surrounding the benefits of routine surveillance in ulcerative colitis (Collins et al. 1987), it is even harder to justify such a recommendation for Crohn's disease.

Colorectal Cancer with Schistosomiasis

Schistosomiasis is known to be endemic in millions of people in China and adjacent countries, so that the possible link to cancer is of vital importance, as the mortality resulting from such an association could be considerable. Evidence for the association of S. japonicum with colorectal cancer is somewhat tenuous but has been suggested by four sources of information: (a) the frequent occurrence of both diseases in areas of China where schistomiasis is endemic (Chen et al. 1981; Ming-Chai et al. 1980, 1981; Zhang 1985); (b) numerous case reports of schistosomal cysts within colorectal cancer specimens (Hashimoto et al. 1986); (c) similarities of clinicopathological features of schistosomiasis to ulcerative colitis (Ming-Chai et al. 1980, 1981); and (d) development of dysplasia with schistosomiasis (Chen et al. 1981). Schistosomiasis is also associated with colonic strictures (Iyer et al. 1985) and polyposis coli (Hussein et al. 1983; Zuckerman et al. 1983), but the link of these two entities to cancer is tenuous at best.

Ming-Chai et al. (1980, 1981) have studied 454 colorectal cancers in China, 28% of which were associated with schistosomiasis. Their observations point to several analogies between ulcerative colitis-related and schistosomiasis-related cancers: a disease duration of 10 years or more, the tendency to form pseudopolyps and ectopically regenerating glands, and the multicentricity of cancers in the colon. Furthermore, Chen et al. (1981) reviewed surgical specimens from 60 patients with schistosomal granulomatous disease without cancer and found mild to severe dysplasia in 36, or 60%. The dysplasia was either focal or diffuse and, as in ulcerative colitis, occurred in flat mucosa. The authors feel that these dysplastic changes are the pathological basis for the malignant potential of schistosomal colitis, as they are thought to be in long-standing ulcerative colitis. Just as ulcerative colitis-related cancers have features distinctive from those of de novo colorectal cancer, Dimette et al. (1956) have also reported significant differences between 17 schistosoma-related and 81 de novo cancers in Egypt. The male preponderance was much greater in the former (16:1 versus 4:1), the mean age less (38 versus 47 years), and the pathological type more often ulcerative (47% versus 27%).

On the other hand, some epidemiological studies do not support an association between schistosomiasis and cancer. Zhang et al. (1985) found 75 cancers among 200 000 patients with schistosomiasis, a rate of only 37.5/100 000, and concluded that there was no relationship between the two diseases (Zhang 1985). Xu and Su 1984 likewise found no increase in relative risk of colon cancer among patients with schistosomiasis.

Surveillance for Cancer Versus Prevention of Schistosomiasis

As schistosomiasis is an endemic disease in large areas of Asia and Africa, control of this infection by public health measures is the most effective way of eliminating the long-term cancer risk. Colonoscopy with multiple biopsies, removal of polyps and pseudopolyps, and examination of histological slides for dysplasia could theoretically help in identifying the patients at risk and in detecting early colorectal cancers. This approach, however, would not be a cost-effective measure in populations with an endemic disease in the poorer countries of the world. Zhang Shi-Quin described a screening and prevention program carried out in 1977–1978 in Haining County, in the People's Republic of China (Zhang 1985). This study found history, physical examination, rectal examination, and occult blood study to be of no value in detecting cancers; sigmoidoscopy was the only useful method of detection.

Conclusions

The incidence of colorectal cancer is increased in inflammatory bowel disease – unequivocally in ulcerative colitis, probably in Crohn's disease, and possibly in schistosomal colitis. The absolute numbers of patients developing such malignancies in the non-specific forms of disease are low compared to overall cancer rates in the general population, but because of higher relative risks, younger ages of onset, distinctive clinicopathological features, and the difficulties of making a diagnosis, it is important that this complication of inflammatory bowel disease be widely appreciated. In specific areas of Asia, schistosomiasis-related colorectal cancer is potentially a major epidemiological problem because it affects such a large population.

The prognosis today is no worse for colorectal cancers in ulcerative colitis or Crohn's disease (except for those occurring in excluded bowel), nor even for those occurring in schistosomiasis, than for de novo cancers of the large bowel (see Table 1). Surveillance has been advised for ulcerative colitis-related colorectal cancers, but there is still doubt as to whether it will be cost effective or how it will affect prognosis and survival. There is even greater doubt concerning its role in monitoring patients with Crohn's disease for either colorectal or small bowel cancers. Prevention of schistosomiasis by public health measures, rather than surveillance by colonoscopy, is the preferred solution to the problem of schistosomiasis-related colorectal cancer.

Acknowledgement. The authors thank Jean DiCarlo for her excellent assistance in the preparation of this chapter and Devaprasad Reuben for the diligent and meticulous work that made systematic collection of our data possible.

References

Alexander-Williams J (1976) Inflammatory disease of the bowel. The risk of cancer. Dis Colon Rectum 19:579–581

Alexis R, Domingo J (1986) Schistosomiasis and adenocarcinoma of prostate: a morphologic study. Hum Pathol 18:757–760

Allan R, Steinberg DM, Dixon K, Cooke WT (1975) Changes in the bidirectional sodium flux across the intestinal mucosa in Crohn's disease. Gut 15:201–204

Atwell JD, Duthie HL, Goligher JC (1965) The outcome of Crohn's disease. Br J Surg 52:966–972

Baker WNW, Glass RE, Ritchie JK, Aylett SO (1978) Cancer of the rectum following colectomy and ileorectal anastomosis for ulcerative colitis. Br J Surg 65:862–868

Blackstone MO, Ridell RH, Rogers BHC, Levin B (1981) Dysplasia-associated lesion or mass (DALM) detected by colonoscopy in long-standing ulcerative colitis: an indication for colectomy. Gastroenterology 80:366–374

Bonnevie O, Binder V, Anthonisen P, Riis P (1974) The prognosis of ulcerative colitis. Scand J Gastroenterol 9:81–91

Brown N, Weinstein VA, Janowitz HD (1970) Carcinoma of the ileum 25 years after bypass for regional enteritis: a case report. Mt Sinai J Med 27:675–678

Buchmann P, Allan RN, Thompson H, Alexander-Williams J (1980) Carcinoma in a recto-vaginal fistula in a patient with Crohn's disease. Am J Surg 140:462–463

Butt JH, Morson BC (1981) Dysplasia and cancer in inflammatory bowel disease (Editorial). Gastroenterology 80:865–868

Butt JH, Lennard-Jones JE, Ritchie JK (1980) A practical approach to the risk of cancer in inflammatory bowel disease. Med Clin North Am 64:1203–1220

Chen MC, Chang PY, Chuang CY, Chen YJ, Wang FP, Tang YC, Chou SC (1981) Colorectal cancer and schistosomiasis. Lancet 1:971–973

Church JM, Weakley FI, Fazio VW, Sebek BA, Achkar E, Carwell M (1985) The relationship between fistulas in Crohn's disease and associated carcinoma. Report of four cases and review of the literature. Dis Colon Rectum 28:361–366

Clemmensen T, Johansen A (1972) A case of Crohn's disease of the colon associated with adenocarcinoma extending from cardia to the anus. Acta Pathol Microbiol Scand [A] 80:5–8

Collins RH, Feldman M, Fordtran JS (1987) Colon cancer, dysplasia, and surveillance in patients with ulcerative colitis. N Engl J Med 316:1654–1658

Colp R (1934) Case of non-specific granuloma of terminal ileum and cecum. Surg Clin North Am 14:443–449

Cooper DJ, Weinstein MA, Korelitz BI (1984) Complications of Crohn's disease predisposing to dysplasia and cancer of the intestinal tract: considerations of a surveillance program. J Clin Gastroenterol 6:217–224

Crohn BB (1966) Granulomatous colitis: an attempt at clarification. Mt Sinai J Med 33:503–515

Crohn BB, Rosenberg H (1925) The sigmoidoscopic picture of chronic ulcerative colitis (non-specific). Am J Med Sci 170:220–227

Crohn BB, Ginzburg L, Oppenheimer GD (1932) Regional ileitis. A pathologic and clinical entity. JAMA 99:1323–1329

Crucioli V (1967) Rectal biopsy in Crohn's disease. Rendiconti Gastroenterol 4:73–76

Dalziel TK (1913) Chronic interstitial enteritis. Br Med J 2:1068–1070

Darke SG, Parks AG, Grogono JL, Pollock DJ (1973) Adenocarcinoma and Crohn's disease: a report of two cases and analysis of the literature. Br J Surg 60:169–175

deDombal FT, Watts JMcK, Watkinson G, Goligher JC (1966) Local complications of ulcerative colitis: stricture, pseudopolyposis, and carcinoma of colon and rectum. Br Med J 1:1442–1447

Deschner EE, Winawer SJ, Long FC, Boyle CC (1977) Early detection of colonic neoplasia in patients at high risk. Cancer 40:2625–2631

Devroede G (1980) Risk of cancer in inflammatory bowel disease. In: Winawer S, Schottenfeld D, Sherlock P (eds) Colorectal cancer, prevention, epidemiology and screening. Raven, New York, pp 325–334

Devroede GJ, Taylor WF, Sauer WG et al. (1971) Cancer risk and life expectancy of children with ulcerative colitis. N Engl J Med 285:17–21

Dimmette RM, Elwi AM, Sproat HF (1956) Relationship of schistosomiasis to polyposis and adenocarcinoma of large intestine. Am J Clin Pathol 26:266–276

Dobbins WO (1977) Current status of the precancer lesion in ulcerative colitis. Gastroenterology 73:1431–1433

Edwards FC, Truelove SC (1964) The course and prognosis of ulcerative colitis. IV. Carcinoma of the colon. Gut 5:15–22

Faust EC, Meleny HE (1924) Studies on schistosomiasis japonica. Am J Hyg (Monographic series no 3)

Ferguson R, Allan RN, Cooke WT (1975) A study of the cellular infiltrate of the proximal jejunal mucosa in ulcerative colitis and Crohn's disease. Gut 15:205–208

Fielding JF, Prior P, Waterhouse JA, Cooke WT (1972) Malignancy in Crohn's disease. Scand J Gastroenterol 7:3–7

Fleming KA, Pollock AC (1975) A case of "Crohn's carcinoma." Gut 16:533–537

Frank JD, Shorey BA (1973) Adenocarcinoma of the small bowel as a complication of Crohn's disease. Gut 14:120–124

Fresco D, Lazarus SS, Dotan J, Reingold M (1982) Early presentation of carcinoma of the small bowel in Crohn's disease ("Crohn's carcinoma"): case reports and review of the literature. Gastroenterology 82:783–789

Ghoneim MA, Ashamalla A, Gaballa MA, Ibrahim EI (1985) Cystectomy for carcinoma of the bilharzial bladder. 126 patients 10 years later. Br J Urol 57:303–305

Ginzburg L, Schneider KM, Dreizin DH, Levinson C (1956) Carcinoma of the jejunum occurring in a case of regional enteritis. Surgery 39:347–351

Goligher JC (1968) Ulcerative colitis. In: Goligher JC, deDombal FI, McWatts J, Watkinson G (eds) Williams and Wilkins, Baltimore, p 4

Goodman MJ, Skinner JM, Truelove SC (1976) Abnormalities in the apparently normal bowel mucosa in Crohn's disease. Lancet 1:275–278

Greenstein AJ, Sachar DB, Kark AE (1975) Stricture of the anorectum in Crohn's disease involving the colon. Ann Surg 181:207–212

Greenstein AJ, Sachar D, Pucillo A, Kreel I, Geller S, Janowitz HD, Aufses AH (1978) Cancer in Crohn's disease after diversionary surgery: a report of seven carcinomas occurring in excluded bowel. Am J Surg 135:86–90

Greenstein AJ, Sachar DB, Smith H, Pucillo A, Papatestas AE, Kreel I, Geller SA, Janowitz HD, Aufses AH (1979a) Cancer in universal and left-sided ulcerative colitis: factors determining risk. Gastroenterology 77:290–294

Greenstein AJ, Sachar DB, Pucillo A, Vassiliades G, Smith H, Kreel I, Geller SA, Janowitz HD, Aufses AH (1979b) Cancer in universal and left-sided ulcerative colitis: clinical and pathologic features. Mt Sinai J Med 46:25–32

Greenstein AJ, Sachar DB, Smith H, Janowitz HD, Aufses AH (1980) Patterns of neoplasia in Crohn's disease and ulcerative colitis. Cancer 46:403–407

Greenstein AJ, Sachar DB, Smith H, Janowitz HD, Aufses AH (1981) A comparison of cancer risk in Crohn's disease and ulcerative colitis. Cancer 48:2742–2745

Greenstein AJ, Gennuso R, Sachar DB, Heimann T, Smith H, Janowitz HD, Aufses AH (1985) Extraintestinal cancers in inflammatory bowel disease. Cancer 56:2914–2921

Greenstein AJ, Slater G, Heimann TM, Sachar DB, Aufses AH (1986) A comparison of multiple synchronous colorectal cancer in ulcerative colitis, familial polyposis coli, and de novo cancer. Ann Surg 203:123–128

Greenstein AJ, Meyers S, Szporn A, Slater G, Janowitz HD, Aufses AH (1987) Colorectal cancer in regional ileitis. Q J Med 237 (New Series 62): 33–40

Grundfest SF, Fazio V, Weiss RA et al. (1981) The risk of cancer following colectomy and ileorectal anastomosis for extensive mucosal ulcerative colitis. Ann Surg 193:9–14

Gyde SN, Prior P, Macartney JC, Thompson H, Waterhouse JAH, Allan RN (1980) Malignancy in Crohn's disease. Gut 21:1024–1029

Hamilton SR (1985) Colorectal carcinoma in patients with Crohn's disease. Gastroenterology 89:398–407

Hammerberg C, Slezak P, Tribukait B (1984) Early detection of malignancy in ulcerative colitis: a flow cytometric DNA analysis. Cancer 53:291–295

Hanauer SB, Wong KK, Frank PH, Sweet DL, Kirsner JB (1982) Acute leukemia following inflammatory bowel disease. Dig Dis Sci 27: 545–548

Hashimoto Y, Muratani A, Nishiyama H, Ashida H, Kurogo F, Souno K, Murao S, Maeda S (1986) A case of colon cancer associated with schistosomiasis japonica. 32: 815–818

Hinton JM (1966) Risk of malignant change in ulcerative colitis. Gut 7: 427–432

Hughes RH, Hall TJ, Block GE, Levin B, Moossa AR (1978) The prognosis of carcinoma of the colon and rectum complicating ulcerative colitis. Surg Gynecol Obstet 146: 46–48

Hussein AM, Medany S, Abou el Magd AM, Sherif SM, Williams CB (1983) Multiple endoscopic polypectomies for schistosomal polyposis of the colon. Lancet 1: 637–674

Itzkowitz SH, Lee H, Hanauer SM, Goldenberg A, Kion YS (1987) New biochemical markers associated with dysplasia in ulcerative colitis (Abstract). Gastroenterology 92: 1449

Iyer HV, Abaci IF, Rehnke EC, Enquist IF (1985) Intestinal obstruction due to schistosomiasis. Am J Surg 149: 409–411

Katzka I, Brody RS, Morris E, Katz S (1983) Assessment of colorectal cancer risk in patients with ulcerative colitis: experience from a private practice. Gastroenterology 85: 22–29

Keighley MRB, Thompson H, Alexander-Williams J (1975) Multifolcal colonic carcinoma and Crohn's disease. Surgery 78: 534–537

Kewenter J, Ahlman H, Hulten L (1978) Cancer risk in extensive ulcerative colitis. Ann Surg 188: 824–828

Kim U, Klein M, Baek S, Richman A, Aufses AH (1976) Carcinoma of the small intestine in Crohn's disease – occurrence in a bypassed loop. Mt Sinai J Med 43: 461–466

Kojiro M, Kakizoe S, Yano H, Tsumagari J, Kenmochi K, Nakashima T (1986) Hepatocellular carcinoma in schistosomiasis japonica. A clinicopathologic study of 59 autopsy cases of hepatocellular carcinoma associated with chronic schistosomiasis japonica. Acta Pathol Jpn 36: 525–532

Korelitz BI (1983) Carcinoma of the intestinal tract in Crohn's disease: Results of a survey conducted by the National Foundation for Ileitis and Colitis. Am J Gastroenterol 78: 44–46

Lavery IC, Chiulli RA, Jagelman DG, Fazio DW, Weakley FL (1982) Survival with carcinoma arising in mucosal colitis. Ann Surg 195: 508–512

Lennard-Jones JE, Morson BC, Ritchie JK, Shove DC, Williams CB (1977) Cancer in colitis assessment of the individual risk by clinical and histological criteria. Gastroenterology 73: 1280–1289

Lennard-Jones JE, Morson BC, Ritchie JK et al. (1983) Cancer surveillance in ulcerative colitis. Lancet 2: 149–152

Lightdale CJ, Sternberg SS, Posner G, Sherlock P (1975) Carcinoma complicating Crohn's disease: report of seven cases and review of the literature. Am J Med 59: 262–268

Ming-Chai C, Chi-Yuan C, Pei-Yu C, Jen-Chun H (1980) Evolution of colorectal cancer in schistosomiasis. Cancer 46: 1661–1675

Ming-Chai C, Chi-Yuan C, Fu-Pan W, Pei-Yu C, Yi-Jen C, Yang-Chuan T, Shun-Chuan C (1981) Colorectal cancer and schistosomiasis. Lancet 1: 971–973

Morson BC, Pang LSC (1967) Rectal biopsy as an aid to cancer control in ulcerative colitis. Gut 8: 423–434

Nugent FW, Haggitt RC (1984) Results of a longterm prospective surveillance program for dysplasia in ulcerative colitis (Abstract). Gastroenterology 86: 1197

Ohman ULF (1982) Colorectal carcinoma in patients with ulcerative colitis. Am J Surg 144: 344–349

Perrett AD, Truelove SC, Massarella GR (1968) Crohn's disease and carcinoma of colon. Br Med J 2: 466–468

Prior P, Gyde SN, Macartney JC, Thompson H, Waterhouse JAH, Allan RN (1982) Cancer morbidity in ulcerative colitis. Gut 23: 490–497

Riddell RH, Goldman H, Ransohoff DF et al. (1983) Dysplasia in inflammatory bowel disease: standardized classification with provisional clinical applications. Hum Pathol 14: 931–968

Ritchie JK, Hawley PR, Lennard-Jones JE (1981) Prognosis of carcinoma in ulcerative colitis. Gut 22: 752–755

Sachar DB, Greenstein AJ (1981) Cancer in ulcerative colitis: good news and bad news (Editorial). Ann Intern Med 95: 642–644

Shorter RG (1983) Risks of intestinal cancer in Crohn's disease. Dis Colon Rectum 26: 686–689

Slaney G, Brooke BN (1959) Cancer in ulcerative colitis. Lancet 2: 694–698

Slater G, Greenstein AJ, Aufses AH (1984) Anal carcinoma in patients with Crohn's disease. Ann Surg 199: 348–350

Thompson EM, Clayden G, Price AB (1983) Cancer in Crohn's disease – an "occult" malignancy. Histopathology 7: 365–376

van Heerden JA, Beart RW (1980) Carcinoma of the colon and rectum complicating chronic ulcerative colitis. Dis Colon Rectum 23: 155–159

Warren R, Barwick KW (1983) Crohn's colitis with carcinoma and dysplasia. Report of a case and review of 100 small and large bowel resections for Crohn's disease to detect incidence of dysplasia. Am J Surg Pathol 7: 151–159

Warren S, Sommers SC (1948) Cicatrizing enteritis (regional enteritis) as a pathologic entity: analysis of one hundred and twenty cases. Am J Pathol 24: 475–501

Weedon DD, Shorter RG, Ilstrup DM, Huizenga KA, Taylor WF (1973) Crohn's disease and cancer. N Engl J Med 289: 1099–1102

Xu Z, Su D (1984) Schistosoma japonicum and colorectal cancer: an epidemiological study in the People's Republic of China 34: 315–318

Zhang SQ (1985) Screening and prevention of colorectal cancer in Haining County. Dis Colon Rectum 28: 300–304

Zinkin LD, Brandwein C (1980) Adenocarcinoma in Crohn's colitis. Dis Colon Rectum 23: 115–117

Zuckerman MJ, Goldfarb JP, Cho KC, Molnar JJ (1983) An unusual pedunculated polyp of the colon association with schistosomiasis. J Clin Gastroenterol 5: 169–172

Biomarkers in the Identification of High-Risk Groups

M. Lipkin

Memorial Sloan-Kettering Cancer Center, 1275 York Avenue, New York, NY 10021, USA

Contents

Introduction

Studies of the proliferation and differentiation of cells within the gastrointestinal tract have now identified stages of abnormal development that are associated with increased susceptibility to gastrointestinal cancer. In the large intestine, and in the esophagus and stomach of human subjects with either genetic predisposition to cancer, or whose susceptibility is believed due mainly to dietary factors, modifications of epithelial cell proliferation and differentiation occur in disorders that predispose individuals to this desease. In early stages before the development of gastrointestinal neoplasia, proliferative cell-cycle control mechanisms become modified, leading to continued DNA synthesis in maturing cells and a delayed onset of normal terminal differentiation. In more advanced stages of precancerous disease, more extensive changes occur in gastrointestinal cells which exhibit progressively increasing degrees of abnormally delayed maturation.

In humans with this disease, and in rodents after treatment with chemical carcinogens, among the earliest modifications that develop in gastrointestinal epithelial cells is increased proliferative activity in a basal region of epithelium that has been referred to as the "proliferative compartment." This expansion of cell proliferation develops in all cancer-prone regions of the gastrointestinal tract that have been studied both in humans and in rodent models – in the esophagus, stomach, and colon. Eventually excessive numbers of proliferating cells accumulate in the epithelium without undergoing normal terminal differentiation (reviewed in Lipkin 1987, 1988). This chapter will describe the findings that develop in the large intestine of human subjects, and comparisons will be made with similar findings in the human esophagus and stomach, and in the gastrointestinal tract of rodents treated with chemical carcinogens. Recent applications of a biomarker of increased cancer susceptibility to studies in the field of cancer prevention also will be given.

Diseases of the Large Intestine

In diseases of the large intestine that lead to increased frequencies of human colorectal cancer, *expansions of cell proliferation* in the epithelial lining have been found. This is summarized in Table 1. This expansion of the compartment of proliferative cells occurs in familial polyposis (Deschner et al. 1963; Bleiberg et al. 1972; Lipkin 1974; Deschner and Lipkin 1975; Iwama et al. 1977; Lipkin et al. 1983, 1984), in individuals who have had sporadic adenomas (Cole and McKalen 1963; Maskens et al. 1982; Lipkin et al. 1985 b; Terpstra et al. 1987), or previous familial and nonfamilial colon cancers (Lipkin et al. 1983, 1984, 1985; Terpstra et al. 1987; Maskens and Deschner 1977; Romagnoli et al. 1984; Lipkin 1987 a), and in ulcerative colitis (Bleiberg et al. 1970; Eastwood and Trier 1973; Serafini et al. 1981; Deschner et al. 1983 a; Lehy et al. 1983; Biasco et al. 1984). In the flat colonic mucosa of individuals having colonic carcinoma, DNA content in cells in the upper third of colonic crypts was also increased, a finding not observed in colonic mucosa of normal subjects (Suzuki et al. 1985). In ulcerative colitis, it was possible to identify subpopulations of hyperproliferating cells that expressed an antigen normally decreased in maturing cells (Biasco et al. 1984).

Benign colonic adenomas are believed to be an intermediate stage between normal colonic epithelial cells and carcinoma; the probability of carcinoma developing in benign colonic adenomas increases directly as adenomas increase in size (Morson and Bussey 1970). In the colonic adenomas of familial polyposis, in addition to an expansion of the proliferative compartment of epithelial cells, a marked shift of the entire proliferative region to the surface of the adenomas has been found (Lightdale et al. 1982).

Table 1. Expansion of the proliferative compartment of epithelial cells in human subjects

Organ	Disease	References
Large intestine	Familial polyposis	Deschner et al. (1963) Bleiberg et al. (1972) Lipkin et al. (1974) Deschner et al. (1975) Iwama et al. (1977) Lipkin et al. (1983, 1984)
	Sporadic adenomas	Cole et al. (1963) Maskens et al. (1982) Lipkin et al. (1985 b) Terpstra et al. (1987) Lipkin et al. (1987)
	Colon cancer	Maskens et al. (1977) Romagnoli et al. (1984) Lipkin et al. (1983, 1984)
	Ulcerative colitis	Bleiberg et al. (1970) Eastwood et al. (1973) Serafini et al. (1981) Deschner et al. (1983) Lehy et al. (1983) Biasco et al. (1984)

Table 2. Biomarkers of abnormal differentiation of gastrointestinal epithelial cells

Organ	Biomarker	References
Large intestine	Development of colonic adenomas	Gardner (1951) Morson et al. (1970) Bussey (1975) Lipkin et al. (1980) Winawer et al. (1986)
	Histopathology of inflammatory diseases	Morson and Bussey (1970)
	Cytokeratin expression in polyposis	Garin Chesa et al. (1987)
	Blood group antigens	Sakamato et al. (1986) Cordon-Cardo et al. (1986) Abe et al. (1986) Kim et al. (1986)
	Modified gene expression	Royston et al. (1983) Garin Chesa et al. (1987) Augenlicht et al. (1987)
	Modified response to growth factors	Friedman (1981) Friedman et al. (1984) Coffey et al. (1986)

Other abnormal properties have also been observed in colonic adenomas. Among these are the modulation of secretion of plasminogen activator by tumor promoters (Friedman 1981; Friedman et al. 1984) and abnormal retrograde migration of adenomatous epithelial cells away from the surface of the mucosa deep into the crypts (Lightdale et al. 1982), as occurs with malignant cells; however, benign adenomatous epithelial cells do not invade through the basal layer.

During the *abnormal differentiation of colonic epithelial cells* in precancerous diseases further changes occur. These are summarized in Table 2. Thus, blood group-related antigens of the ABH and Lewis (Le) systems become modified, with neosynthesis of ABH specificities appearing in tumor cells together with accumulation of precursor antigens (Sakamoto et al. 1986; Cordon-Cardo et al. 1986; Abe et al. 1986; Kim et al. 1986). Increased expression of Le antigens, especially y and extended y determinants, has been found, the latter not being found in normal colonic mucosa, and having a restricted pattern of distribution in normal tissues. Le_y expression in polyps was further correlated with histological type and degree of dysplasia (Abe et al. 1986). Of importance, extended or trifucosyl Le_y antigen expression was limited exclusively to premalignant adenomatous polyps and was invariably absent from nonpremalignant or hyperplastic polyps. Among adenomatous polyps, extended Le_y antigen expression tended to correlate with three known parameters of malignant potential: larger polyp size, villous histology and severe dysplasia. Therefore, in human colon the Le_y hapten appears to be an oncodevelopmental cancer-associated antigen, and extended Le_y antigens may be specific markers for premalignancy and malignancy (Abe et al. 1986; Kim et al. 1986).

Further changes occur in colonic epithelial cells during abnormal differentiation, and, as neoplasms develop; these include modifications of cytokeratin expression (Garin Chesa et al. 1986), the expression of abnormal carbohydrate antigens, and morphological, immunological, and biochemical modifications in the cells (Wolman and Mastromarino 1984; Wolman 1987). Alterations of gene structure and expression also occur in the hereditary disease familial polyposis, and in carcinogen-induced and sporadic colonic cancer as colonic cells undergo abnormal differentiation and develop into adenomas and carcinomas (Bodmer et al. 1987; Augenlicht et al. 1987a).

Among modifications in gene expression, the c-*myc* oncogene has been implicated in the processes of normal cell proliferation and differentiation. In normal colonic mucosa, c-*myc* oncogene product was expressed maximally in the normal mid-zone region of differentiating cells, and in dysplastic areas of adenomatous polyp cells (Garin Chesa et al. 1987). Expression of the *ras* gene was found highest in the most differentiated cells in the upper region of normal colonic crypts, and a high level of Ha-*ras* expression appeared to be a marker for a differentiated state of colonic carcinoma cells involving mucin production (Augenlicht et al. 1987b). Colonic carcinoma cells also secrete transforming growth factor (TGF)alpha and TGFbeta. As in keratinocytes, these may contribute to differentiation of the epithelial cells, and an imbalance of these two endogenous growth modifiers to aberrant development of preneoplastic cells (Coffey et al. 1986).

Diseases of the Esophagus

Interesting comparisons can be made between findings noted in the colon and those developing in esophagus in diseases leading to increased frequencies of esophageal cancer. In several diseases of the esophagus that lead to increased frequencies of cancer, the numbers of proliferating epithelial cells in the esophageal basal layer increase as the proliferative compartment expands. Barrett's disease of the esophagus leads to a marked increase in the incidence of esophageal cancer and may account for a large fraction of the esophageal cancer occurring in the United States (Naef et al. 1975). In this disease increased numbers of immature epithelial cells accumulate in the esophageal lining and some undergo metaplastic changes; proliferative cells sometimes reach the surface of the esophageal lining, and their numbers increase as the proliferative compartment expands (Herbst et al. 1978; Pellish et al. 1980).

In Linxian, China, an exceptionally high incidence of and mortality from esophageal cancer have been found to occur. Cumulative esophageal cancer death rates to age 75 have been reported to be as high as 33% for males and 20% for females (Lim et al. 1983). In this high-risk region of China, and in other geographical regions of high esophageal cancer incidence, the squamous epithelial lining gradually undergoes morphological changes from normal to hyperplastic and to dysplastic before the onset of cancer. In precancerous esophageal disease in Linxian, it has been noted that as hyperplasia and dysplasie develop, the proliferative compartment progressively increases in size, and the absolute numbers of proliferative cells markedly increase (Muñoz et al. 1985; Yang et al. 1987). When esophageal epithelial cells develop increasing degrees of dysplasia and preinvasive carcinoma, the DNA content of individual cells increases with increased ploidy (Avtandilov et al. 1985).

Further changes similarly occur during the abnormal differentiation of esophageal epithelial cells. As normal esophageal squamous epithelial cells undergo differentiation, they express other biomarkers including different molecular species of keratins, as do colonic epithelial cells and squamous epidermal cells (Sun and Green 1976, 1978). However, when esophageal epithelial cells become malignant, they express keratin species not present in normal esophageal cells (Scaramuzzino et al. 1986). Esophageal carcinoma cells also develop various ectopic tumor-associated antigens, including human chorionic gonadotropin, human placental lactogen, alpha-fetoprotein, carcinoembryonic antigen and nonspecific cross-reacting antigen (Burg-Kurland et al. 1986). These cells also contain lower quantities of surface epidermal growth factor (EGF) receptors with much higher affinity than normal esophageal cells, as modulation of cell growth is altered during abnormal development (Banks-Schlegel and Quintero 1986).

Diseases of the Stomach

In diseases of the stomach that lead to increased frequencies of human gastric cancer, characteristic changes in cell proliferation and differentiation also occur. The development of gastric carcinoma is preceded by increased proliferative activity of gastric epithelial cells, and by intermediate stages of abnormal cell differentiation, including metaplasia of the small and large intestinal types and dysplasia. In these diseases, proliferating epithelial cells fail to differentiate normally as they migrate to the surface of the mucosa, and immature cells line the gastric surface, directly contacting the contents of the stomach.

Thus, in chronic atrophic gastritis, a hyperproliferative condition develops as increased numbers of cells undergo replication more rapidly than normal and migrate more rapidly than normal to the surface of the epithelial lining where immature epithelial cells are then exuded from the surface. In gastric atrophy, the immature proliferative epithelial cell compartment also expands, and other metabolic functions increase (Winawer and Lipkin 1969; Deschner et al. 1972; Sizikov and Azykbekov 1981; Lipkin et al. 1985a; Bell et al. 1967; Willems and Bleiberg 1978).

Recent findings in peptic ulcer disease (Sizikov and Azykbekov 1981) have shown that levels of gastric epithelial cell proliferation are similar to those of mild gastritis without atrophy and of minimal gastric atrophy. However, cell proliferation progressively increases with increasing gastric atrophy, reaching a peak in severe atrophy and gastritis as cells with impaired terminal differentiation cover the mucosa.

In Colombia, South America, a well-characterized population has been studied, consisting of individuals having chronic atrophic gastritis who develop gastric cancer with very high frequency. Three findings were noted: (a) an expansion of the proliferative compartment of epithelial cells; (b) a grossly hyperproliferative state with excessive numbers of replicating cells in the gastric lining; and (c) a failure of cells to undergo normal maturation (Lipkin et al. 1985a). The last was shown both by morphological evidence of immature cells covering the surface of the stomach, and by increased expression of an antigen in hyperproliferating cells that is normally decreased in maturing cells (Lipkin et al. 1985a).

After surgical resection of part of the stomach to treat peptic ulcer disease, the susceptibility of individuals to develop gastric cancer in the remaining stomach increases significantly. Studies of changes that develop in the gastric epithelium after partial gastrectomy have shown progressive expansions of the proliferative compartment of epithelial cells extending to the surface of the stomach with increasing dysplasia and accumulations of increasing numbers of abnormally proliferating cells (Hansen et al. 1978; Assad and Eastwood 1980; Offerhaus et al. 1985).

During development of the abnormal intermediate stage of cell differentiation known as "metaplasia," which is associated with an increased frequency of stomach cancer, other changes develop in gastric epithelial cells. Intestinal metaplasia is increased in the gastric mucosa of patients with cancer compared to individuals with gastric ulcer, implying again that metaplasia is an indicator of precancerous disease. Differences in expression of intestinal enzymes in gastric mucosa have been used to classify metaplastic glands as "complete," i.e., containing all or most small-intestinal enzymes, or "incomplete" with fewer enzymes expressed than in normal small-intestinal mucosa (Correa 1984); the latter is considered closer to dysplasia and carcinoma. In early and more mature metaplasia, the neutral mucin of normal gastric cells is replaced by sialomucin (small-intestinal type), while in advanced metaplasia sulphomucins of the colonic type are seen and are considered a marker of dysplasia (Correa 1984; Matsukura et al. 1980; Jass and Filipe 1980; Nardelli et al. 1983). In metaplastic gastric epithelium, normal gastric antigens are also lost; in well-differentiated lesions they are replaced by normal intestinal antigens, and in less well-differentiated lesions by embryonic antigens (Bara et al. 1980). In chronic atrophic gastritis, hyperproliferating epithelial cells increase the expression of an antigen that is normally decreased in maturing gastric cells (Lipkin et al. 1985a).

Thus, as noted above throughout the gastrointestinal tract in humans, in diseases that lead to increased frequencies of cancer, expanding populations of proliferating epithelial cells have been found before the development of observable tumors. Throughout the entire gastrointestinal tract, therefore, the normal mucosa is a comparatively *quiescent* mucosa in terms of cell proliferation, and fully mature cells are able to develop in order to function, to cover, and to protect the surface of the gastrointestinal tract. As cells progress through different stages of premalignancy, newer studies have begun to show expression, and modified responses of the cells to growth factors and tumor promoters that may further contribute to abnormal cell development.

In *animal models,* the progression of gastrointestinal cells to malignancy has also been studied: chemical carcinogens have induced similar expansions of the compartment of proliferative cells (Table 3), together with abnormal differentiation and modified gene expression (Royston and Augenlicht 1983) in rodent gastrointestinal epithelial cells. In experimental animal models, whose results closely imitate the empirical findings in humans, progressive changes have been initiated by the adminstration of chemical carcinogens that include: in *esophagus* N-methyl-N-nitrosoaniline, N-methyl-N-benzylnitrosamine, dimethylnitrosamine, and N-methyl-N-amylnitrosamine (Napalkov and Pozharisski 1969; Stinson et al. 1978; Schrager et al. 1986; Rubio 1983; Kuwayama and Eastwood 1988); in *stomach* N-methyl-N'-nitro-N-nitrosoguanidine (MNNG) (Deschner et al. 1979; Kuwayama and Tomino 1985); in *colon* dimethylhydrazine, MNNG, N-methyl-N-nitrosourea, and azoxymethane (Wiebecke et al. 1969; Thurnherr et al. 1973; Richards 1977; Chang 1978; Pozharisski et al. 1979; Deschner et al. 1983b; Heitman et al. 1983; Suzuki and Umehara 1986;

Table 3. Expansion of the proliferative compartment of epithelial cell studies of rodents treated with chemical carcinogens

Organ	Chemical carcinogen	References
Esophagus	N-Methyl-N-nitrosoaniline	Napalkov Pozharisski (1969)
	N-Methyl-N-benzylnitrosamine	Stinson et al. (1978)
		Schraeger et al. (1986)
	Dimethylnitrosamine	Rubio (1983)
	N-Methyl-N-amylnitrosamine	Kuwayama and Eastwood (1978)
Stomach	N-Methyl-N'-nitro-N-nitrosoguanidine	Deschner et al. (1979)
		Kuwayama and Tomino (1985)
Large intestine	1,2-Dimethylhydrazine	Wiebeckie et al. (1969)
		Thurnherr et al. (1973)
		Richards (1977)
		Chang (1978)
		Pozhariski et al. (1979)
		Deschner et al. (1983)
		Heitman et al. (1983)
		Suzuki and Umehara (1986)
	N-Methyl-N'-nitro-N-nitrosoguanidine	Kikkawa (1974)
	N-Methyl-N-nitrosourea	Cohen et al. (1980)

Kikkawa 1974; Cohen et al. 1980; Matthews and Cooke 1986); and in epithelium of *cervix* 3,4-benzpyrene and 20-methylcholanthrene (Rubio and Lagerlof 1974; Hasegawa et al. 1976). In precancerous diseases of the human cervix, an expansion of the proliferative compartment of epithelial cells and modifications of cell differentiation also occur (Wilbanks et al. 1967; Chi et al. 1977; Schubert et al. 1983). In the colon, as carcinogenesis progressed after azoxymethane, DNA content also increased in proliferative and functional cells and in adenomas, reflecting increased numbers of proliferative cells at higher positions in the colonic crypts (Matthews and Cooke 1986).

Application of Biomarkers to Studies of Cancer Prevention in Human Subjects

It has recently been suggested that biomarkers of abnormal gastrointestinal cell proliferation could assist studies in the field of cancer prevention (Lipkin 1987, 1988). Although genetic predisposition contributes to the evolution of gastrointestinal neoplasia, components of the ingested diet are believed to have a major influence on the incidence rates both of adenomas and colon cancer in human popoulations with widely differing frequencies of cancer in different parts of the world. Because of this, many studies have been carried out in animal models where the appearance of tumors can be measured over short time periods; these have indicated that specific dietary factors can inhibit the induction and development of a wide variety of tumors, including those arising in the gastrointestinal tract.

Thus, it has been pointed out that compounds belonging to over 20 different classes of chemicals have potential capability for chemoprevention; some of these are naturally occurring constituents of food. The chemopreventive agents can be classified into two broad categories (reviewed in Wattenberg 1985): inhibitors effective against the formation or activation of tumor-initiating agents (i.g., genotoxic agents), or against tumor promoters.

Thus, new rationales for dietary intervention have emerged from epidemiological studies and from studies of animal models that might warrant evaluation in human populations. Since epithelial cell proliferation is increased in the colon, stomach, and esophagus of human subjects with increased susceptibility to gastrointestinal cancer before the appearance of tumors, analysis of gastrointestinal cell hyperproliferation was recently considered for possible application to this problem. An example of an application of this type is found in recent studies involving oral calcium administration to individuals at increased risk for colonic cancer.

In animal models bile acids and fatty acids have increased colonic cell proliferation, and supplemental dietary calcium decrease colonic cell proliferation induced by bile acids and fatty acids (Wargovich et al. 1983, 1984; Bird et al. 1986). Supplemental dietary calcium also lowered the compensatory increase in colonic cell proliferation occurring after partial resection of the small intestine in an animal model and the yield of carcinogen-induced colonic tumors in several animal models (Appleton et al. 1986, 1987; Pence and Buddingh 1987).

In human subjects at increased risk for familial colon cancer, the biomarker of colonic epithelial cell hyperproliferation has recently been studied before and after oral dietary supplementation with calcium (Lipkin and Newmark 1985, 1988; Lipkin et al. 1987b; Rozen et al. 1987). Following calcium supplementation epithelial cell proliferation in the group as a whole was significantly reduced, yielding an altered colonic crypt profile approaching that previously observed in subjects at low risk for colon cancer. It is important to note that reductions were greatest in individuals having pronounced hyperproliferation of colonic epithelial cells, while other individuals whose proliferation was close to normal remained unchanged. Dietary supplementation with calcium also increased the numbers of maturing cells in the crypts as in characteristic of low-risk populations (Lipkin and Newmark 1985, 1988; Lipkin et al. 1987b; Rozen et al. 1987).

Direct exposure of normal human colonic epithelial cells to physiological amounts of calcium in vitro also showed the cells capable of responding with decreased proliferation; however, when the neoplastic transformation of colonic cells progressed to adenomas and carcinomas, the cells were unresponsive to calcium in vitro (Buset et al. 1986). Calcium has also induced a more quiescent proliferative state in normal epithelial cells of many other tissues including keratinocytes, mammary epithelial cells, esophageal epithelium, bronchial epithelium and urothelium, and led to terminal differentiation together with growth inhibition in some of the cell systems (reviewed in Buset et al. 1986). Hyperproliferation of mammary epithelial cells induced by increased dietary fat intake was also decreased by supplemental dietary calcium in serveral animal models (Zhang et al. 1987; Jacobson et al. 1987).

Thus in the various studies cited above, measurements of the proliferation and differentiation of epithelial cells have provided "intermediate biomarkers" that permit measurement of early effects of nutritional intervention in the cells of both human subjects and animal models. In the further application of biomarkers to the field of cancer prevention it appears that this approach may permit many more nutritional and pharmacological intervention studies to be carried out in human subjects as future attempts to inhibit the development of neoplasia increase.

References

Abe K, Hakomori S, Ohshiba S (1986) Differential expression of difucosyl type 2 chain (LeY) defined by monoclonal antibody AH6 in different locations of colonic epithelia, various histological types of colonic polyps, and adenocarcinomas. Cancer Res 46:2639–2644

Appleton GVN, Bristol JB, Williamson RCN (1986) Increased dietary calcium and small bowel resection have opposite effects on colonic cell turnover. Br J Surg 73:1018–1021

Appleton GVN, Davies PW, Bristol JB, Williamson RCN (1987) Inhibition of intestinal carcinogenesis by dietary supplementation with calcium. Br J Surg 74:523–525

Assad RT, Eastwood GL (1980) Epithelial proliferation in human fundic mucosa after antrectomy and vagotomy. Gastroenterology 79:807–811

Augenlicht LH, Wahrman MZ, Halsey H, Anderson L, Taylor J, Lipkin M (1987a) Expression of cloned sequences in biopsies of human colonic tissue and in colonic carcinoma cells induced to differentiate in vitro. Cancer Res 47:6017–6021

Augenlicht LH, Augeron C, Yander G, Laboisse C (1987b) Overexpression of *ras* in mucus-secreting colon carcinoma cells of low tumorigenicity. Cancer Res 47:3763–3765

Avtandilov G, Zhavoronkov AA, Sakhipov N (1985) Concentration of DNA in nuclei of the epithelium of the esophageal mucosa in chronic esophagitis, precancer and cancer (comparative microspectrophotometric study). Arkh Patol 47(12):33–37

Banks-Schenkel SP, Quintero J (1986) Human esophageal carcinoma cells have fewer, but higher affinity epidermal growth factor receptors. J Biol Chem 261:4359–4362

Bara J, Loisillier F, Burtin P (1980) Antigen gastric and intestinal mucous cells in human colonic tumors. Br J Cancer 41:209–221

Bell B, Almy TP, Lipkin M (1967) Cell proliferation kinetics in the gastrointestinal tract of man. III. Cell renewal in esophagus, stomach and jejunum of a patient with treated pernicious anemia. J Natl Cancer Inst 38:615–628

Biasco G, Lipkin M, Minarini A, Higgins P, Miglioli M, Luigi B (1984) Proliferative and antigenic properties of the rectal cells in patients with chronic ulcerative colitis. Cancer Res 44:5450–5454

Bird RP, Schneider R, Stamp D, Bruce WR (1986) Effect of dietary calcium and cholic acid on the proliferative indices of murine colonic epithelium. Carcinogenesis 7:1657–1661

Bleiberg H, Mainguet P, Galand P, Chretien J, Dupont-Mairesse N (1970) Cell renewal in the human rectum: in vitro autoradiographic study on active ulcerative colitis. Gastroenterology 58:851–855

Bleiberg H, Mainguet P, Galand P (1972) Cell renewal in familial polyposis: comparison between polyps and adjacent healthy mucosa. Gastroenterology 63:240

Bodmer WF, Bailey CJ, Bodmer J, Bussey HJR, Ellis A, Gorman P, Lucibello VA, Murday VA, Rider SH, Scambler P, Sheer D, Solomon E, Spurr NK (1987) Localization of the gene for familial adenomatous polyposis on chromosome 5. Nature 328:614–616

Burg-Kurland CL, Purnell DM, Combs JW, Hillman EA, Harris CC, Trump BF (1986) Immunocytochemical evaluation of human esophageal neoplasms and prenoeplastic lesions for beta-chorionic gonadotropin, placental lactogen, alphafetoprotein, carcinoembryonic antigen, and non specific cross-reacting antigen. Cancer Res 46:2936–2943

Buset M, Lipkin M, Winawer S, Swaroop S, Friedman E (1986) Inhibition of human colonic epithelial cell proliferation in vivo and vitro by calcium. Cancer Res 46:5426–5430

Bussey HJR (1975) Familial polyposis coli. Johns Hopkin University Press, Baltimore

Chang WWL (1978) Histogenesis of symmetrical 1,2-dimethylhydrazine-induced neoplasms of the colon in the mouse. J Natl Cancer Inst 60:1405–1418

Chi CH, Rubio CA, Lagerlof B (1977) The frequency and distribution of mitotic figures in dysplasia and carcinoma in situ. Cancer 39:1218–1223

Coffey RJ, Shipley GD, Moses HL (1986) Production of transforming growth factors by human colon cancer lines. Cancer Res 46: 1164–1169

Cohen BI, Raicht RF, Deschner EE, Takahashi M, Sarwal AN, Fazzini E (1980) Effect of cholic acid feeding on N-methyl-N-nitrosourea-induced colon tumors and cell kinetics in rats. J Natl Cancer Inst 64: 573–578

Cole JW, McKalen A (1963) Studies on the morphogenesis of adenomatous polyps in the human colon. Cancer 16: 998–1002

Cordon-Cardo C, Lloyd KO, Sakamoto J, McGroarty ME, Old LI, Melamed MR (1986) Immunohistologic expression of blood group antigens in normal human gastrointestinal tract and colonic carcinoma. Int J Cancer 37: 667–676

Correa P (1984) Chronic gastritis as a cancer precursor. Scand J Gastroenterol 19(104): 131–136

Deschner EE, Lipkin M (1975) Proliferative patterns in colonic mucosa in familial polyposis. Cancer 34: 413–418

Deschner EE, Lewis CM, Lipkin M (1963) In vitro study of human rectal epithelial cells. I. Atypical zone of H[3] thymidine incorporation in mucosa of multiple polyposis. J Clin Invest 42: 1922–1928

Deschner EE, Winawer SJ, Lipkin M (1972) Patterns of nucleic acid and protein synthesis in normal human gastric mucosa and atrophic gastritis. J Natl Cancer Inst 48: 1567–1574

Deschner EE, Tamura K, Bralow SP (1979) Early proliferative changes in rat pyloric mucosa induced with MNNG. Front Gastrointest Res 4: 25–31

Deschner EE, Winawer SJ, Katz S, Kahn E (1983a) Proliferative defects in ulcerative colitis patients. Cancer Invest 1: 41–47

Deschner EE, Long FC, Hakissian M, Herrmann SL (1983b) Differential susceptibility of AKR, C57BL/6J, and CF1 mice to 1,2-dimethylhydrazine-induced colonic tumor formation predicted by proliferative characteristics of colonic epithelial cells. J Natl. Cancer Inst 70: 279–282

Eastwood GL, Trier JS (1973) Epithelial cell renewal in cultured rectal biopsies in ulcerative colitis. Gastroenterology 64: 383–390

Friedman E (1981) Differential response of premalignant epithelial cell classes to phorbol ester tumor promoters and to deoxycholic acid. Cancer Res 4: 4588–4599

Friedman E, Gillin S, Lipkin M (1984) 12-O-tetradecanoylphorbol-13-acetate stimulation of DNA synthesis in cultured preneoplastic familial polyposis colonic epithelial cells but not in normal colonic epithelial cells. Cancer Res 44: 4078–4086

Gardner EJ (1951) Am J Hum Genet 3: 167–176

Garin Chesa PG, Rettig WJ, Melamed MR (1986) Expression of cytokeratins in normal and neoplastic colonic epithelial cells – implications for cellular differentiation and carcinogenesis. Am J Surg Pathol 10: 829–835

Garin Chesa P, Rettig WJ, Melamed MR, Old LJ, Niman HL (1987) Expression of p21 ras in normal and malignant tissues, lack of association with proliferation and malignancy. Proc Natl Sci USA (in press)

Hansen OH, Larsen JK, Svendsen LB (1978) Changes in gastric mucosal cell proliferation after antrectomy or vagotomy in man. Scand J Gastroenterol 13: 947–952

Hasegawa K, Matsuura Y, Tojo S (1976) Cellular kinetics and histological changes in experimental cancer of the uterine cervix. Cancer Res 36: 359–634

Heitman DW, Grubbs BG, Heitman TO, Cameron IL (1983) Effects of 1,2-dimethylhydrazine treatment and feeding regimen on rat colonic epithelial cell proliferation. Cancer Res 43: 1153–1162

Herbst JJ, Berenson MM, McCloskey DW, Wiser WC (1978) Cell proliferation in esophageal columnar epithelium (Barret's esophagus). Gastroenterology 75: 683–687

Iwama T, Utsunomiya J, Sasaki J (1977) Epithelial cell kinetics in the crypts of familial polyposis of colon. Jpn J Surg 7: 230–234

Jacobson EA, Russell R, Newmark HL, Amer MA, Carroll KK (1987) Fat, calcium and tumor development in dimethyl-benz(A)antracene (DMBA)-treated rats. Proc Can Fed Biol Soc 30: 112

Jass JR, Filipe MI (1980) Sulfomucins and precancerous lesions of the human stomach. Histopathology 4: 271–279

Kikkawa N (1974) Experimental studies on polypogenesis and carcinogenesis of the large intestine. Med J Osaka Univ 24: 293–314

Kim YS, Yuan M, Itzkowitz SH, Sun QB, Kaizu T, Palekar A, Trump BF, Hakomori S (1986) Expression of LeY and extended LeY blood group-related antigens in human malignant, premalignant, and nonmalignant colonic tissues. Cancer Res 46:5985–5992

Kuwayama H, Eastwood GL (1988) Light and electron microscopic and autoradiographic studies on N-methyl-N-amylinitrosamine induced rat esophageal carcinogenesis. Dig Dis Sci (in press)

Kuwayama H, Tomino Y (1985) Effect of sodium chloride on epithelial proliferation in MNNG-treated rat antrum. Jpn J Cancer Res 30:200

Lehy T, Mignon M, Abitbol JL (1983) Epithelial cell proliferation in the rectal stump of patients with ileorectal anastomosis for ulcerative colitis. Gut 24:1048–1056

Lightdale C, Lipkin M, Deschner E (1982) In vivo measurements in familial polyposis: kinetics and location of proliferating cells in colonic adenomas. Cancer Res 42:4280–4283

Lim P et al. (1983) Precancerous lesions of the esophagus: a review. Chin J Oncol 5:391–395

Lipkin M (1974) Phase 1 and phase 2 proliferative lesions of colonic epithelial cells in diseases leading to colonic cancer. Cancer 34:878–888

Lipkin M (1987) Biomarkers of increased susceptibility to gastrointestinal cancer. Their development and application to studies of cancer prevention. Gastroenterology 92:359–364

Lipkin M (1988) Biomarkers of increased susceptibility to gastrointestinal cancer: new application to studies of cancer prevention in human subjects. Cancer research, perspectives in cancer research 48:235–245

Lipkin M, Newmark H (1985) Effect of edded dietary calcium on colonic epithelial cell proliferation in subjects at high-risk for familial colon cancer. N Engl J Med 313:1381–1384

Lipkin M, Newmark H (1988) Application of intermediate biomarks and the prevention of cancer of the large intestine. In: Basic and clinical perspectives of colorectal polyps and cancer. Liss, New York 1988, pp 135–150

Lipkin M, Sherlock P, De Cosse S (1980) Risk factors and preventive measures in the control of cancer of the large intestine. Curr Prob Cancer 4:1–57

Lipkin M, Blattner WE, Fraumeni JF, Lynch HT, Deschner EE, Winawer S (1983) Tritiated thymidine ($^\Phi$p, $^\Phi$h) labeling distribution as a marker for hereditary predisposition to colon cancer. Cancer Res 43:1899–1904

Lipkin M, Blattner WA, Gardner EJ, Burt RW, Lynch H, Deschner E, Winawer S, Fraumeni JF (1984) Classification and risk assessment of individuals with familial polyposis, Gardner syndrome and familial non-polyposis colon cancer from [^{3}H]dThd-labeling patterns in colonic epithelial cells. Cancer Res 44:4201–4207

Lipkin M, Correa P, Mikol YB, Higgins PJ, Cuello C, Zarama G, Fontham E, Zavala D (1985a) Proliferative and antigenic modifications in epithelial cells in chronic atrophic gastritis. J Natl Cancer Inst 75:613–619

Lipkin M, Uehara K, Winawer S, Sanchez A, Bauer C, Phillips R, Lynch HT, Blattner WA, Fraumeni JF Jr (1985b) Seventh-Day Adventist vegetarians have quiescent proliferative activity in colonic mucosa. Cancer Lett 26:139–144

Lipkin M, Enker WF, Winawer SJ (1987a) Tritiated-thymidine labeling of rectal epithelial cells in "non-prep" biopsies of individuals at increased risk for colonic neoplasia. Cancer Lett 37:153–161

Lipkin M, Friedman E, Winawer S, Newmark H (1987b) Colonic epithelial cell proliferation in responders and nonresponders to supplemental dietary calcium. Cancer Res 49:248–254

Maskens AP, Deschner EE (1977) Tritiated thymidine incorporation into epithelial cells of normal-appearing colorectal mucosa of cancer patients. J Natl Cancer Inst 58:1221–1224

Maskens AP, Meersseman F, Beckers C (1982) In vitro radioautographic study of adenomatous polyp and hyperplasia of the rectocolic mucosa in man. Scand J Gastroenterol 7:43

Matsukura N, Susuki K, Kawachi T, Aoyagi M, Sugimura T, Kitaoka H, Numajiri H, Shirota A, Itabashi M, Hirota T (1980) Distribution of marker enzymes and mucin in intestinal metaplasia in human stomach and relation to complete and incomplete types of intestinal metaplasia to minute gastric carcinomas. J Natl Cancer Inst 65:231–240

Matthews J, Cooke T (1986) Changes in crypt cell DNA content during experimental colonic carcinogenesis. Br J Cancer 53:787–791

Morson BC, Bussey JR (1970) Predisposing causes of intestinal cancer. Curr Probl Surg 1–46

Muñoz N, Lipkin M, Crespi M, Wahrendorf J, Grassi A, Lu S (1985) Proliferative abnormalities of the oesophageal epithelium of Chinese populations at high and low risk for oesophageal cancer. Int J Cancer 36: 187:189

Naef AP, Savary M, Ozzello L (1975) Columnar lined lower esophagus: an acquired lesion with malignant predisposition. Report on 140 cases of Barrett's esophagus with 12 adenocarcinoma. J Thorac Cardiovasc Surg 70: 826–835

Napalkov PN, Pozharisski KM (1969) Morphogenesis of experimental tumors of the esophagus. J Natl Cancer Inst 42: 922–940

Nardelli J, Bara J, Rosa B, Burtin PJ (1983) Intestinal metaplasia and carcinomas of the human stomach: an immunohistologic study. J Histochem Cytochem 31: 366–375

Offerhaus GJA, van de Stadt J, Samson G, Tytgat GNJ (1985) Cell proliferation kinetics in the gastric remnant. Eur J Cancer Clin Oncol 2: 73–79

Pellish LJ, Hermos JA, Eastwood GL (1980) Cell proliferation in three types of Barrett's epithelium. Gut 21: 26–31

Pence BC, Buddingh F (1987) Inhibition of dietary fat promotion of colon carcinogenesis by supplemental calcium or vitamin D. Proc Am Assoc Cancer Res 28: 154

Pozharisski KM, Likhachev AJ, Llimashevski VF, Shaposhnikov JD (1979) Experimental intestinal cancer research with reference to human pathology. Adv Cancer Res 30: 165–237

Richards TC (1977) Early changes in the dynamics of crypt cell populations in mouse colon following administration of 1,2-dimethylhydrazine. Cancer Res 37: 1680–1685

Romagnoli P, Filipponi F, Bandettini L, Brugnola D (1984) Increase of mitotic activity in the colinic mucosa of patients with colorectal cancer. Dis Colon Rectum 27: 305–308

Royston ME, Augenlicht LH (1983) Biotinated probe containing a long-terminal repeat hybridized to a mouse colon tumor and normal tissue. Science 222: 1339–1341

Rozen P, Fireman Z, Wax Y, Ron E (1987) Oral calcium supresses increased colonic mucosal proliferation of persons at risk for colorectal neoplasia. Gastroenterology 92 (2): 1603

Rubio CA (1983) Epithelial lesions antedating oesophageal carcinoma. I. Histologic study in mice. Pathol Res Pract 176: 269–275

Rubio CA, Lagerlof B (1974) Autoradiographic studies of experimentally induced atypias in the cervical epithelium of mice. Acta Pathol Microbiol Scand [A] 82: 475–482

Sakamoto J, Furukawa K, Gordon-Cardo C, Yin BWT, Rettig WJ, Oettgen HF, Old LJ, Lloyd KO (1986) Expression of Lewis[a], Lewis[b], X, and Y blood group antigens in human colonic tumors and normal tissue and in human tumor-derived cell lines. Cancer Res 46: 1553–1561

Scaramuzzino D, Stoner GD, Goldblatt PJ (1986) Keratin protein expression in nontumorigenic and tumorigenic rat esophageal epithelial cells. Proc Am Assoc Cancer Res 27: 69

Schrager TF, Busey WF, Goldman ME, Newberne PM (1986) Enhancement of methylbenzyl-nitrosamine-induced esophageal carcinogenesis in zinc-deficient rats: effects on incorporation [³H]-thymidine into DNA of esophageal epithelium and liver. Carcinogenesis 7: 1121–1126

Schubert B, Kunz J, Banaschak A (1983) Labelling patterns of carcinomas of the cervix and their precancerous stages after ³H-thymidine incorporation. Acta Histochem 27: 111–115

Serafini EP, Kirk AP, Chambers TJ (1981) Rate and pattern of epithelial cell proliferation in ulcerative colitis. Gut 22: 648–652

Sizikov AI, Azykbekov R (1981) Histoautoradiographic study of gastric epithelial DNA synthesis in precancerous lesions of the stomach. Vopr Onkol 27(10): 19–22

Stinson SF, Squire RA, Sporn MB (1978) Pathology of esophageal neoplasms and associated proliferative lesions induced in rate by N-methyl-N-benzylnitrosamine. J Natl Cancer Inst 61: 1471–1475

Sun T-T, Green H (1976) Differentiation of the epidermal keratinocyte in cell culture. Formation of the cornified envelope. Cell 9: 511–521

Sun T-T, Green H (1978) Keratin filaments of cultured human epidermal cells. Formation of intermolecular disulfide bonds during terminal differentiation. J Biol Chem 253: 2053–2060

Suzuki H, Umehara N (1986) Early mucosal changes in dimethylhydrazine-induced colonic carcinogenesis in rats. Jpn J Surg 16: 140–143

Suzuki H, Honda E, Matsumoto K, Iriyama K (1985) Tissue CEA determination and cytophotometric DNA analysis of colorectal mucosa in patients with colorectal cancer. Jpn J Surg 15: 449–454

Terpstra OT, van Blankenstein M, Dees J, Eilers GAM (1987) Abnormal pattern of cell prolife-
    ration in the entire colonic mucosa of patients with colon adenoma of cancer. Gastro-
    enterology 92: 704–748
Thurnherr N, Deschner EE, Stonehill EH, Lipkin M (1973) Induction of adenocarcinomas of
    the colon in mice by weekly injections of 1,2-dimethylhydrazine. Cancer Res 33: 904–945
Wargovich MJ, Eng VWS, Newmark HL, Bruce WR (1983) Calcium ameliorates the toxic effect
    in deoxycholic acid on colonic epithelium. Carcinogenesis 4: 1205–1207
Wargovich MJ, Eng VWS, Newmark HL, Bruce WR (1984) Calcium inhibits the damaging and
    compensating proliferative effects of fatty acids on mouse colon epithelium. Cancer Lett
    23: 253–258
Wattenberg LW (1985) Chemoprevention of cancer. Cancer Res 45: 1–8
Wiebecke B, Lohrs U, Gimmy J, Eder M (1969) Erzeugung von Darmtumoren bei Mäusen
    durch 1,2-Dimethylhydrazin. Z Gesamte Exp Med 53: 239–243
Wilbanks GD, Richart RM, Terner JY (1967) DNA content of cervical intraepithelial neoplasia
    studied by two-wavelength Feulgen cytophotmetry. Am J Obstet Gynecol 98: 792–799
Willems G, Bleiberg H (1978) Proliferative changes in the gastric mucosa of patients with
    pernicious anemia. In: Gerard A (ed) Gastrointestinal tumors: a clinical and experimental
    approach. Pergamon, New York, p 39
Winawer SJ, Lipkin M (1969) Cell proliferation kinetics in the gastrointestinal tract of man. IV.
    Cell renewal in the intestinalized gastric mucosa. J Natl Cancer Inst 42: 9
Winawer SJ, Ritchie MT, Diaz BJ et al. (1986) The National Polyp Study: aims and organiza-
    tion. In: Rozen P, Winawer SJ (eds) Secondary prevention of colorectal cancer. pp 216–225
    (Gastrointestinal research, vol 10)
Wolman SR (1987) Genetic markers of colonic neoplasia. Semin Surg Oncol 3: 120–125
Wolman SR, Mastromarino AJ (1984) Markers of colonic cell differentiation: a summary. In:
    Mastromarino AJ, Brattain MG (eds) Markers of cell differentiation. Raven, New York,
    pp 131–139
Yang GC, Lipkin M, Yang K, Wang GQ, Li TY, Yang CS, Winawer SJ, Newmark H, Blot W,
    Fraumeni JF Jr (1987) Proliferation of esophageal epithelial cells in individuals in Linxian,
    China. J Natl Cancer Inst 79: 1241–1246
Zhang L, Bruce WR, Bird RP (1987) Influence of dietary fat and calcium on the proliferative
    indices of mouse mammary glands. Proc 46: 436

Dietary Factors in the Pathophysiology of Colorectal Cancer

Dietary Fat and Colorectal Cancer: Experimental Evidence for Tumor Promotion

P. M. Newberne[1] and S. Sahaphong[2]

[1] Department of Pathology, Boston University School of Medicine, 784 Massachusetts Ave., Boston, MA 02118, USA
[2] Department of Pathobiology, Faculty of Science, Mahidol University, Rama VI Road, Bangkok, 10400 Thailand

Contents

Introduction

Investigations into colorectal cancer during the past three decades have suggested that genetic variation accounts for only a small percentage of the approximately 500 000 new cases of this type of cancer worldwide each year (Muir and Parkin 1985). It is becoming more apparent that environmental factors, particularly dietary constituents, are important and are causally implicated in a significant percentage of colorectal cancer.

Epidemiologic data suggest that the incidence of colon cancer is associated with the consumption of diets high in fat and in protein (Armstrong and Doll 1975; Doll and Peto 1981; Committee on Diet, Nutrition and Cancer 1982). Knox (1977) and others have reported, from epidemiologic studies, a strong correlation between mortality and cancer of the large intestine and per capita total fat intake, but some investigators have described varying results from other epidemiologic studies in relation to cancer of the large bowel and fat intake, with correlations largely based on international studies.

Studies from individual countries have been less convincing than inter-country investigations and, generally, have not shown a significant correlation between total fat intake and large bowel cancer (Bingham et al. 1979; Lyon and Sorenson 1978; Kolonel and Marchand 1986). Nevertheless, suggestions are sufficiently convincing for many clinical investigators to be urging intervention trials.

The diets of Danish residents are associated with a high risk and that of the Finns with a low risk for colon cancer, based on food fat contents. Phillips (1975) has also reported a direct association between colon cancer and the frequent consumption of high-fat food in studies of Seventh Day Adventists in the United States. Dales et al. (1978) observed a direct association between colon cancer and frequent consumption of foods high in saturated fat, the association stronger for those who not only consumed diets high in saturated fat, but also low in fiber content.

Numerous investigations clearly point to a suggestion for fat and colon cancer interactions, but many of the data are conflicting and difficult to interpret (Howell 1975; Haenszel et al. 1973, 1980; Bjelke 1978; Graham et al. 1978). Enstrom (1975) has pointed out that trends in beef intake (and thus fat intake) in the United States over the past five decades do not correlate with trends in the incidence of colorectal cancer, either from incidence or from mortality data.

Because the human studies have been less than conclusive, animal investigations have been used in attempts to clarify effects of fat on induced colon cancer. These models have provided information on the pathogenesis of tumors, on genetic, environmental (including diet), and other influences on tumor development and on many other aspects of the disease.

The Rodent Model for Colon Cancer

Two types of chemicals have been used to induce rodent tumors for dietary studies. One is a direct-acting carcinogen, N-methyl-N-nitrosourea (MNU), which requires no activation; and the other one, dimethylhydrazine (DMH), requires metabolic activation. Chemicals of the second group may be activated in the colon or partially activated in the liver, transported to the target intestinal mucosa by the blood or fecal stream, and undergo final activation by microbial flora in the bowel lumen or by the mucosa itself. In colon mucosa, as in other tissues, active carcinogens alkylate or form adducts with DNA, alter cell division, and induce preneoplastic biochemical and morphologic changes (Wargovich et al. 1983). There are preferred sites in the rodent colon for tumor development and for occurrence of certain histologic types of tumor. A characteristic of some preferred sites is the presence of sub- and intramucosal lymphoid aggregates, a normal component of the bowel wall, similar to the small-intestinal Peyer's patches. However, the functional activities of the colon aggregates may differ in some respects from Peyer's patch lymphoid cells (Nauss et al. 1984a, b, 1986, 1987; Newberne and Nauss 1986).

Species and strain in rodents influence susceptibility to intestinal carcinogenesis: males are generally more susceptible than females, but the differences may not be marked. Nutrients and other components of diets, drugs, and other chemicals exert significant modulation effects on chemical carcinogenesis in the colon with modulation related to alteration of carcinogen metabolism by fecal stream enzymes or by enzymes of the mucosa. In addition, there may be increased or decreased tissue antioxidant capacity, changes in bile constituents or other components of the fecal stream, alteration of immunologic responses or differences in nucleic acid metabolism, and gene expression in the target cells or initiated cells, all of which can influence carcinogenesis. Investigation of the modulating influences on carcinogenesis as well as of pathogenesis and biology of colon tumors in rodent models can be expected to provide data that will contribute to control of the disease in human populations.

Rodent models for investigation of the association of intestinal cancer and inflammatory bowel disease have not been as useful as the tumor model but they are being pursued (Devroede 1980; Lightdale and Sherlock 1980; Sinclair et al. 1983; Yardley et al. 1983). The increased risk of cancer in patients with inflammatory bowel disease is sufficienty great for experimental animal models to be needed to identify the factor(s) responsible for increased risk. Hill et al. (1987) have recently reported on the increased bile acids in patients with ulcerative colitis at the outset of the trial who later develop colon cancer. The postulated interactions of infection, genetic predisposition, the immune system, and other factors in the etiology of inflammatory bowel disease (Lightdale and Sherlock 1980), and the numerous putative causes and modulating factors for intestinal carcinogenesis are amendable to studies in the rodent model.

Histologic studies of progressive epithelial changes in the rodent models are already contributing to evaluation of the relative significance of potential precursor lesions in humans, identified in the repeated rectal and colonic biopsies being studied in attempts to define patients at significant risk for cancer (Morson 1980; Yardley et al. 1983). Characterization of inflammatory, immunologic, dietary, and other factors that influence carcinogenesis in the animal models and definition of the period(s) in the progression of the disease at which they act can define questions to be examined in studies of the human disease. The influence of dietary fat interacting with other risk factors for colon cancer is one of many disease entities where rodent models are proving useful.

Chemical Induction of Colon Cancer

Before proceeding to the matter of the promoting effects of dietary fat on experimental rodent colon cancer, a description of the models and their histologic and metabolic characteristics would be useful. Rats and mice treated with symmetrical DMH or its metabolites azoxymethane (AOM) or methylazoxymethanol acetate (MAMA) develop cancer of the large bowel in a predictable manner, in frequency and incidence. DMH and its two derivatives are procarcinogens, highly specific for intestinal mucosal cells. Their relative potencies are determined by their chemical reactivity and metabolism to the ultimate carcinogen in the target cell. Toxicity is avoided by use of small doses that are still highly effective in inducing tumors which have a short latent period compared to carcinogens for many other organs.

Metabolism of Carcinogen

DMH is activated in vivo via azomethane (AM), AOM, and methylazoxymethanol (MAM) to yield the ultimate carcinogen (Weisburger and Fiala 1983). Both AOM and MAM (in the stabilized acetate form) are specific colon carcinogens in rodents (Ward et al. 1973; Weisburger and Fiala 1983) and are more effective than DMH on a molar basis. Spontaneous decomposition of MAM can occur in vivo, but the organo-specificity of DMH and kinetic analysis of its metabolism support the hypothesis that unidentified enzymatic reactions in target tissues also play important roles in converting MAM to the ultimate carcinogen (Weisburger and Fiala 1983).

The liver is the primary site for oxidation of DMH to MAM which is then transported via the blood to the colon and other organs. The importance of the liver in DMH metabolism was emphasized by Druckrey et al. (1967) who observed increased toxicity and tumorigenesis when high doses of the carcinogen were adminstered by i.g. gavage compared to the s.c. route. DMH metabolism varies with dose and route of administration; when administered continuously in the drinking water at both low (Druckrey et al. 1967) and high (Toth and Patil 1982) doses, DMH induces angio-sarcomas rather than intestinal tumors. Druckrey postulated that at low doses of carcinogen, DMH might be metabolized to monomethylhydrazine, a compound which produces endothelial cell tumors in the liver.

DMH metabolism has been further elucidated by studying inhibition of carcino-genesis. Compounds that block DMH induction of tumors inhibit DMH activation, i.e., disulfiram. This compound inhibits DMH and, to a lesser extent, AOM-induced carcinogenesis (Wattenberg 1983); it also inhibits the N-oxidation of AM and the C-oxidation of AOM. Pyrazole, an inhibitor of alcohol dehydrogenase, blocks MAM intestinal tumorigenesis (Zedeck and Tan 1978), but the incidence of skin and renal tumors is increased (Notman et al. 1982). In this case it is likely that the intestinal metabolism of MAM is blocked and the compound shunted to other organs where it is activated by enzymes other than alcohol dehydrogenase.

Selenium supplementation appears to inhibit DMH-induced colon carcinogenesis by a number of mechanisms that act at several stages of tumorigenesis, one of which is by blocking the oxidation of AM (Jacobs 1983).

The first step in DMH-induced colon carcinogenesis appears to be alkylation of target organ DNA (Maskens 1980). Both N-7-methylguanine (7-MeG) and O-6-methylguanine (O^6 MeG) have been isolated from colonic mucosal DNA of rats injected with [^{14}C] DMH (Hawks and Magee 1974; Rogers and Pegg 1977; Swenberg et al. 1979) and in cultured rat colon after incubation with labeled DMH (Autrup and Williams 1983). Levels of O^6 MeG are initially higher in some non-target organs than in the colon (Rogers and Pegg 1977; Swenberg et al. 1979). However, because the rate of repair in the colon is slow, the miscoding adduct persists for a longer period of time (Swenberg et al. 1979).

Disulfiram and pyrazole, compounds that inhibit DMH metabolism, decrease O^6 MeG formation in rat colonic DNA while other inhibitors, such as selenium, have no effect on O^6 MeG levels and appear to act via different mechanisms (Bull et al. 1981). The extent of colonic DNA alkylation in mice and rats appears to be proportional to susceptibility to DMH-induced colon carcinogenesis (Cooper et al. 1978; Pollard and Luckert 1980) but not by some other carcinogens (James and Autrup 1983).

Genesis and Location of Rodent Colon Tumors

Tumors arise in greatest numbers in the distal colon and grow as sessile polyps or as intramural tumors. In the rat, sessile, often mucinous, invasive adenocarcinomas tend to be localized in the proximal colon (Ward 1974; Shamsuddin and Trump 1981; Shamsuddin 1983) while polypoid tumors are more often found distally. Tumor location in mice is predominantly in the distal large bowel. Ulceration and bleeding are common, particularly in the polypoid tumors, and both types may obstruct the colon with intussusception as a terminal event. Metastases are not common but may range from 5% to 36% involvement of mesenteric lymph nodes (Fisher et al. 1981; Pozharisski et al. 1979).

Histologic Characteristics of Induced Colon Cancer

DMH-induced colon adenocarcinomas are similar histologically to human colon tumors. A few adenomas have been diagnosed, and progression from benign to malignant lesions has been described (Madara et al. 1983). The adenomas are similar to, but do not entirely mimic, tubular or tubulovillous polyps in the human. The evidence for progression is not strong since malignant tumors are found as early as or earlier than adenomas (Maskens and Dujardins-Loits 1981; Shamsuddin 1983). However the high dose of carcinogen used in most studies may have precluded observation of the sequence of dysplasia, adenoma, and carcinoma that appears to occur in the development of at least some colon tumors in humans.

Adenocarcinomas in the animal models vary in architectural and cytologic characteristics. Most produce little mucin, show well-developed glands, and tend to grow exophytically. Other tumors produce a large amount of mucin, are partially or entirely composed of signet ring cells with little or no gland formation, and tend to invade the bowel wall early. The tumors grow circumferentially and often metastasize to regional nodes and to the liver. The mucin-producing tumors tend to occur in rats given higher doses of DMH or AOM (Rogers and Gildin 1975; Fisher et al. 1981; Nauss et al. 1984a, b).

The localization of colon tumors in rats over lymphoid aggregates has been recognized for many years (Rogers et al. 1973a; Garmaise et al. 1975; Ward 1974; Nauss et al. 1984b). Similar localization has been reported in mice. In the lower small bowel, also, tumors are frequently found associated with Peyer's patches. The colon epithelium over lymphoid aggregates is largely surface type with little or no crypt formation. It is composed of two types of epithelial cells that may take up and digest bacteria or other antigens from the lumen and pass them on to the adjacent lymphoid cells. This epithelium appears to be analogous to the small-intestinal epithelium observed over Peyer's patches of the small gut (Bland and Britton 1984). The lymphoid tissue is considered by some investigators to have a dierect role in modulating the induction and growth of colon tumors.

The effects of gut bacterial populations and other local factors on colon carcinogenesis have been investigated, with comparisons between conventional and germ-free rats and of antibiotic-treated and untreated rats. Germ-free or antibiotic-treated rats do not develop tumors induced by DMH in as high an incidence as do conventional rats, but germ-free rats have increased tumor incidence when treated with AOM or N-methyl-N'-nitro-N-nitrosoguanidine (MNNG) (Goldin and Gorback 1981, 1983).

In some experiments in rats given DMH, defunctionalized colon loops removed from the fecal stream were at the same or even greater risk of developing tumors as colon loops exposed to the fecal stream (Rubio and Nylander 1981). In other experiments using a different preparation, tumors were reduced but not absent in the defunctionalized segment. This suggests that components of the fecal stream are not required for tumorigenesis by DMH, and that its metabolites reach the colon via the blood. Transposition experiments have demonstrated specific susceptibility of colon, compared to small-intestinal mucosa, to the carcinogenicity of DMH (Celik et al. 1981) and AOM (Gennaro et al. 1973).

Surgical resection or bypass of the small intestine after completion of DMH administration resulted in an increased incidence and number of colon tumors, an indication that promoting factors, such as bile acids and conjugates, may be present in the fecal stream. Similar results have been reported using AOM as the carcinogen (Williamson et al. 1980).

Carcinogens that do not require metabolic activation induce tumors at the site of application in the colon or rectum (Narisawa et al. 1981; Narisawa and Weisburger 1975). Intrarectal administration of either MNNG of MNU induces colon adenomas, adenocarcinomas, sarcomas, and hyperplastic polyps depending on the dose and species of animal used. High doses (8–32 mg per rat) result in a preponderance of sessile tubulopapillary carcinomas, while polypoid adenocarcinomas are the typical lesion at lower doses (4–8 mg per rat) (Ward et al. 1978; Nauss et al. 1984b). Weese et al. (1983) have demonstrated a progression of MNU-induced tumors in Sprague-Dawley (SD) rats from initial intraepithelial dysplasia and in situ carcinomas to intramural and transmurally invasive adenocarcinoma and eventually to lymph node metastases. At low doses MNU-induced neoplasms are rarely associated with colonic lymphoid aggregates (Nauss et al. 1984a), but the model has been used quite effectively to study the modifying effect of environmental factors, including diet, on colon tumorigenesis (Cohen et al. 1982).

Influence of Dietary Fat on Colon Cancer in Rodents

A number of studies in animals have indicated that colon tumorigenesis is enhanced by high-fat diets when the tumors are induced with DMH, AOM, MAMA, MNU, and dimethylbenzanthracene (DMBA) (Bansal et al. 1978; Nigro et al. 1973, 1975; Reddy 1979; Reddy 1986; Reddy et al. 1974; Rogers and Newberne 1980; Bull et al. 1979; Broitman et al. 1979).

One of the earlier demonstrations that dietary fat might have an effect on colon carcinogenesis was a report by Nigro et al. (1973), who demonstrated that rats treated with AOM under the conditions of their study developed more intestinal tumors when fed a diet containing 35% added beef fat, compared to those fed a regular "chow-type" control diet that contained considerably less fat. These data are difficult to interpret because the laboratory chow used in these studies was an ill-defined diet with varied components, and one cannot precisely distinguish the influence of calories and other factors from fat on tumorigenesis.

Reddy et al. (1977a) and Reddy (1986) have produced a number of reports regarding large bowel carcinogenesis induced by DMH or AOM and the effects of quality and quantity of fat on incidence and multiplicity of tumors. These

Table 1. The effect of dietary fat on colon tumorigenesis

Animal	Diet	Effect of high-fat diet on colon tumorigenesis	Reference
No carcinogen			
CF7BL/1	0% vs. 10% added corn oil[a]	Increased incidence	El-Khatib and Cora (1981)
1,2-Dimethylhydrazine			
Male and female Fischer rat	5% vs. 20% corn oil or lard[b]	Increased incidence and frequency of tumors	Reddy et al. (1977 a, b)
Male Sprague-Dawley rat	5% vs. 20% coconut oil[b]	Increased frequency	Broitman et al. (1977)
Male Fischer rat	5% vs. 20% beef fat[b]	Increased incidence and frequency of colon adenomas	Reddy et al. (1977 a, b)
Male W/Fu rat	5% vs. 30% corn oil[b]	Increased incidence and metastase; decreased latency time	Bansal et al. (1978)
Male Sprague-Dawley rat	15% corn oil vs. 30% beef fat	Increased cumulative probability of death	Rogers et al. (1980)
Male Sprague-Dawley rat	5% mixed fat vs. 24% corn oil or 24% beef fat or 24% Crisco[c]	None	Nauss et al. (1984 a, b) Newberne and Nauss (1987)
Male BALB/c mouse	5% mixed fat vs. 30% mixed fat[d]	None	Nutter et al. (1983)
Male Sprague-Dawley rat	5% corn oil vs. 24% corn oil[c]	None	Nauss et al. (1987)
Azoxymethane			
Male Sprague-Dawley rat	5% vs. 30% beef fat[b]	Increased frequency	Bull et al. (1979)
Male Sprague-Dawley rat	low fat vs. 35% beef fat[a]	Increased frequency and incidence	Nigro et al. (1975)
Methylazoxymethanol acetate			
Male Fischer rat	5% vs. 20% beef fat[a]	Increased incidence and frequency of adenomas	Reddy et al. (1977 a, b)
N-Methyl-N-nitrosourea			
Male Fischer rat	5% vs. 20% beef fat[b]	Increased incidence and frequency of adenomas	Reddy et al. (1977 a, b)
Male Sprague-Dawley rat	5% mixed fat vs. 24% corn oil or 24% beef fat or 24% Crisco[c]	None	Nauss et al. (1984 a)
3,2-Dimethyl-4-aminobiphenyl			
Male Fischer rat	5% vs. 23% beef fat[c]	Increased incidence and frequency in conventional but not germ-free rats	Reddy and Ohmori (1981)

Types of diets:
[a] Natural product.
[b] Semipurified, nonisocaloric.
[c] Semipurified, isocaloric.
[d] Mixed semipurified and natural product.

investigators have reported that rats fed 20% beef fat had a significantly increased incidence of colon tumors compared to those fed 5% fat. In some of these studies it did not appear to matter whether the fat was saturated or unsaturated, it was associated with about the same tumor incidence. It appeared from these studies that the animals ate the same quantity of diet, but, since the caloric density of low- and high-fat diet differed, those eating the high-fat diets received more calories. Other investigators have also reported on the effects of dietary fat on carcinogenesis in rodents, but much of the data are equivocal. When examined in detail as to the dietary composition, the effect of fats on colon carcinogenesis is inconclusive (Broitman 1981), as described below.

To date, there have been approximately 30 different trials in animals published from nine laboratories which have examined the influence of dietary fat on chemically induced colon cancer in rodents. Representative data are summarized in Tables 1 and 2. In some of these studies, there was a concomitant lipotrope deficiency (Rogers and Newberne 1973, 1980), or the excess fat was added to laboratory chow (Nigro et al. 1975), or to purified diets, with the results that the diets were not isocalorically balanced (Bansal et al. 1978; Reddy et al. 1977a, b; Bull et al. 1979). There is decreased consumption of nutrients by animals fed high-fat diets that are not properly balanced for the increased caloric density unless the diet is modified to correct imbalances. These nutritional imbalances, rather than fat itself, may have altered colon tumorigenesis.

In examining the data listed in Table 1 as well as additional studies not shown, it is clear that fat had a positive effect in many of the studies but not in all of them. Table 2 shows that in about half of the studies, high levels of dietary fat increased either the incidence or frequency of colon tumors, but in about 37% of the studies there was no effect of high dietary fat.

As noted above, Nigro et al. (1975) demonstrated that if beef tallow was added to laboratory animal chow the frequency of AOM-induced intestinal tumors in rats was increased (Table 3, Study 1). Since the total dose of carcinogen was high, all treated rats developed intestinal tumors, and incidence rates could not be analyzed. Multiple tumors (five to ten per rat) were produced, and animals fed the high-fat diet had a 114% increase in small-intestinal tumors and a 48% increase in colon tumors. Histopathologic examination of representative tumors indicated that they were all carcinomas.

Reddy et al. (1977a, b) induced intestinal tumors using DMH which is a precursor of AOM (Table 3, Study 2). Since the total dose of carcinogen was lower than that

Table 2. Effect of high levels of dietary fat on experimental colon carcinogenesis

Type of fat	Studies n	Increased frequency	Increased incidence	No change
Polyunsaturated vegetable fat	14	3	6	5
Saturated vegetable fat	3	1	0	2
Saturated animal fat	13	5	4	4
	30	9	10	11

Table 3. Two studies demonstrating an enhancing effect of dietary fat on colon cancer in rats

Study	Basal diet	Fat level (%)	Carcinogen	Colon tumor incidence (%)	Tumors/tumor-bearing rat				
					Total	Colon	Small intestine	Adeno-carcinoma	Adenoma
Study 1									
Nigro et al. (1975)	Chow	5	AOM	100	5.9	3.1	2.8	ND	ND
	Chow[a]	35	AOM	100	10.5	4.6	6.0	ND	ND
P value				NS	0.01	0.05	0.025		
Study 2									
Reddy et al. (1977a)	Semipurified	5	DMH	23	1.14	ND	ND	0.57	0.57
	Semipurified[b]	20	DMH	60	1.33	ND	ND	0.28	1.06
P value				0.05	NS	—	—	NS	NS

[a] Fat added to chow.
[b] Fat substituted for carbohydrate.
AOM, azoxymethane; DMH, 1,2-dimethylhydrazine; ND, not determined; NS, not significant.

used in Study 1, not all animals developed intestinal tumors and overall incidence data could be evaluated. Colon tumor incidence was significantly higher ($P < 0.05$) in animals fed 20% beef tallow compared to those fed 5% tallow. However, there were no significant differences in tumor frequency. The histopathologic data indicated that adenomas rather than adenocarcinomas accounted for the increased number of tumors in animals fed the high-fat diets. No data were presented regarding the incidence of adenocarcinomas. These two studies demonstrate that more attention must be directed to developing a uniform system of assessing experimental tumorigenesis which would include histopathologic classification of all masses as well as appropriate statistical analysis of tumor incidence and frequency.

The results from several studies in our laboratory have failed to support the hypothesis that dietary fat, quality or quantity, alone influence experimental colon cancer (Nauss et al. 1984a, b; Locniskar et al. 1985). There are suggestions, however, that other factors, interacting with dietary fat, may participate in the potential for susceptibility to colon cancer (Newberne and Nauss 1986). Some of the salient features of our studies are described below.

Male weanling rats of SD [Crl:CD (SD) BR] and Fischer (CDF-F344/Crl BR; F344) strains were obtained from the Charles River Breeding Laboratories Inc. (Wilmington, MA), systematically randomized, and assigned to experimental groups of the various studies. They were housed individually in stainless steel wire mesh suspended cases in climate-controlled quarters ($22 \pm 2\,°C$) with a 12-h light/dark cycle. They were given distilled water and one of the several diets described below.

We used diets, defined in every detail, which contained fats varying in quality and quantity (Table 4). Generally, the diets used 5% as the low level and either 20% or 24% as the high level. In all cases, the diets were isocaloric and balanced with respect to nutrient to caloric ratio. The levels of fat are shown in the various tables. The carcinogens were used at different levels and according to different protocols. Tumor incidences and differences in food consumption and in weight gain were compared by the χ^2 test or by analysis of variance.

Table 4. Isocalorically balanced high-fat diets[a]

	5% Mixed fat (g)	24% Beef tallow (g)	24% corn oil (g)	24% crisco (g)
Casein	20.0	24.0	24.0	24.0
Sucrose	21.0	12.0	12.0	12.0
Dextrose	21.0	12.0	12.0	12.0
Dextrin	21.0	12.0	12.0	12.0
Vitamin mix	2.0	2.4	2.4	2.4
Salts	5.0	6.0	6.0	6.0
Cellulose	4.0	5.0	5.0	5.0
Beef tallow	1.6	22.0	–	–
Corn oil	1.6	2.0	24.0	–
Crisco	1.6	–	–	24.0

[a] All diets were balanced with the same nutrient/caloric ratios, regardless of the source and amount of fat.

Routine necropsy procedures were used, except that all tumors or suspicious lesions were carefully identified as to location in the colon, measurements were made of those of 1 mm or more in size, and all were carefully categorized histologically.

Results

The results of three different trials using an indirect carcinogen (DMH) or the direct-acting MNU are shown in Table 5. A comparison is also shown of i.g. and s.c. administration of DMH. There were no significant differences in colon tumor incidences, frequency, or cumulative probability of death between rats fed 5% fat or those which received 24% fat diets.

In view of these negative results we considered the possibility that an enhancing effect of dietary fat might be related to special aspects of experimental conditions including the strain of rat. We used two different strains of rats, the F344 and SD, and diets of different nutrient composition; the differences in fat were 5% or 20% beef fat with or without added corn oil.

There are three methods of adding fat to an experimental diet, the choice of which can have a profound effect on animal nutrient consumption. If extra fat is added to a chow or natural product diet, there is an overall dilution of nutrients. The substitution of fat for carbohydrate alters the concentration of calories and other nutrients in the diet; the animals fed the high-fat diets will consume less protein, fiber, vitamins and minerals, all of which have been implicated as risk factors in colon cancer (Committe on Diet, Nutrition and Cancer 1982).

We prepared two semipurified diets which differed in the method of fat addition as well as in the concentration of certain micronutrients. The first diet, which was

Table 5. Three studies demonstrating no effect of dietary fat on chemically induced colon cancer in rats

Dietary fat		Study 1 [a] DMH i.g.		Study 2 [d] MNU i.r.		Study 3 [e] DMH (i.g. vs. s.c.) i.g.		s.c.	
		Inci-dence [b] (%)	Fre-quency [c] (%)	Inci-dence (%)	Fre-quency	Inci-dence (%)	Fre-quency	Inci-dence (%)	Fre-quency
Mixed fat	(5)	77	1.6	55	1.6	–	–	–	–
Corn oil	(5)	–	–	–	–	63	1.4	58	1.3
Beef tallow	(24)	68	1.5	63	1.4	–	–	–	–
Corn oil	(24)	63	1.4	55	1.2	68	1.3	48	1.6
Crisco	(24)	55	1.5	38	1.1	–	–	–	–

[a] Nauss et al. (1983); total dose = 75 mg DMH · 2 HCl/kg body weight.
[b] Incidence = percentage of animals in group bearing colon tumors ($n = 40$).
[c] Frequency = number of tumors per tumor-bearing rat.
[d] Nauss et al. (1984a); total dose MNU = 6 mg/rat.
[e] Locniskar et al. (1985); total dose = 150 mg DMH · 2 HCl/kg body weight.
DMH, 1,2-dimethylhydrazine; MNU, N-methyl-N-nitrosourea.

Table 6. Effect of DMH on colon tumor induction: strain and body weight differences

Dietary fat (%)	Nutrient to calorie ratio	Vitamins and minerals	Final body weight ($\bar{X} \pm SD$)	Tumor incidences (%)	Tumors/ TBR
Sprague-Dawley rat strain					
5	Balanced	Supplemented	495 ± 38	27	1.5
20	Balanced	Supplemented	580 ± 27	57	1.5
5	Not balanced	Not supplemented	412 ± 30	30	1.1
20	Not balanced	Not supplemented	467 ± 35	33	1.2
Significance (P)			< 0.01	< 0.07	NS
Fischer-344 rat strain					
5	Balanced	Supplemented	342 ± 20	27	1.6
20	Balanced	Supplemented	373 ± 23	37	1.1
5	Not balanced	Not supplemented	221 ± 12	27	1.4
20	Not balanced	Not supplemented	236 ± 14	33	1.0
Significance (P)			< 0.01	NS	< 0.06

DMH (200 mg DMH · 2 HCl/kg) administered s.c. (10 mg/kg per week for 20 weeks). Animals killed 10 weeks after the last dose of carcinogen. TBR, tumor-bearing rat; NS, not significant.

isocalorically balanced, was identical to the diet used in our earlier studies. It contained levels of some of the vitamins and minerals in excess of the recommended requirement for normal growth according to the American Institute of Nutrition (1977). Except for the addition of agar, the composition of the second diet was the same as that used in studies where an enhancing effect of dietary fat on DMH-induced colon tumors was reported (Table 3, Study 2). It was not isocalorically balanced.

The salient features of this study are shown in Table 6. Although the dose of DMH was adjusted on a body weight basis, the response of an animal to the toxic effects of the carcinogen was dependent on strain and diet composition. F344 rats were more sensitive to the toxic effects of DMH, and the deficit in weight gain was greatest for animals fed the non-isocalorically balanced diet with the lowest concentration of certain vitamins and minerals. This same trend was evident in SD rats.

The effect of the four different diets on colon tumorigenesis as presented in Table 6 demonstrates that in the SD group, colon tumor incidence was 57% in rats fed diet 1 which contained 20% fat, compared to 27%–33% in the other three groups. When the four groups were compared by a χ^2 test, the effect was not significant ($P = 0.07$ level). When the diet 1–5% group was compared to the diet 1–20% group, the P value was 0.02. If multiple comparisons are made, it is generally recommended that the value for significance be lowered, making the effect of marginal significance. There were no significant effects on tumor frequency (number of tumors per tumor-bearing rat). Dietary treatment had no significant effect on colon tumor incidence or frequency in F344 rats. In neither strain were differences observed in tumor size, degree of differentiation or extent of invasion through the colon wall.

SD and F344 rats differ significantly in rate of weight gain and final body mass, so it was of interest to examine the relationship between food consumption and colon tumorigenesis in these two strains. One way to examine the data is to determine mean food consumption and energy intake in tumor-bearing and tumor-free animals. We carried out such calculations for rats in each strain at time periods as follows: (a) prior to DMH treatment; (b) during treatment (2 and 3 months) and (c) immediately prior to the terminal sacrifice. For SD rats (Fig. 1) there were no significant differences in mean body weight of tumor-bearing and tumor-free animals. Food intake is expressed as kcal/100 g body weight daily. When the food efficiency ratio was calculated, no differences were seen in body weight, caloric intake, or food efficiency ratio between tumor-bearing and tumor-free rats (Fig. 2).

Visek and Clinton (1983) had observed that if animals were ranked according to their caloric intake, breast tumor incidence and frequency were higher in SD rats ranked in the upper two-thirds according to calories consumed. We therefore did a similar analysis of the data from our most recent study. Colon tumor incidence and frequency in SD rats increased as one moved from the lower to the upper levels of food intake (Fig. 3). A significant and interesting aspect of these data were the 1-month intake data, prior to carcinogen treatment; these data showed that SD rats, which were eating more prior to DMH treatment, were more likely to develop tumors. Similar results were obtained for the 3- and 5-month intake data (data not shown).

When we carried out the same calculations for F344 animals, however (Fig. 4), no association was observed between level of caloric intake and colon tumorigenesis. It may be that the effect of calories is more pronounced in a rapidly growing strain than in more slowly growing, leaner animals.

Results from three separate long-term trials in our own laboratory with SD rats as noted above showed no effect of dietary fat on DMH- or MNU-induced colon

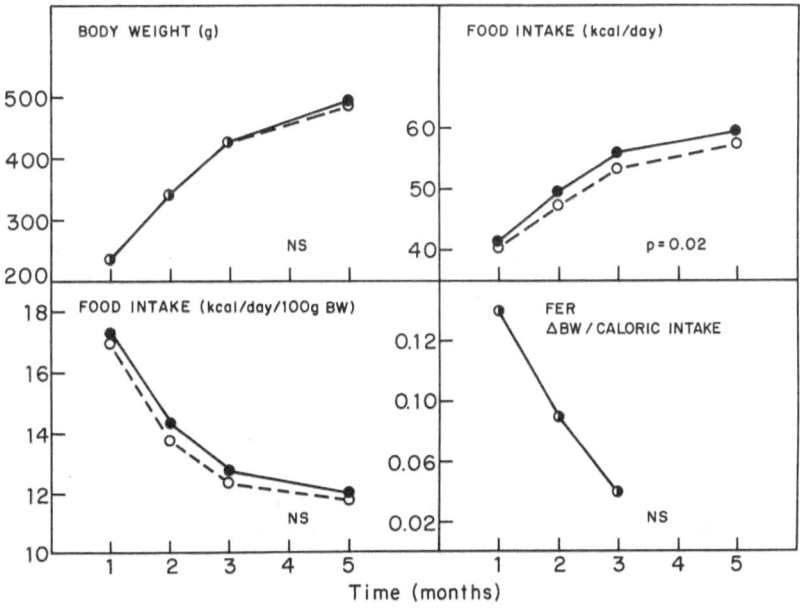

Fig. 1. Food intake and body weight gain in tumor-bearing (*open circles*) and tumor-free (*solid circles*) SD rats

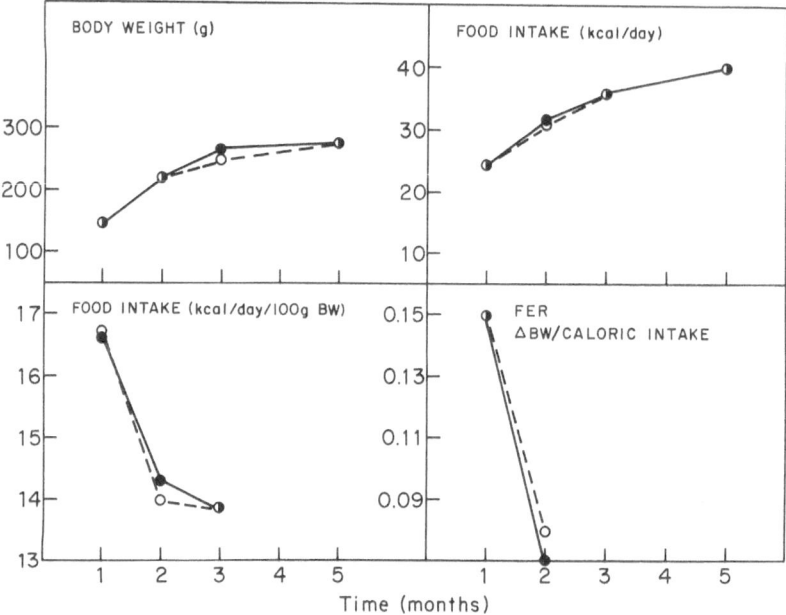

Fig. 2. Food intake and body weight gain in tumor-bearing (*open circles*) and tumor-free (*solid circles*) F-344 rats

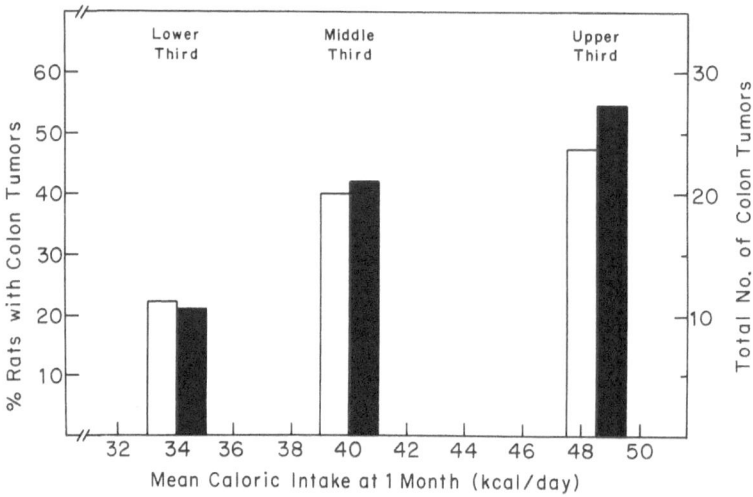

Fig. 3. Caloric intake and DMH-induced colon tumors in SD rats. *Open columns*, percentage of rats with colon tumors; *solid columns*, total number of colon tumors

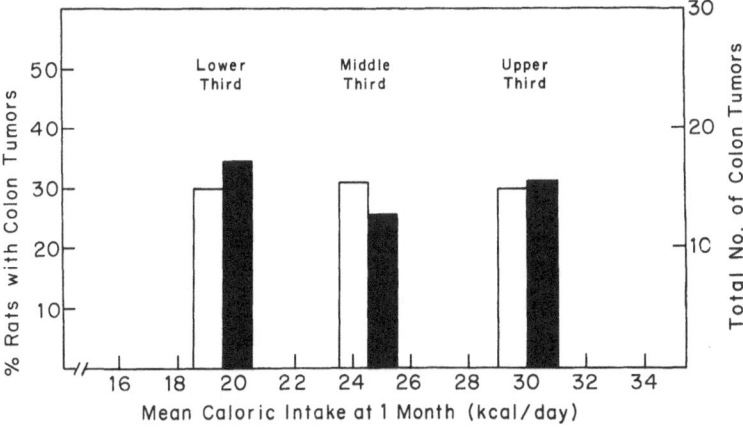

Fig. 4. Caloric intake and DMH-induced colon tumors in F-344 rats. *Open columns,* percentage of rats with colon tumors; *solid columns,* total number of colon tumors

tumorigenesis. In our most recent trial using a longer carcinogen treatment procedure, 20% beef fat did not increase colon tumorigenesis in F344 rats. The effect of dietary fat in SD rats was mixed. The more significant factor was total caloric intake and this was strain dependent. Animals fed a diet which promoted optimal growth had a barely significant increase in colon tumor incidence but not in frequency or size. This effect was not observed using a second diet which resulted in slower growth.

Influence of Interactions of Fat and Other Factors

Because the evidence for fat alone promoting colon cancer in animal models is conflicting and inconclusive, but as there is evidence for a linkage in some human studies, we proceeded to pursue two additional lines of research. These were designed to elucidate what appears to be a complex interaction between dietary fat and other factors as well as caloric intake per se.

Since caloric intake appears to have significant bearing on risk for tumors, diets which differ in calories and which modify food intake must be taken into consideration. Human and animal studies have shown that consumption of high-fiber diets is associated with increased fecal loss of fat and nitrogen and therefore a reduced availability of calories (Nyman and Asp 1982; Cummings 1983; Isaksson et al. 1984; Kaur et al. 1985; Nauss et al. 1987). Much remains to be done to clarify this issue but more evidence is accumulating in animal and human studies to suggest that excess calories increase risk. Increased caloric intake, from fat or from other sources, could modify the human or animal metabolism early in life to increase risk later. This would be especially significant in the case of imprinting patterns for enzyme systems involved in carcinogen activation and deactivation early in life. These may remain more active in late life. We demonstrated years ago (Newberne and Young 1973) that high nutrient intake early in life had a profound effect much later in life even though the excess was imposed only during the early perinatal period. With the foregoing data in mind, it seemed appropriate to ask whether or not calories per se may not be a significant factor, if not a primary influence, on risk for some forms of cancer. The more convincing epidemiologic information appears more often than not to involve increased calories with interactions with fat and protein mentioned most frequently.

An additional point to be raised is with regard to caloric intake at critical times in the lifespan of an individual. A highly critical period to be exposed to excess calories is during the period of most rapid growth when certain metabolic patterns may be established which can influence risk later in life. It has been pointed out (Gortner 1975) that per capita intake of fat (and thus, calories) has steadily increased over the past 50 years in the United States, and that dietary fat intake peaks in the 12–14 age group for women and falls fairly steadily thereafter thoughout life. By contrast, however, men do not reach their maximal fat intake until near the end of adolescence (15–20 years), with the amount of fat consumed dropping off only after age 20. These two age periods coincide with periods of most rapid rates of growth for both sexes. One may therefore ask, with respect to colon cancer risk and the above-noted caloric intake during periods of most rapid growth, does this food habit equate causally with the age-adjusted death rates for cancer per 100,000 for colon and rectum in the United States of 25.1 and 18.2 for male and female, respectively in 1980–1981? (Cancer Statistics 1986).

An argument can be made for increased fat and calories during the early period of life increasing risk for colon cancer later in life. Males consume more fat and more calories early on, compared to females, and their colon cancer death rate is correspondingly higher. This appears to be even more the case in the black population of the United States. Overweight, high blood pressure, colorectal cancer, and other degenerative diseases afflict black males more than their female counterparts or the white population of both sexes.

In addition to the above-noted rat strain effect, where the more rapidly growing SD rat was at greater risk when consuming larger amounts of calories, we have just completed exploratory studies, the results of which bear on the hypothesis that calories per se are significant in risk for colon cancer. The data in Tables 7 and 8 suggest that the early postnatal period, when growth is most rapid, is an important time for establishing risk if caloric intake is increased during this critical period of growth and development.

Table 7 lists results of reducing the number of pups in litters to either 4 for group 2 or eight group 1 at birth, the latter a conventional litter size. Aside from litter size, nothing differed among the groups from birth to weaning. This provided significantly increased calories in the form of milk during the first 3 weeks of life in the group with litter size of four. This was also the case for group 3. At weaning, group 3 was given per individual rat the amount of food provided the paired mate in conventional litter size of eight. While all rats were essentially the same size at birth, the smaller litters of four each had significantly increased body weights at weaning. Moreover, group 3, which consumed the same as group 1 after weaning never dropped back to the weight of group 1 to which they were pair-fed.

Table 8 shows the number of rats with colon tumors in each group. Clearly, increased caloric intake, even only during the period of lactation (group 3) increased risk for developing a tumor. The number of tumors per tumor-bearing rat, malignancy, degree of invasiveness, and other factors important to a correct interpretation

Table 7. Influence of postnatal caloric intake on body weight

Group		Sex	Body weight (g) post-DMH			
No.	Treatment		At birth (g±SD)	At weaning (g±SD)	At 1 week (g±SD)	At 4 months (g±SD)
1	Normal weanlings, eight per litter from birth	M	·5.8±0.50	43±4	430±30	685±62
		F	5.5±0.11	37±3	296±14	488±60
2	Weanlings from litters reduced to four at birth	M	5.2±0.41	61±4	549±26	780±71
		F	5.1±0.20	50±3	389±18	569±19
3	Weanlings from litters reduced to four at birth, pair-fed to group 1 after weaning	M	5.6±0.30	59±5	466±20	710±63
		F	5.2±0.09	48±2	341±16	536±31

Table 8. Influence of caloric intake on colon tumor incidence

Group		Sex	Mean caloric intake		Rats with tumor	
No.	Treatment		1 week after DMH (Kcal per day)	4 months after DMH (Kcal per day)	(n)	(%)
1	Normal weanlings, eight per litter from birth	M	47±5.1	51±5.2	12/25	48
		F	41±3.2	46±2.8	10/24	42
2	Weanlings from litters reduced to four at birth	M	69±5.2	68±4.2	34/40	85
		F	46±4-1	48±3.8	10/40	50
3	Weanlings from litters reduced to four at birth pair-fed to group 1 after weaning	M	46±4.7	50±4.3	19/25	75
		F	42±3.6	46±2.7	13/31	42

supported the concept that increased calories during early periods of life influence risk later in life.

Inasmuch as dietary fat alone is associated with variable results with respect to risk for colon cancer, we have pursued another line of research, examining the influence of interactions of high fat and variable vitamin A. In earlier studies with animal models we observed a significant effect of vitamin A on induced colon cancer in rats (Newberne and Suphakarn 1977; Rogers et al. 1973). Since vitamin A plays an important role in the maintenance of the integrity of the colon, as well as other surface epithelia, we induced tumors of the colon in rats fed varying dietary concentrations of dietary fat and vitamin A. Table 9 lists results of one recently completed study. The data in Table 9 strongly suggest that not only is vitamin A important in risk for colon cancer, but that interactions between high dietary fat and vitamin A concentrations can have profound effects on colon cancer risk. Thus, while dietary fat alone may influence risk for colon cancer in human, it is likely that the apparent promoting influence of fat may be more than quality or quantity alone; interactions of fat and other dietary constituents may be more important in determining risk.

Table 9. Variable fat and vitamin A on color cancer

Treatment	Vitamin A	Corn oil	Rats with colon tumors	
	(mg/kg)	(%)	(n)	(%)
Control A, low fat[a]	10	5	12	40
Low A, low fat[a]	3	5	15	50
High A, low fat[a]	30	5	8	24
Control A, high fat[b]	10	24	15	50
Low A, high fat[b]	3	24	26	86
High A, high fat[b]	30	24	13	43

[a] Diets contained low level of fat (5% by weight).
[b] Diets contained high level of fat (24% by weight).

Discussion

The hypothesis that high dietary fat intake enhances colon tumorigenesis receives support from international studies demonstrating a correlation between per capita fat disappearance from the market place and mortality from colon cancer (Armstrong and Doll 1975), but findings from case-control studies on more accurate fat intake have been contradictory (Byers and Graham 1984). In a 15-year prospective study, Stemmerman et al. (1984, 1986) actually found no differences in colon cancer and saturated fat intake compared to controls. In a more recent prospective study involving 8006 Hawaiian Japanese men, these investigators found no association between total fat intake and colon cancer, confirming their earlier findings.

Animals studies from a number of laboratories have produced equivocal results regarding the influence of dietary fat on experimentally induced colon carcinogenesis. No two investigators have used exactly the same diet formulation or carcinogen treatment protocol, making comparisons among these various studies difficult or impossible. An enhancing or promoting effect of dietary fat on experimentally induced colon tumors in rodents is generally observed in models where additional fat was added to chow or natural product diets, a procedure which results in an overall dilution and imbalance of nutrients with consequent imprecise interpretation of results. An improved formulation was provided by semipurified diets where excess fat was substituted for carbohydrate on a weight basis. Although such diets do not take into account the increased caloric density of the high-fat diets and the reduction in nutrient intake by animals consuming such diets, they are an improvement over chow-type diets. Isocaloric formulations increased the levels of protein, fiber, vitamins, and minerals in the high-fat diets to maintain a constant nutrient-to-calorie ratio. Even these designs are subject to criticism because the values used for available energy of fat may have been underestimated (Donato and Hegsted 1985).

Since caloric intake appears to have a significant bearing on risk for tumors, diets which differ in calories and which modify food intake must be taken into consideration. Human and animal studies have shown that consumption of much fiber and nitrogen and, therefore, a reduced availability of calories (Nyman and Asp 1982;

Cummings et al. 1988; Isaksson et al. 1984) reduce risk for colon cancer. Much remains to be done, however, to clarify this issue, but more evidence is accumulating in animal and human studies to suggest that a complex phenomenon is operating in the case of risk for colon cancer and that many factors interact to produce a much more complex situation that just a single dietary variable.

The studies reported here have shown that dietary variables, other than fat level, do have profound effects on the response of animals to a colon carcinogen. When diets are not isocalorically balanced the levels of protein, fiber, vitamins, and minerals consumed by animals in a high-fat group may be inadequate under stressful conditions, such as periods of long-term carcinogen administration. We observed this effect to be more pronounced in F344 rats than in SD animals. Failure to recognize the importance of marginal nutrition and the variable responses of different rodent strains to carcinogen administration may explain, in part, the inconsistencies in the literature regarding the effect of dietary fat on experimentally induced colon tumorigenesis. Other concerns include failure to carefully categorize the lesions by accurate histopathology with lymphoid aggregates counted as tumors.

Vitamin A has, among other characteristics, a role as scavenger of free radicals in biologic systems. With high fat in the diet, particularly unsaturated fat, free radicals in tissue in the colon would be significantly higher than in tissues of individuals consuming a low-fat diet and, perhaps, a low, saturated fat diet. Free radicals have been documented to cause tissue injury, particularly where unsaturated fats are available in the tissues for peroxidation.

The question of enhancement or promotion of colon tumors by dietary fat is yet to be answered. Since dietary total fat (quality and quantity) has been associated by some investigators with increased risk for colon cancer in humans and experimental animals, and results from various laboratories and between investigators are highly variable and subject to differences in interpretation, it seems likely that effects attributed to fat are a result of much more complex interactions of fat and other dietary factors and nutrients.

We must begin to dissect the complexity by addressing interactions and other factors which affect overall growth and development and the promotion of initiated cells to neoplasia. This is not to infer, however, that dietary fat is not important as a risk factor in human colon. Available data suggest that it is a significant factor. Most likely, however, it is acting in concert with other dietary variables. We also believe that there is sufficient evidence to suggest to populations at high risk for colon cancer to reduce their fat intake, even though we do not know now the exact nature of, or mechanisms for, fat effects and the interactions of fat and other variables. Fundamental research in experimental animals and carefully designed and conducted human studies should provide some of these answers.

References

American Institute of Nutrition (1977) Report of the AIN ad hoc committee on standards for nutritional studies. J Nutr 107:1340–1348

Armstrong B, Doll R (1975) Environmental factors and cancer incidence and mortality in different countries with special reference to dietary practices. Int J Cancer 15:617–631

Autrup H, Williams GM (1983) Carcinogenesis studies in human gastrointestinal epithelium. In: Autrup H, Williams GM (eds) Experimental colon carcinogenesis. CRC, Boca Raton, pp 95–106

Bansal BR, Rhoads JE, Bansal SC (1978) Effects of diet on colon carcinogenesis and the immune system in rats treated with 1,2-dimethylhydrazine. Cancer Res 38:3293–3303

Bingham S, Williams DRR, Cole TJ, James WPT (1979) Dietary fibre and regional large-bowel cancer mortality in Britain. Br J Cancer 40:456–463

Bjelke E (1978) Dietary factors and the epidemiology of cancer of the stomach and large bowel. Aktuel Ernaehrungsmed Klin Prax (Suppl 2): 10–17

Bland PW, Britton DC (1984) Morphological study of antigen-sampling structures in the rat large intestine. Infect Immun 43:693–699

Broitman SA (1981) Cholesterol excretion and colon cancer. Cancer Res 41:3738–3740

Broitman SA, Vitale JJ, Vavrousek-Jakuba E, Gottlieb LS (1977) Polyunsaturated fat, cholesterol and large bowel tumorigenesis. Cancer 40:2455–2463

Bull AW, Soullier BK, Wilson PS, Hayden MT, Nigro ND (1979) Promotion of azoxymethane-induced intestinal cancer by high-fat diet in rats. Cancer Res 39:4956–4959

Bull AW, Burd AD, Nigro ND (1981) Effect of inhibitors of tumorigenesis on the formation of O^6-methylguanine in the colon of 1,2-dimethylhydrazine-treated rats. Cancer Res 41: 4938–4941

Byers T, Graham S (1984) The epidemiology of diet and cancer. In: Klein G, Weinhouse S (eds) Advances in Cancer Research. Academic, New York, pp 1–16

Cancer Statistics (1986) Ca-A Cancer journal for clinicians. American Cancer Society, New York, 36:16–27

Celik C, Mittelman A, Paolini NS, Lewis D, Evans JT (1981) Effects of 1,2-symmetrical dimethyl-hydrazine on jejunocolic transposition in Sprague-Dawley rats. Cancer Res 41:2908–2911

Cohen B, Racht RF, Faccini E (1982) Reduction N-nitrosourea induced colon tumors in the rat by cholesterol. Cancer Res 42:5050–5052

Committee on Diet, Nutrition, and Cancer (1982) Assembly of Life Sciences. National Research Council. Diet, nutrition, and cancer. National Academy Press, Washington

Cooper HK, Buecheler J, Kleihues P (1978) DNA alkylation in mice with genetically different susceptibility. Cancer Res 38:3063–3065

Cummings JH (1983) Fermentation in the human large intestine: evidence and implications for health. Lancet 1:1206–1211

Dales LG, Friedman GD, Ury HK, Grossman S, Williams SR (1978) A case-control study of relationships of diet and other traits to colorectal cancer in American Blacks. Am J Epidemiol 109:132–144

Devroede G, Winawer S, Schottenfield D, Sherlock P (eds) (1980) Risk of cancer in inflammatory bowel disease. In: Colorectal cancer: prevention, epidemiology and screening. Raven, New York, pp 325–344

Doll R, Peto R (1981) The causes of cancer. Oxford University Press, Oxford

Donato K, Hegsted DM (1985) Efficiency of utilization of various sources of energy for growth. Proc Natl Acad Sci USA 82:4866–4870

Druckrey H, Preussman S, Ivanbovic D, Schmahl J, Afbham G, Blum HD, Mennel M, Muller M, Petropoulos P, Schneider H (1967) Organotropic carcinogenic effects of 65 different N-nitroso compounds on BD rats. Z Krebsforsch 69:103–201

El Khatib SM, Cora EM (1981) Role of high fat diet in tumorigenesis in C57BL/1 mice. JNCI 66:297–301

Enstrom JE (1975) Colorectal cancer and consumption of beef and fat. Br J Cancer 32:432–439

Fisher ER, Paulson J, McCoy M (1981) Genesis of 1,2-dimethylhydrazine-induced colon cancer. Arch Pathol Lab Med 105:29–37

Garmaise ABK, Rogers AE, Saravis C, Zamcheck N, Newberne P (1975) Immunologic aspects of 1,2-dimethylhydrazine-induced colon tumors in rats. J Natl Cancer Inst 54:1231–1235

Gennaro AR, Villanueva R, Sukonthaman Y, Vathanopas V, Rosemond GP (1973) Chemical carcinogenesis in transposed intestinal segments. Cancer Res 33:536–541

Goldin B, Gorbach SL (1981) Effect of antibiotics on rat intestinal tumors induced by 1,2-dimethylhydrazine dihydrochloride. J Natl Cancer Inst 67:877–880

Goldin B, Gorbach SL (1983) Activation of carcinogens by bacterial and microsomal enzyme systems. Gastroenterology 85:200–201

Gortner WA (1975) Nutrition in the United States 1900–1974. Cancer Res 35: 3246–3253

Graham S, Dayal H, Swanson M, Mittleman A, Wilkinson G (1978) Diet in the epidemiology of cancer of the colon and rectum. J Natl Cancer Inst 61: 709–714

Haenszel W, Berg JW, Segi M, Krihara M Locke FB (1973) Large-bowel cancer in Hawaiian Japanese. J Natl Cancer Inst 51: 1765–1779

Haenszel W, Locke FB, Segi M (1980) A case-control study of large bowel cancer in Japan. J Natl Cancer Inst 64: 17–22

Hawks A, Magee DM (1974) The alkylation of nucleic acids in the rat and mouse in vivo by the carcinogen 1,2-dimethylhydrazine. Br J Cancer 30: 440–447

Hill MJ et al. (1987) Faecal bile acids, dysplasia and carcinoma in ulcerative colitis. Lancet ii: 185–186

Howell MA (1975) Diet as an etiological factor in the development of cancers of the colon and rectum. J Chronic Dis 29: 67–80

Isaksson G, Lundquist I, Akesson B, Ihse I (1984) Effect of pectin and wheat bran on intraluminal pancreatic enzyme activities and on fat absorption as examined with the triolein breath test in patients with pancreatic insufficiency. Scand J Gastroenterol 19: 457–473

Jacobs MM (1983) Selenium inhibition of 1,2-dimethylhydrazine-induced colon carcinogenesis. Cancer Res 43: 1646–1649

James JT, Autrup H (1983) Methylated DNA adducts in the large intestine of ICR/HA and C57BL/HA mice given 1,2-dimethylhydrazine. J Natl Cancer Inst 70: 541–546

Kaur AP, Bhat CM, Grewal RB (1985) Effect of cellulose incorporation in a low fiber diet on fecal excretion and digestibility of nutrients in adolescent girls. Nutr Rep Int 32: 383–390

Knox EG (1977) Foods and diseases. Br J Prev Soc med 31: 71–80

Kolonel LN, Marchand LL (1986) The epidemiology of colon cancer and dietary fat. In: Ip C, Birt DF, Rogers AE, Metlin C (eds) Dietary fat and cancer. Liss, New York, pp 69–92

Lightdale CJ, Sherlock P (1980) Cancer in Crohn's disease: Memorial Hospital experience and review of the literature. In: Winawar S, Schottenfeld D, Sherlock P (eds) Colorectal cancer: prevention, epidemiology, and screening. Raven, New York, pp 341–346

Locniskar M, Nauss KM, Kaufmann P, Newberne PM (1975) Interaction of dietary fat and route of carcinogen administration on 1,2 DMH-induced colon tumorigenesis in rats. Carcinogenesis 6: 349–354

Lyon JL, Sorenson AW (1978) Colon cancer in a low-risk population. Am J Clin Nutr 31: 5227–5230

Madara JL, Harte P, Deasey J et al. (1983) Evidence for adenoma carcinoma progression in DMH-induced rat neoplasm. Am J Pathol 110: 230–235

Maskens AP (1980) Confirmation of the two-step nature of chemical carcinogenesis in the rat colon adenocarcinoma model. Cancer Res 41: 1240–1245

Maskens AP, Dujardins-Loits R (1981) Experimental adenomas and carcinomas of the large intestine behave as distinct entities: most carcinomas arise de novo in flat mucosa. Cancer 47: 81–89

Morson BC (1980) Use of dysplasia as an indicator of risk for malignancy in patients with ulcerative colitis. In: Winawer S, Schottenfeld D, Sherlock P (eds) Colorectal cancer: prevention, epidemiology, and screening. Raven, New York, pp 341–346

Muir CS, Parkin DM (1985) The world cancer burden: prevent on perish. Br Med J 1: 5–6

Narisawa T, Weisburger JH (1975) Colon cancer induction in mice by intrarectal instillation of N-methylnitrosourea. Proc Soc Exp Biol Med 148: 166–172

Narisawa T, Sata M, Tani M, Kudo T, Takahashi T, Goto A (1981) Inhibition of development of methylnitrosourea-induced rat colon tumors by indomethacin treatment. Cancer Res 41: 1954–1957

Nauss KM, Locniskar M, Newberne PM (1983) Effects of alterations in quantity and quality of dietary fat on 1,2-DMH-induced colon tumorigenesis in rats. Cancer Res 43: 4083–4090

Nauss KM, Locniskar M, Pavlina T, Newberne PM (1984a) Morphology and distribution of 1,2-dimethylhydrazine dihydrochloride-induced colon tumors and their relationship to gut-associated lymphoid tissue in the rat. J Natl Cancer Inst 73: 915–924

Nauss KM, Locniskar M, Sondergaard D, Newberne PM (1984b) Lack of effect of dietary fat on N-nitrosomethylurea (NMU)-induced colon tumorigenesis in rats. Carcinogenesis 5: 255–260

Nauss KM, Jacobs LR, Newberne PM (1986) Dietary fat and fiber: relationship to caloric intake, body growth, and colon tumorigenesis. Am J Clin Nutr 45 (Suppl 1): 149–372

Nauss KM, Bueche D, Newberne PM (1987) Effect of beef fat on DMH-induced colon tumorigenesis: influence of rat strain and nutrient composition. J Nutr 117: 739–747

Newberne PM, Nauss KM (1986) Dietary fat and colon cancer: variable results in animal models. In: Ip C, Birt DF, Rogers AE, Mettlin C (eds) Dietary fat and cancer. Liss, New York, pp 311–330

Newberne PM, Suphakarn V (1977) Preventive role of vitamin A in colon carcinogenesis in rats. Cancer 40: 2553–2556

Newberne PM, Young VR (1973) Marginal maternal vitamin B_{12}: long term effects. Nature 242: 263–270

Nigro ND, Bhadrachari N, Chomchai C (1973) A rat model for studying colon cancer. Effect of cholestyramine on induced tumors. Dis Colon Rectum 16: 438–443

Nigro ND, Sigh DV, Campbell RL, Pak MS (1975) Effect of dietary fat on intestinal tumors. J Natl Cancer Inst 54: 439–442

Notman J, Tan QH, Zedeck MS (1982) Inhibition of methylazoxymethanol-induced intestinal tumors in the rat by pyrazole with paradoxical effects on skin and kidney. Cancer Res 42: 1774–1780

Nutter RL, Gridley DS, Kettering JD, Goude AG, Slater JM (1983) BALB/c mice fed milk or beef protein. JNCI 71: 867–875

Nyman M, Asp N-G (1982) Fermentation of dietary fiber components in the rat intestinal tract. Br J Nutr 47: 357–364

Phillips RL (1975) Role of life-style and dietary habits in risk of cancer among Seventh-Day Adventists. Cancer Res 35: 3513–3522

Pollard M, Luckert P (1980) Indomethacin treatment of rats with dimethylhydrazine-induced intestinal tumors. Cancer Treat Rep 64: 1323–1327

Pozharisski KM, Likhachev A, Klimashevski V, Shaposhnikov J (1979) Experimental intestinal cancer research with special reference to human pathology. Adv Cancer Res 30: 165–237

Reddy BS (1979) Nutrition and colon cancer. Adv Nutr Res 2: 199–218

Reddy BS, Weisburger JH, Wynder EL (1974) Effects of dietary fat level and dimethylhydrazine on fecal acid and neutral sterol excretion and colon carcinogenesis in rats. J Natl Cancer Inst 52: 507–511

Reddy BS, Watanabe K, Weisburger JH (1977a) Effect of high-fat diet on colon carcinogenesis in F344 rats treated with 1,2-dimethylhydrazine, methylazoxymethanol acetate, or methylnitrosourea. Cancer Res 37: 4156–4159

Reddy BS, Watanabe K, Weisburger JH, Wynder EL (1977b) Promoting effect of bile acids in colon carcinogenesis in germ-free and conventional F344 rats. Cancer Res 37: 3238–3242

Reddy BS, Cohen LA, McCoy GD, Hill P, Weisburger JH, Wynder EL (1980) Nutrition and its relationship to cancer. Adv Cancer Res 32: 237–345

Reddy BS, Ohmori T (1981) Effect of intestinal microflora and dietary fat on colon carcinogenesis in F344 rats. Cancer Res 451: 1363–1367

Reddy BS (1986) Amount and type of dietary fat and colon cancer: animal model studies. In: Ip C, Birt DF, Rogers AE, Mettlin C (eds) Dietary fat and cancer. Liss, New York, pp 295–309

Rogers AE (1975) Variable effects of a lipotrope-deficient, high-fat diet on chemical carcinogenesis in rats. Cancer Res 35: 2469–2474

Rogers AE, Gildin J (1975) Effect of BCG on dimethylhydrazine induction of colon tumors in rats. J Natl Cancer Inst 55: 385–391

Rogers AE, Newberne PM (1973) Dietary enhancement of intestinal carcinogenesis by dimethylhydrazine in rats. Nature 246: 491–492

Rogers AE, Newberne PM (1980) Lipotrope deficiency in experimental carcinogenesis. Nutr Cancer 2: 104–112

Rogers KJ, Pegg AE (1977) Formation of O^6-methylguanine by alkylation of rat liver, colon, and kidney DNA following administration of 1,2-dimethylhydrazine. Cancer Res 37: 4082–4087

Rogers AE, Herndon BJ, Newberne PM (1973) Induction by dimethylhydrazine of intestinal carcinoma in normal rats and rats fed high or low level of vitamin A. Cancer Res 33: 1003–1009

Rubio CA, Nylander G (1981) Further studies on the carcinogenesis of the colon and the rat with special reference to the absence of intestinal contents. Cancer 48: 951–953

Shamsuddin AKM (1983) In vivo induction of colon cancer: dose and animal species. In: Autrup H, Williams GM (eds) Experimental colon carcinogenesis. CRC, Boca Raton, pp 51–79

Shamsuddin AKM, Trump BF (1983) Colon epithelium. II. In vivo studies of colon carcinogenesis. Light microscopic, histochemical, and ultrastructural studies of histogenesis of azoxymethane-induced colon carcinomas in Fischer 344 rats. J Natl Cancer Inst 66: 389–401

Sinclair TS, Brunt PW, Mowat NA (1983) Nonspecific proctocolitis in northeastern Scotland: a community study. Gastroenterology 85: 1–11

Stemmerman GN, Nomura AM, Heilbrun LK (1984) Dietary fat and the risk of colorectal cancer. Cancer Res 44: 4633–4637

Stemmerman GN, Nomura AM, Heilbrun LK (1986) Cancer risk in relation to fat and energy intake among Hawaiian Japanese. A prospective study. In: Hayashi Y, Nagoo M, Sugimura T et al. (eds) Diet, nutrition and cancer. Japan Scientific Society Press, Tokyo, pp 265–274

Swenberg JA, Cooper HK, Bucheler J, Kleihues P (1979) 1,2-Dimethylhydrazine-induced methylation of DNA bases in various rat organs and the effect of pretreatment with disulfiram. Cancer Res 39: 465–467

Toth B, Patil K (1983) Enhancing effect of vitamin E on murine intestinal tumorigenesis by 1,2-dimethylhydrazine dihydrochloride. J Natl Cancer Inst 70: 1107–1111

Visek WJ, Clinton SK (1983) Dietary fat and breast cancer. In: Perkins EG, Visek WJ (eds) Dietary fats and health. American Oil Chemists Society, Champaign, IL, pp 721–728

Ward JM (1974) Morphogenesis of chemically induced neoplasms of the colon and small intestine in rats. Lab Invest 30: 505–513

Ward JM, Yamamoto RS, Brown CA (1973) Pathology of intestinal neoplasms and other lesions in rats exposed to azoxymethane. J Natl Cancer Inst 51: 1029–1039

Wargovich MJ, Medline A, Bruce WR (1983) Early histopathologic events of evolution of colon cancer in C57BL/6 and CF1 mice treated with 1,2-dimethylhydrazine. J Natl Cancer Inst 71: 125–131

Wattenberg LW (1983) Inhibition of neoplasia by minor dietary constituents. Cancer Res 43 (Suppl): 2448–2453

Weisburger JH, Fiala ES (1983) Experimental colon carcinogenesis and their mode of action. In: Autrup H, Williams GM (eds) Experimental colon carcinogenesis. CRC, Boca Raton, pp 27–50

Williamson RCN, Bauer FLR, Terpstra OT, Ross JS, Malt RA (1980) Contrasting effects of subtotal enteric bypass, enterectomy, and colectomy on azoxymethane-induced intestinal carcinogenesis. Cancer Res 40: 538–543

Yardley JH, Ransohoff D, Riddell RH, Goldman H (1983) Incidence of inflammatory bowel disease: going up or down? Gastroenterology 85: 196–203

Zedeck MS, Tan Q (1978) P-effect of pyrazole in tumor induction by MAM. Pharmacologist 20: 174–181

Cholesterol, Neutral Sterols and Colorectal Cancer

J. P. Cruse

Department of Histopathology, Royal Free Hospital and Medical School, Rowland Hill Street, London NW3 2PF, U.K.

Contents

Introduction

Colorectal cancer is a serious public health problem on which improved diagnosis and treatment have made little impact over several decades. This relative lack of progress indicates a fundamental weakness in the strategies with which we are attacking the disease as diagnosis and treatment are both focused on the established cancer and ignore its primary cause(s).

Using examples such a cholera, medical history has taught us that diseases can be prevented long before their causes are fully identified or understood. In the past, all that was needed was sufficient evidence to implicate key causal factors which, when removed, broke the chain of events leading to disease (Doll 1967).

What we are searching for to prevent colorectal cancer therefore falls far short of a comprehensive understanding of the molecular events underlying its carcinogenesis. We simply need sufficient evidence upon which to act. Here it is argued that we already have sufficient information to implicate dietary cholesterol, and its endogenously derived metabolites neutral sterols, as cocarcinogens during the development of colorectal cancer.

Rationale for Cancer Prevention

The induction of most human cancers is thought to be a multi-step process (Peto 1977), and there is good evidence to support this idea in colorectal carcinogenesis (Hill et al. 1978). The existence of several steps in the cause of a disease is important. It enables us to deduce that each step may have different causes and allows us to focus our preventive attention on the weakest links in the causative chain of events leading to cancer.

Current concepts envisage the early (initiation) stages of carcinogenesis being caused by inherited or acquired somatic mutations, the latter as a result of exposure to genotoxic mutagens (Peto 1977). Since environmental mutagens are ubiquitous and act rapidly and irreversibly in damaging DNA (Miller 1978), the initiation stages do not seem to present a practical target for preventive action.

Experimental research has shown that the later, post-initiation stages of carcino-genesis (e.g. promotion) occur slowly, require long-term, continuous exposure to non-genotoxins and are susceptible to modulation (Berenblum 1978). These later stages may therefore be a more feasible point at which to attempt to break the causative chain.

With this rationale in mind, the strategy for preventing human colorectal cancer by removing, reducing or inhibiting exposure to a putative cocarcinogen (dietary choles-terol and neutral sterols) can now be assessed.

Epidemiological Evidence Implicating Dietary Factors in Human Colorectal Carcinogenesis

Three decades of epidemiological research have identified a large number of dietary and non-dietary risk factors associated with the development of colorectal cancer. It is well established that the disease has its greatest impact in urbanised, affluent Western societies (Correa and Haenszel 1978). Differences in the geographical distri-bution of the disease have now been clearly accounted for by differences in diet. While there is still some debate about the precise dietary subcomponents implicated, the strongest positive correlations of risk are with a high intake of animal fats and cholesterol (Doll and Peto 1981; Committee on Diet, Nutrition and Cancer 1982).

In examining the evidence implicating any given dietary subcomponent, it is worth remembering that human diets are complex mixtures of chemicals and that the risk of a given type of diet may well be the sum of all the various cocarcinogenic and protective factors. Similarly, fat-rich Western diets are often also high in cholesterol, so it is difficult to unravel the relative contributions of different types of animal fats.

As a framework for assessing the available information on cholesterol and colo-rectal cancer, Table 1 lists some criteria to be fulfilled by putative dietary colorectal cocarcinogens in human studies. Although not exhaustive, the table provides some "rules of evidence" for implicating a cocarcinogen. Any dietary constituent which stands up to similarly rigorous analysis is a worthy candidate for preventive action. The criteria could equally well be applied to any of the putative cocarcinogens discussed in this book, as well as to other, yet unrecognised candidates.

Table 1. Criteria to be fulfilled by putative dietary colorectal cocarcinogens in human studies

---

1. Epidemiological

The following should show a significant correlation with dietary intake of the cocarcinogen:

a. Variation among countries
   Intercountry variations in disease distribution
   Disease time trends
   Changes following population migration
b. Variation within countries
   Urban-rural differences
   Socioeconomic gradients in risk
   Religious or cultural differences in risk
c. Variations in individual risk factors
   Patients with a family history of CRC
   Patients with premalignant colorectal diseases, e.g. FAP, adenomatous polyps

2. Metabolic Epidemiology

a. Biochemical concentrations of the cocarcinogen (or its precursors or metabolites) in the blood, faeces or other body fluids should differ significantly in patients with CRC and in high-risk groups compared to controls.
b. There should be a dose-response relationship between the intake, body fluid levels or excretion of the cocarcinogen and all gradations of risk for CRC.
c. Biochemically plausible and testable carcinogenic mechanism(s) should exist to explain how the cocarcinogen causes CRC.
d. The physiological conditions necessary for cocarcinogenesis should be demonstrated in humans (cocarcinogen reaches target organ, levels of pH, eH, etc.).

3. Interventional

Prospective interventional studies should show changes in risk of CRC following deliberate dietary or pharmacological alterations designed to remove, reduce or inhibit the action of the cocarcinogen.

CRC, colorectal cancer.

Dietary Cholesterol

Human Studies

The role of dietary and endogenous cholesterol in human cancer has received scientific attention for several decades (Cruse 1980). The suspicion that excessive cholesterol intake may be a risk factor for colorectal cancer was stimulated by the observation of a strong positive correlation between international mortality rates for colorectal cancer and those for atherosclerotic heart disease (Wynder and Shigematsu 1967). Since cholesterol-rich diets were already causally implicated in coronary heart disease (Royal College of Physicians Report 1976), this suggested shared aetiological factors.

Using criteria broadly similar to those outlined in Table 1, it has been argued (Cruse et al. 1979) that the striking geographical variations observed in the worldwide distribution of human colorectal cancer between and within countries can be accounted for by differences in dietary cholesterol intake. This hypothesis is controversial (Hill 1980), and it would be fair to concede that the epidemiological information available to date neither refutes the idea nor permits the conclusion that cholesterol-rich diets are the cause of colorectal cancer.

The large amount of epidemiological information linking dietary fat and cholesterol to colorectal cancer has been reviewed in detail by several workers (Lilienfeld 1981; Committee on Nutrition, Diet and Cancer 1982; McMichael et al. 1984; Broitman 1986). Most authors have commented at length on the wide variations in the statistical methods used in this type of research and on the difficulty of studying the effect of a single dietary variable such as cholesterol. However, the salient fact to emerge from these major reviews is how few studies have specifically addressed the cholesterol question.

One of the few international studies to focus on the question of whether dietary cholesterol intake increases the risk of developing colon cancer was the correlational analysis reported by Liu et al. (1979). They found a highly significant correlation between colon cancer mortality and cholesterol-rich diets in 20 industrialised countries (Table 1, criterion 2a). The possible effects of dietary fat and fibre intake in colon carcinogenesis were studied by performing partial correlation and cross-classification analyses. The authors provided statistical support for their conclusion that "cholesterol intake is more important in the aetiology of colon cancer than is dietary fat or fibre intake". To date, neither this publication nor its conclusions have been seriously challenged.

This observation was extended by a Canadian case-control study involving multivariate analysis of major nutrient intake in 348 cases of colon cancer and 194 cases of rectal cancer compared with age- and sex-matched controls (Jain et al. 1980). This showed a significant increase in risk of colorectal cancer associated with increasing cholesterol intake which was dose related (Table 1, criterion 2b). However, this study suffers from the limitation that it relied on a dietary history questionnaire, which is thought to be a suboptimal means of measuring nutrient intake.

Other case-control studies, such as that of Kolonel et al. (1981), have assessed the relationship between dietary cholesterol and cancers at as many as 15 sites and found no significant association between dietary fat or cholesterol and colon or rectal cancer. In this study, only carcinomas of the lung and larynx were significantly associated with dietary cholesterol, a somewhat surprising conclusion. This illustrates the inherent problems of sorting out the facts from the "noise" in epidemiological research, particularly when the hypothetical net is cast too widely.

Commenting that too few studies have been designed to test whether the consumption of specific fats (such as cholesterol) is associated with colon cancer, the Committee on Diet, Nutrition and Cancer (1982) has concluded that the relationship is not yet clear. The position remains so today, and more epidemiological work clearly needs to be done.

Animal Studies

While human epidemiological studies rarely produce clear-cut answers to questions linking diet and cancer, it is possible, by good design and sufficient repetition, to be virtually certain of the relationship between cause and effect in animal experiments (Doll 1963). Table 2 summarises some important criteria to be fulfilled in assessing the roles of putative cocarcinogens in such experiments.

Table 2. Criteria to be fulfilled by putative dietary colorectal cocarcinogens in animal studies

1. Irrespective of the animal model used, the feeding of a diet containing the putative cocarcinogen should significantly augment the development, growth or spread of large bowel cancer.

2. Diets completely lacking the cocarcinogen should show significant protective effects (increased latent period and survival; or reduced incidence, multiplicity or size of large bowel tumours).

3. A dose–response relationship should be demonstrable between dietary intake of the cocarcinogen and the cocarcinogenic effect.

4. A biochemically testable mechanism of cocarcinogenic action should be postulated, tested and demonstrated.

5. The physiological conditions necessary for cocarcinogenesis should be present in the animals.

6. The biochemical levels of the putative cocarcinogen should be significantly different in the body fluids of carcinogen-treated animals fed the cocarcinogen compared to controls.

7. The removal, inhibition or reduction of the cocarcinogen in the diet should be associated with a corresponding reduction in the cocarcinogenic effect.

Colon cancer can be induced in rodents and other animals by a variety of chemical and other carcinogens. Irrespective of the carcinogen used, carcinogenesis in most such models is susceptible to dietary modification (LaMont and O'Gorman 1978). This is fortunate for the researcher as it not only fulfils the first criterion in Table 2, but also points to the fundamental importance of diet in carcinogenesis.

Four independent laboratories have specifically studied the effects of dietary cholesterol on chemically induced colon carcinogenesis in rodents (Broitman et al. 1977; Cruse et al. 1978; Hiramatsu et al. 1983; Klurfeld et al. 1983). Despite the differences in strains of rats used, types of chemical carcinogen employed and standard died fed, all found that the presence of dietary cholesterol enhanced colon carcinogenesis.

This effect could be measured using several different end points, including significantly increased numbers and incidence of large bowel tumours (Broitman et al. 1977; Hiramatsu et al. 1983), increased tumour size (Klurfeld et al. 1983), increased percentage of invasive carcinomas (Klurfeld et al. 1983), increased metastases (Cruse et al. 1978; Hiramatsu et al. 1983), and reduced latent period and lifespan (Cruse et al. 1978). Control animals fed cholesterol-free diets in these experiments showed corresponding reductions in these parameters, so satisfying the second criterion in Table 2. The only detraction is that the cholesterol diets in two of the experiments (Broitman et al. 1977; Klurfeld et al. 1983) also confoundingly contained bile salts to aid cholesterol absorption.

Faecal Cholesterol and Neutral Sterols

Human Studies

It is now widely believed that environmental factors are of paramount importance in the cause(s) of human cancers (Doll and Peto 1981). Since the local environment of the colorectum is largely determined by the faeces within its lumen, research workers have intensively studied the biochemistry and microbiology of the faecal contents to search for metabolic clues to the causes of colorectal cancer.

The physiology and potential role of cholesterol and faecal neutral sterols in colorectal carcinogenesis have been reviewed by Owen and Hill (1982). Cholesterol enters the lumen of the large bowel by several routes, including that derived from the diet and from endogenous sources such as bile and exfoliated intestinal epithelial cells. As it is poorly absorbed, any excess of cholesterol from any source, particularly the diet, is eventually excreted via the colon. The colonic epithelial cells of Western people consuming cholesterol-rich diets are therefore constantly exposed to high levels of faecal cholesterol and its metabolites (Table 1, criterion 2d).

Raised levels of faecal cholesterol and its metabolites are associated with all gradations of risk for colorectal cancer (Table 1, criterion 2a). Healthy high-risk Americans consuming a mixed Western diet excrete greater levels than low-risk rural South African Blacks (Salyers et al. 1977). The same is true in international comparisons between other high- and low-risk groups (Hill et al. 1971), even within the same country (Reddy and Wynder 1973).

The relationship between risk of colon cancer and faecal neutral sterol excretion includes individual patients as well as populations. Patients with colon cancer (Reddy and Wynder 1977) and those with all predisposing diseases, namely familial adenomatous polyposis (Reddy et al. 1976), adenomatous polyps (Reddy and Wynder 1977), ulcerative colitis (Reddy et al. 1977) and Gardiner's syndrome (Core and Watne 1974) all excrete more faecal cholesterol and metabolites than appropriate controls.

Faecal Cholesterol Degradation Patterns

Most cholesterol in faeces is excreted after bacterial degradation as the neutral sterol metabolites coprostanone and coprostanol, with minor amounts as unchanged cholesterol. Metabolic studies have shown significant differences between people in the extent to which faecal cholesterol is converted to its metabolites (Owen and Hill 1982).

Patients with familial adenomatous polyposis (FAP) have the greatest overall lifetime risk for developing large bowel cancer, and their colonic metabolism must hold some clues as to why they are so prone to this disease. Several research groups have studied their faecal sterol excretion patterns (Bone et al. 1975; Reddy et al. 1976; Watne et al. 1976; Lipkin et al. 1981) and discovered that they were relatively unable to degrade faecal sterols, excreting most of their faecal cholesterol unchanged.

FAP is an autosomally dominant inherited disease, and one would expect about half of the children of patients with the disease to be similarly affected. Bone et al. (1975) found that 34 out of 74 of the offspring of the FAP patients also showed the low cholesterol conversion pattern and that 25 of these developed FAP, while 38 out of 40 children with normal cholesterol conversion patterns did not. This is as expected and firmly implicates the low cholesterol conversion pattern as a risk factor.

Non-degradation of faecal cholesterol is also found in a minority of apparently healthy North American individuals (Wilkins and Hackman 1974), but it has not yet been established whether these people are at higher risk for large bowel cancer. Such biochemical tests may turn out to be useful markers for risk of developing colorectal cancer in both individuals and populations. However, it is not yet understood how these differences in metabolism arise or how they translate biochemically into risk for cancer.

Animal Studies

Cholesterol-fed rats show a 20-fold greater faecal excretion of neutral sterols compared to animals fed control diets (Hiramatsu et al. 1983). Carcinogen treatment also increased faecal neutral sterol output in some studies (Reddy et al. 1974) but not in others (Hiramatsu et al. 1983).

Faecal cholesterol degradation patterns have been studied in only a few experiments. Hiramatsu et al. (1983) found that cholesterol-fed rats had a low conversion pattern compared to controls. Since cholesterol feeding of carcinogen-treated animals significantly enhanced colon carcinogenesis, the results suggest that increased excretion of unchanged faecal cholesterol may be more harmful than an excess of cholesterol metabolites. The parallel with the low conversion pattern in humans with FAP is striking.

In passing, it is worth noting the observation of Reddy and Watanabe (1979) that direct intrarectal administration of cholesterol or its metabolites to rats treated with the colon carcinogen N-methyl-N-nitro-N-nitrosoguanidine (MNNG) did not lead to tumour-promoting activity. Unlike dietary cholesterol, intrarectal cholesterol is therefore insufficient to promote cancer. This illustrates the importance of ingestion as the correct route for cocarcinogenic action and, by implication, the requirement for the correct physiological conditions within the intestinal lumen for successful cocarcinogenesis (Table 2).

Serum Cholesterol

Human Studies

Serum cholesterol is one the most intensively studied variables in medical science, and readers are referred to the major reviews for details of individual publications relating serum cholesterol specifically to colorectal cancer (Feinlieb 1981; Lilienfeld 1981; McMichael et al. 1984; Broitman 1986).

Since affluent Western populations are at risk for both heart disease and colorectal cancer and since elevated serum cholesterol is a risk factor for the former, one would logically also expect there to be a positive correlation between serum cholesterol and large bowel cancer. It turns out that what is true for populations does not automatically apply for individuals with colon cancer.

Observational studies have assessed the risk of cancers at various sites in individuals in relation to their serum cholesterol levels and produced the surprising finding that colorectal cancer cases have significantly lower mean serum cholesterol levels than non-cancer controls. This unexpected inverse relationship has been confirmed in over a dozen independent studies in many different countries, most notably the Whitehall study of Rose and Shipley (1980) and the study of Kark et al. (1980) in Evans County,

Georgia, United States. Although seven studies (analysed in detail by Feinlieb 1981 and McMichael et al. 1984) found no inverse association, the overall consensus among epidemiologists seems to be that the association is true, and the debate now centres on the possible explanations and implications of the finding (Jacobsen and Thelle 1987).

Feinlieb (1981) has systematically considered the alternative explanations, including chance, coincidence, confounding and competing risk of death from heart disease. The most important explanations from the public health point of view are a causal association (i.e. that low serum cholesterol contributes to the increased individual risk) and the alternative that the presence of cancer lowers the serum cholesterol (the so-called preclinical cancer effect; Rose and Shipley 1980).

The possibility that low serum cholesterol levels may increase the risk of colon cancer has aroused concern about the clinical use of cholesterol-lowering drugs in the primary prevention of ischaemic heart disease (Oliver 1979). The published results of all the major trials involving diet and cholesterol-lowering drugs such as clofibrate have been reviewed (McMichael et al. 1984; Anonymous 1988) with the reassuring conclusion that cancer incidence and mortality, although slightly increased, were not significantly different between treatment and control groups. It therefore seems that drug-induced lowering of serum cholesterol is not associated with increased risk of cancer, while naturally occurring low levels are (Broitman 1986).

The preclinical cancer effect, whereby the presence of cancer lowers the blood cholesterol (Rose and Shipley 1980) seems plausible. However, subsequent analysis of the large Framingham study (Sorlie and Feinlieb 1982) makes it unlikely. These authors performed time-trend analyses and found that in some cancer cases the serum cholesterol was already low as long as 16–18 years before cancer diagnosis. A similar conclusion was reached by the authors of a large epidemiological follow-up study (Schatzkin et al. 1987) who found that the serum cholesterol level was lower in men 6 or more years before the diagnosis of cancer.

Reports have also recently been published showing a strong positive correlation between serum cholesterol and both colon and rectal cancer in men (Tornberg et al. 1986), and the frequency of colorectal adenoma formation (Mannes et al. 1986).

Such apparent contradictions have been termed the "cholesterol conundrums" by Broitman (1986) who suggests a hypothesis which goes some way towards explaining the facts. He postulates that individuals who maintain low serum cholesterol while consuming high-fat, cholesterol-rich Western diets may be metabolically different from other people and that this phenomenon may provide a marker for those at increased risk for the development of large bowel cancer. This is considered further in the Discussion below.

Animal Studies

Serum cholesterol levels were studied in several of the dietary cholesterol experiments already discussed. Broitman et al. (1977) designed an experiment to compare the effects of altering the disposition of dietary cholesterol between the vascular and intestinal compartments in rats treated with dimethylhydrazine (DMH). Rats fed cholesterol-rich diets with saturated fats (to enhance cholesterol absorption) developed increased serum cholesterol levels, increased vascular lipidosis but reduced colon tumorigenesis. Conversely, rats fed cholesterol-rich diets with polyunsaturated fats (which inhibit cholesterol absorption) developed lower serum cholesterol levels and increased numbers of colon tumours. This seems to indicate that the differential distribution of ingested cholesterol within the body can determine the degree of tumorigenesis in the large bowel.

Cholesterol-fed rats in three other experiments (Hiramatsu et al. 1983; Klurfeld et al. 1983; Barton et al. 1987) showed elevated serum cholesterol levels in association with a cocarcinogenic effect of dietary cholesterol (Table 2, criterion 6). In the latter experiment, rats with DMH-induced colon carcinoma showed significant increases in serum free and percentage-free cholesterol compared to tumour-free animals or rats with adenomas. It is remarkable that it should be possible to demonstrate clear relationships between serum cholesterol levels and the presence or absence of large bowel cancer in animals, even if the direction of the change is not identical to that observed in man.

Possible Mechanisms of Cholesterol Cocarcinogenesis

There are many hypothetical or actual means whereby dietary factors may affect the incidence of cancer (Doll and Peto 1981). Theoretical mechanisms whereby cholesterol can be cocarcinogenic have been postulated (Cruse et al. 1979). These are broadly based on Berenblum's (1978) outline of preparative, permissive, promoting and conditional types of cocarcinogenic action.

The available evidence strongly favours a promotional role for dietary cholesterol during colorectal carcinogenesis. This is in keeping with the generalisation that most dietary fats act as promoters during experimental carcinogenesis (Carroll and Khor 1975). This has been specifically substantiated by an experiment (Cruse et al. 1984) which showed that cholesterol prefeeding was not cocarcinogenic, and that delayed exposure to dietary cholesterol delayed the onset of experimental colon cancer, in the manner of a classical tumour promoter.

While the theoretical knowledge that cholesterol is a colon tumour promoter is extremely useful in terms of preventive action, logic and good science require that biochemically plausible molecular mechanisms exist to explain how any putative cocarcinogen participates in causing large bowel cancer (Tables 1 and 2).

Fortunately for the scientist, there is no shortage of suitable biochemical mechanisms whereby cholesterol can accelerate the carcinogenic process (Sabine 1977; Chen et al. 1978). Cholesterol is a precursor of all the steroid hormones, and differential cocarcinogenesis in men and women may explain the observed differences in the sex incidence of the disease (Correa and Haenszel 1978). Cholesterol is also an essential structural and functional component of all animal cell membranes, and diet-related changes in membrane cholesterol may bioregulate the proliferation of colonic epithelial cells as in leukaemia (Inbar and Shinitzky 1974).

An exogenous supply of cholesterol is essential for clonal cell proliferation (Chen et al. 1978; Chen 1984), which is a fundamental hallmark of carcinogenesis. Cholesterol-rich diets also directly induce intestinal mucosal drug metabolising enzymes (Hietanen and Laitinen 1978) and might therefore accelerate the biotransformation of carcinogens and mutagens (Hoensch and Hartman 1981). These are merely some of the biochemical mechanisms which could explain how cholesterol may facilitate the development of colorectal cancer.

Discussion

The relationship between diet and large bowel cancer has often been likened to a complex jigsaw puzzle (Burkitt 1975; Bresalier and Kim 1985). We have a substantial number of epidemological pieces telling us that the disease is environmentally determined and that diet, particulary animal fats and cholesterol, plays a critical role. While we have only some of the pieces of the puzzle, the real question is whether we have sufficient pieces of information upon which to act.

In the preceding sections, the human and experimental evidence implicating cholesterol in colorectal carcinogenesis has been reviewed. We know that cholesterol-rich diets increase the population risk of cancer, and that the excretion of excess cholesterol and its metabolites in faeces is associated with all gradations of risk in individuals. Since both eating and excreting excess cholesterol are associated with increased risk, it is what happens in between which requires explanation.

Broitman's (1986) line of reasoning links the disparate observations about dietary, faecal and serum cholesterol into a coherent whole. He argues as follows: we already know that, in any given Western population consuming the usual high fat, high cholesterol diet, there exists a large subgroup destined (? genetically) to develop ischaemic heart disease and a smaller subgroup who will develop colorectal cancer. If diet is the common causative factor, then probably those individuals who manifest hypercholesterolaemia are at risk for heart disease, while those who maintain a low serum cholesterol are at increased risk for developing colorectal cancer.

It is suggested that individuals who remain hypocholesterolaemic on a Western diet (Lin and Connor 1980; Broitman 1986) are either inherently less able to absorb dietary cholesterol (so explaining their lower serum levels), or are more able to excrete the excess as faecal cholesterol and bile acids (thereby explaining their raised faecal levels). This may also account for the low conversion pattern, as an excess of unabsorbed cholesterol may be incompletely degraded by the colonic bacteria.

When the human and experimental evidence linking cholesterol and colorectal cancer is reviewed against the objective criteria summarised in Tables 1 and 2, the sheer weight and coherence of the available information points strongly to a cocarcinogenic role for dietary cholesterol. This dies not deny a similar or synergistic role for other putative cocarcinogens such as bile acids, nor is it incompatible with possible protective effects of certain types of dietary fibre.

If dietary cholesterol is cocarcinogenic during the development of colorectal cancer, then we are in a position to prevent this disease. Cholesterol is not an essential nutrient, and safe and palatable low-cholesterol diets are well established in the primary prevention of ischaemic heart disease, as well as forming part of more healthy eating patterns in Western populations. As has now been demonstrated repeatedly, animals fed on such diets show a greatly reduced tendency to develop large bowel cancer, even when given powerful chemical carcinogens.

While the aetiology of colorectal cancer is complex and multifactorial (Hill 1988), we can do little about many of the non-dietary factors such as inheritance and exposure to environmental mutagens. However, we are able to alter our diets by reducing our intake of animal fats and cholesterol, and this could remove a salient contributory factor to both ischaemic heart disease and colorectal cancer. There are few comparable opportunities for preventing cancer so cheaply, safely and simply.

Conclusion

The concept that dietary fats may be implicated in the cause of human colorectal cancer may have been around for over 6 centuries. John of Arderne, an English surgeon writing about rectal cancer in the fourteenth century, advised against the use of enemas "containing oil or butter or anything fatty; the reason is that all fatty and oily substances nourish the cancer and feed it" (Swain 1983).

Acknowledgements. I wish to thank Dr. M. R. Lewin for critical review of the manuscript and Ms. D. Ayres for editorial assistance.

References

Anonymous (1988) Primary prevention of ischaemic heart disease with lipid-lowering drugs. Lancet 1: 333–334 (editorial)

Barton T, Cruse JP, Lewin MR (1987) Changes in serum lipids related to the presence of experimental colon cancer. Br J Cancer 56: 451–454

Berenblum I (1978) Established principles and unresolved problems in carcinogenesis. J Natl Cancer Inst 60: 723–726

Bone E, Drasar BS, Hill MJ (1975) Gut bacteria and their metabolic activities in familial polyposis. Lancet 1: 1117–1120

Bresalier RS, Kim YS (1985) Diet and colon cancer. N Engl J Med 313: 1413–1414

Broitman SA (1986) Cholesterol conundrums: the relationship between dietary and serum cholesterol in colon cancer. In: Clement IP et al. (eds) Dietary fat and cancer. Liss, New York, pp 435–459

Broitman SA, Vitale JJ, Vavrousek-Jakuba E, Gottlieb LS (1977) Polyunsaturated fat, cholesterol and large bowel tumorigenesis. Cancer 40: 2455–2463

Burkitt DP (1975) Large bowel cancer: an epidemiological jigsaw puzzle. J Natl Cancer Inst 54: 3–6

Carroll KK, Khor HT (1977) Dietary fat in relation to tumorigenesis. Prog Biochem Pharmacol 10: 308–353

Chen HW, Kandutsch AA, Heiniger HJ (1978) The role of cholesterol in malignancy. Prog Exp Tumor Res 22: 275–316

Chen HW (1984) Role of cholesterol metabolism in cell growth. Fed Proc 43: 126–130

Committe on Diet Nutrition and Cancer (1982) Diet, nutrition and cancer. National Academy Press, Washington, DC pp 5-1–5-33

Core SK, Watne AL (1974) Faecal steroids and colon cancer. Fed Proc 33: 260

Correa P, Haenszel W (1978) The epidemiology of large bowel cancer. Adv Cancer Res 26: 1–141

Cruse JP (1980) Dietary studies in experimental colon carcinogenesis. PhD thesis, University of London

Cruse JP, Lewin MR, Ferulano GP, Clark CG (1978) Cocarcinogenic effects of dietary cholesterol in experimental colon cancer. Nature 276: 822–825

Cruse JP, Lewin MR, Clark CG (1979) Hypothesis: dietary cholesterol is cocarcinogenic for human colon cancer. Lancet 1: 752–755

Cruse JP, Lewin MR, Clark CG (1984) An investigation into the mechanism of cocarcinogenesis of dietary cholesterol during the induction of colon cancer in rats by 1,2-dimethylhydrazine. Clin Oncol 10: 213–220

Doll R (1963) Interpretations of epidemiological data. Cancer Res 23: 1613–1623

Doll R (1967) Prevention of cancer: pointers from epidemiology. The Nuffield Provincial Hospitals Trust, UK

Doll R, Peto R (1981) The causes of cancer. J Natl Cancer Inst 66: 1191–1308

Feinlieb M (1981) On a possible inverse relationship between serum cholesterol and cancer mortality. Am J Epidemiol 114: 5–10

Hietanen E, Laitinen M (1978) Dependence of intestinal biotransformation on dietary cholesterol. Biochem Pharmacol 27: 1095–1097

Hill MJ (1980) The aetiology of colorectal cancer. In: Wright R (ed) Recent advances in gastrointestinal pathology. Saunders, London, pp 297–310

Hill MJ (1988) Neoplasms: epidemiology and aetiology. Curr Opin Gastroenterol 4: 3–8

Hill MJ, Drasar BS, Aries V, Crowther JS, Hawkesworth G, Williams REO (1971) Bacteria and the aetiology of cancer of the large bowel. Lancet 1: 95–100

Hill MJ, Morson BC, Bussey HJR (1978) Hypothesis: aetiology of adenoma-carcinoma sequence in large bowel. Lancet 1: 245–247

Hiramatsu Y, Takada H, Yamamura M, Hioki K, Saito K, Yamamoto M (1983) Effect of dietary cholesterol on azoxymethane-induced colon carcinogenesis in rats. Carcinogenesis 4: 553–558

Hoensch HP, Hartmann F (1981) The intestinal enzymatic biotransformation system: potential role in protection from intestinal cancer. Hepatogastroenterology 28: 221–228

Inbar M, Shinitzky M (1974) Cholesterol as a bioregulator in the development and inhibition of leukaemia. Proc Natl Acad Sci USA 71: 4229–4231

Jacobsen BK, Thelle DS (1987) Coffee, cholesterol and colon cancer: is there a link? Br Med J 294: 4–5

Jain M, Cook GM, Davis FG et al. (1980) A case-control study of diet and colorectal cancer. Int J Cancer 26: 757–768

Kark JD, Smith AH, Hames CG (1980) The relationship of serum cholesterol to the incidence of cancer in Evans county, Georgia. J Chron Dis 33: 311–322

Kolonel LN, Hankin JH, Lee J et al. (1981) Nutrient intakes in relation to cancer incidence in Hawaii. Br J Cancer 44: 332–339

Klurfeld DM, Aglow E, Tepper S, Kritchevsky D (1983) Modification of dimethylhydrazine-induced carcinogenesis in rats by dietary cholesterol. Nutr Cancer 5: 16–25

LaMont JT, O'Gorman TA (1978) Experimental colon cancer. Gastroenterology 75: 1157–1169

Lilienfeld AM (1981) The human fog: cancer and cholesterol. Am J Epidemiol 114: 1–4

Lin DS, Connor DS (1980) The longterm effects of dietary cholesterol upon the plasma lipids, lipoproteins, cholesterol absorption and sterol balance in man. J Lipid Res 21: 1042–1052

Lipkin M, Reddy BS, Weisberger JH et al. (1981) Nondegradation of fecal cholesterol in subjects at high risk for cancer of the large intestine. J Clin Invest 67: 304–307

Liu K, Moss D, Persky V et al. (1979) Dietary cholesterol, fat and fiber and colon cancer mortality. Lancet 2: 782–785

Mannes GA, Maier A, Thieme C et al. (1986) Relation between the frequency of colorectal adenoma and the serum cholesterol level. N Engl J Med 315: 1634–1638

McMichael AJ, Jensen OM, Parkin DM, Zaridze DG (1984) Dietary and endogenous cholesterol and human cancer. Epidemiol Rev 6: 192–216

Miller EC (1978) Some current perspectives on chemical carcinogenesis in humans and experimental animals. Cancer Res 38: 1479–1496

Oliver MF (1979) Cholesterol and cancer. Lancet 1: 931–932

Owen RW, Hill MJ (1982) Cholesterol and carcinogenic fecal steroids. In: Beitz D, Hansen RG (eds) Animal products in human nutrition. Academic, London, pp 461–478

Peto R (1977) Epidemiology, multistage models and short-term mutagenicity tests. In: Hiatt HH (ed) Origins of human cancer. Cold Spring Harbor Laboratory, Cold Spring Harbor, New York, pp 1403–1428

Reddy BS, Watanabe K (1979) Effect of cholesterol metabolites and promoting effect of litho-cholic acid in colon carcinogenesis in germ-free and conventional F344 rats. Cancer Res 39: 1521–1524

Reddy BS, Wynder EL (1973) Large bowel carcinogenesis: faecal constituents of populations with diverse incidence rates of colon cancer. J Natl Cancer Inst 50: 1437–1442

Reddy BS, Wynder EL (1977) Metabolic epidemiology of colon cancer; faecal bile acids and neutral sterols in colon cancer patients and patients with adenomatous polyps. Cancer 39: 2533–2539

Reddy BS, Weisburger JH, Wynder EL (1974) Effects of dietary fat level and dimethylhydrazine on faecal acid and neutral sterol excretion and colon carcinogenesis in rats. J Natl Cancer Inst 52: 507–511

Reddy BS, Mastromarino A, Gustafson C et al. (1976) Faecal bile acids and neutral sterols in patients with familial polyposis. Cancer 38: 1694–1698

Reddy BS, Martin CW, Wynder EL (1977) Faecal bile acid and cholesterol metabolites of patients with ulcerative colitis, a high risk group for development of colon cancer. Cancer Res 37: 1697–1701

Rose G, Shipley MJ (1980) Plasma lipids and mortality: a source of error. Lancet 1: 523–526

Royal College of Physicians Report (1976) Prevention of coronary heart disease. J Roy Coll Phys 10: 1–63

Sabine JR (1977) Cholesterol. Dekker, New York, pp 277–288

Salyers AA, Sperry JF, Wilkins TD et al. (1977) Neutral steroid concentrations in the faeces of the North American White and South African Black populations at different risks for cancer of the colon. S Afr Med J 51: 823–827

Schatzkin A, Hoover RN, Taylor PR et al. (1987) Serum cholesterol and cancer in the NHANES I epidemiologic followup study. Lancet 2: 298–301

Sorlie PD, Feinlieb M (1982) The serum cholesterol–cancer relationship: an analysis of time trends in the Framingham study. J Natl Cancer Inst 69: 989–996

Swain CP (1983) A fourteenth century description of rectal cancer. World J Surg 7: 304–307

Tornberg SA, Holm L-E, Carstensen JM et al. (1986) Risks of cancer of the colon and rectum in relation to serum cholesterol and beta-lipoprotein. N Engl J Med 315: 1629–1633

Watne AL, Lai H-Y, Mance MS, Watne S (1976) Faecal steroids and bacterial flora in patients with polyposis coli. Am J Surg 131: 42–46

Wilkins TD, Hackman AS (1974) Two patterns of neutral steroid conversion in the faeces of normal North Americans. Cancer Res 30: 176–181

Wynder EL, Shigematsu T (1967) Environmental factors in cancer of the colon and rectum. Cancer 20: 1520–1561

The Role of Bile Acids in Colorectal Carcinogenesis

B. I. Cohen[1]* and E. E. Deschner[2]

[1] Departments of Surgery, Beth Israel Medical Center, and The Mount Sinai School of Medicine of The City University of New York, First Avenue at 16th Street, New York, New York 10003, USA
[2] Laboratory of Digestive Tract Carcinogenesis, Memorial Sloan-Kettering Cancer Center, 1275 York Avenue, New York, NY 10021, USA

Contents

Introduction

Bile Acids

Structure and Function

Bile acids are formed in the liver of mammals through a series of biochemical reactions starting from the 27-carbon sterol, cholesterol (Fig. 1, I) (Kritchevsky and Nair 1971). The most abundant bile acids possess a 24-carbon atom cyclopentanophenanthrene structure. Two primary bile acids common in man and animals are chenodeoxycholic acid (Fig. 1, II) and cholic acid (Fig. 1, III). These compounds are secreted by the liver into bile where they are present as amidates of either glycine or taurine (Bergstrom and Danielsson 1968; Hofmann 1984; Hofmann and Roda 1984).

Bile acids act as important regulators of bile secretion and cholesterol solubility (Armstrong and Carey 1982; Hofmann et al. 1983). In man, bile acids are concentrated and stored in the gallbladder; in response to a meal they are released into the intestinal tract where they aid in the digestion and absorption of fat (Lack and Weiner 1963). Most bile salts then undergo intestinal reabsorption by either active or passive processes. Bile salts are returned to the liver via the portal blood where they may be reamidated and reexcreted into the bile; thus, the enterohepatic circulation conserves more than 95% of the bile acid pool (Carey 1982).

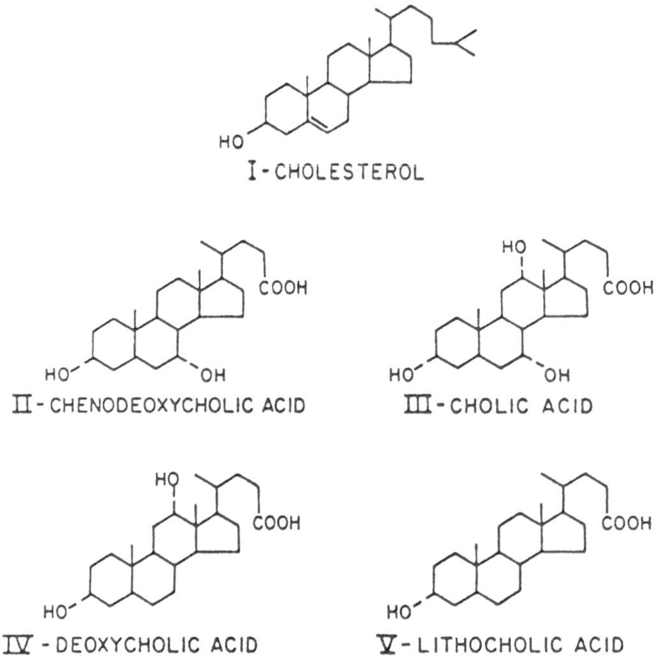

Fig. 1. Structures of cholesterol (*I*) and the major bile acids (*II–V*) of man

Biliary Bile Acids and Fecal Bile Acids

Three bile acids predominate in human bile: cholic acid, chenodeoxycholic acid, and deoxycholic acid (Fig. 1, IV). In contrast, the fecal bile acid profile can be quite complex (Gustafsson 1982; Hylemon and Glass 1983). The most abundant bile acids in feces are formed from the bacterial 7α-dehydroxylation of the primary bile acids; chenodeoxycholic acid → lithocholic acid (Fig. 1, V) and cholic acid → deoxycholic acid. In addition, bile acids can undergo other chemical modifications including dehydrogenation, dehydration, oxidation, and isomerization (Macdonald et al. 1983), producing a wide spectrum of minor fecal bile acids numbering as high as 20–30; bile acids comprise a significant portion of identifiable compounds present in feces. A healthy individual excretes approximately 500–750 mg of bile acids daily (Hofmann 1977). These amounts increase dramatically in individuals with intestinal diseases (Reddy et al. 1976a; Mastromarino et al. 1978; Moskovitz et al. 1979; Mudd et al. 1980; Hill et al. 1983) and in individuals treated with bile acid therapy for dissolution of cholesterol gallstones (Bell et al. 1972; Danzinger et al. 1972; Dowling 1977; Iser and Sali 1981). A number of studies have suggested a causal relationship of bile acids to colonic cancer. This review will summarize recent advances in this field.

Colon Carcinogenesis

Cancer of the colon continues to rank among the dominant forms of cancer and is one of the leading causes of cancer death in North America. To date, early detection and surgical intervention offer the best chance for long-term survival from this cancer. Epidemiological studies have shown that the incidence of colon cancer can vary from continent to continent as well as from population to population in the same locale (Correa and Haenszel 1978; Hill 1981; Zaridze 1983). The diets consumed by individuals in these different populations have been implicated in the etiology of colonic neoplasia (Armstrong and Doll 1975; Hill 1975; Phillips 1975; Reddy et al. 1978; Dales et al. 1979; Haenszel et al. 1980; Jain et al. 1980; Jensen et al. 1982; NCI 1985; Potter and McMichael 1986). It has been shown that individuals consuming diets high in fat (mainly meat-rich diets) (Reddy et al. 1975b; Reddy 1981a; McCay 1983) have an increased incidence of colon cancer compared to populations consuming diets low in fat and protein (vegetarian diets) (Carroll and Khor 1975; Phillips 1975; McCay 1983). Biochemical analyses show that groups of individuals at increased risk for colon cancer, or having the disease, have increased amounts of bile acids in feces (Reddy et al. 1976a; Reddy and Wynder 1977; Reddy et al. 1977b, 1980). A similarity in structure between bile acids and a class of carcinogenic aromatic hydrocarbons (such as, benzo[a]pyrene) led to the hypothesis that bile acids are involved in the etiology of colon cancer (Hill et al. 1983).

Bile Acids in Experimental Colon Cancer

Model systems are essential to explore the development and expression of diseases in man. In vitro as well as in vivo models of colonic neoplasia have been employed to find out whether bile acids affect the course of the disease.

Studies In Vitro

Studies in vitro are designed to simplify the experimental system in order to evaluate a specific question in a more defined environment. However, data obtained in vitro may not necessarily be valid in vivo.

Mutagenicity

Bile acids have been tested for their mutagenic potential using the standard Ames assay (Ames et al. 1975). The 34 bile acids that were tested (including cholic, chenodeoxycholic, lithocholic, and deoxycholic acids) all proved to be negative in this system. Other studies using various saturated bile acids as well as short-chain derivatives (C_{19} and C_{22} bile acids) also proved to have no mutagenic activity. One reason for the failure of the standard Ames test to show mutagenicity for bile acids is the high dose of substrate needed, resulting in inactivation of the assay system (McKillop et al. 1983). At low doses, the test system is too insensitive to detect mutagenicity. A new protocol has revived interest in the mutagenicity and carcinogenicity testing of bile acids (Watabe and Bernstein 1985). Using a fluctuation assay to avoid toxicity, the bile acids deoxycholic acid, cholic acid, chenodeoxycholic acid, but not lithocholic acid, are positive mutagens, with deoxycholic acid exhibiting the highest activity (Watabe and Bernstein 1985). Secondary bile acids, i.e., lithocholic and deoxycholic acids, have been found to act as co-mutagens in the Ames test. The carcinogen 1,2-dimethylhydrazine (DMH) by itself is not mutagenic in vitro; however, when incubated with secondary bile acids, DMH induces transformation of *Salmonella typhimurium*. This finding of a co-mutagenic promotional activity suggests an additional facet in the role of bile acids in the etiology of colon cancer (Wilpart et al. 1983). Deoxycholic acid has been shown to increase colon cancer induced by chemical carcinogen and is probably responsible for increased cellular turnover of the colonic mucosa (Reddy et al. 1976b, 1977c; Deschner et al. 1981; Kelsey 1983; Cohen and Mosbach 1985).

Organ culture

The colon organ culture system was developed to examine chemical carcinogenesis in vitro (Autrup et al. 1978; Mak and Chang 1978; Reiss and Williams 1979; Reiss et al. 1982). Bile acids can be used in these test systems to examine their relationship to colon cancer (Reiss et al. 1987). This methodology employs colon tissue which remains intact when removed from its in vivo environment and freed of intestinal contents. Organ culture provides a link between in vitro and in vivo systems; it also enables investigators to control the development of experimental carcinogenesis and stages of neoplastic expression. A study has shown that N-methyl-N-nitrosourea (MNU) and N-methyl-N'-nitro-N-nitrosoguanidine (MNNG) induce cellular changes in rat colon organ culture that are enhanced by deoxycholic acid and by fecal bile acid extracts (Reiss et al. 1987). While not increasing viability as deoxycholic acid did, small amounts of sodium cholate produce the largest increase in labeling index on DNA synthesis of these colon cultures. This would suggest that cell loss and subsequent compensatory cell replacement is maximized in the presence of cholic acid.

Additional experimental implant studies were carried out to determine whether colon carcinogens (MNU, MNNG) in culture induce neoplastic changes that are enhanced by bile acids. In other words, if colon carcinogenesis is a two-step process (initiation followed by promotion), do bile acids enhance the promotion step of neoplasm development? It has been found that colon cell cultures exposed to carcinogens (initiators) and then to bile acids (deoxycholic acid, a promoter?) survive in a mammary fat pad for as long as 1 year with no tumors formed (Reiss et al. 1987). However, atypias were observed which are enhanced by deoxycholic acid. These results suggest that bile acids can play a role in expression of carcinogen-induced neoplasm, even if the bile acids are not carcinogens themselves. Studies in the organ culture system offer a novel approach to determine whether the minor fecal bile acids are carcinogens or promoters of carcinogenesis.

Studies In Vivo

Animal Models

The use of animal models has contributed to our understanding of the role of bile acids in colon cancer (Reddy et al. 1975a; Bird et al. 1985). With the aid of such models came further proof that the neoplastic process was a two-step phenomenon, initiation followed by promotion (Nigro and Bull 1983). The process of promotion can be influenced by various external factors including diet, age, and environment (Pitot 1983). The role of bile acids in the neoplastic process is believed to be in the promotional step of tumor development. The effect of carcinogen, diet, and bile acid administration on tumor formation will be reviewed.

Carcinogens

Various chemical carcinogens are used to induce colonic cancer in animals (Weisburger 1971; LaMont and O'Gorman 1978; Shamsuddin 1983; Weisburger and Fiala 1983). The most common carcinogen used is DMH; other carcinogens include MNNG and MNU. These carcinogens form colon tumors reproducibly in large numbers in rats and mice, though the dose, route of administration, and strain of animal used may vary. Most neoplastic events occur in the distal colon where early atypias, hyperplasias, adenomatous polyps, and carcinomas are detected after a given time interval. The pathology of the cancers developed in the animals are similar to those in man (Lingeman et al. 1972). In man, however, identification of a chemical carcinogen specific for colon cancer has not been possible so far. It is believed that carcinogens, if they exist in man, are dietary in origin; consequently, many studies have focused on the effects of diet on cancer.

Diet and Cancer

Dietary Fat. Dietary fat appears to exert its effect on the promotional step of colon carcinogenesis (Reddy et al. 1980a, b). Fat is known to increase bile acid secretion into the gut, increase the metabolic activity of gut bacteria, and increase secondary bile acids in the colon that can act as tumor promoters. Presumably, the association of fat and bile acids promote colon cancer (Reddy 1983). For example, more tumors are observed in rats fed a high-fat diet after treatment with the carcinogen azoxymethane (AOM), than before or during AOM administration (Bull et al. 1979). Other studies have also shown an association between increased fat intake and increased incidence of tumors after carcinogen treatment (Reddy et al. 1977a; Reddy and Ohmori 1981). When groups of rats are fed a diet containing either 5% or 20% beef fat, a greater tumor incidence is observed on the diet with the higher fat intake. Thus, an association apparently exists between dietary fat and colon cancer.

Dietary fiber. Dietary fiber is thought to have a protective effect against colon cancer since it is recognized that consumption of a high-fiber diet is related to a low incidence of colon cancer (Weisburger et al. 1980). The fiber may act by increasing fecal bulk and diluting potential carcinogens or promoters (bile acids?), modifying the metabolic activity of the intestinal bacteria, lowering caloric density (Kaur et al. 1985), or modifying the metabolism of carcinogens and/or promoters (Reddy 1983). Dietary fiber alters the enterohepatic circulation of bile acids (Kern et al. 1979). Thus, fiber not only influences bile acid metabolism but may be able to act as a "solvent" for diluting secondary bile acids (Cummings et al. 1979; Dales et al. 1979).

Dietary fibers are a complex group of nutrients often producing mixed effects in experimental systems. In general, insoluble fibers that are poorly fermentable, such as cellulose, lignin, or wheat bran, inhibit colon tumor development (Jacobs 1983; Jacobs and Lupton 1986), whereas soluble fibers which are fermentable, such as pectin (Bauer et al. 1981; Jacobs and Lupton 1986), guar (Jacobs and Lupton 1986), oat bran (Jacob and Lupton 1986), corn bran (Reddy et al. 1983), agar (Glauert et al. 1981), and carrageenan, enhance experimental colon carcinogenesis. Of the latter, pectin, guar, and carrageenan increase cell proliferation (Fath et al. 1984; Jacobs and Lupton 1986). Oat bran and corn bran appear to act by increasing fecal bile acid concentration (Kirby et al. 1981; Reddy et al. 1983) thereby promoting colonic neoplasia.

Bile Acid Administration and Colon Cancer. The initial evidence that bile acids act as tumor promoters in animals was reported by Narisawa et al. (1974), Reddy et al. (1976b, 1977c), and Reddy and Watanabe (1979). In one study, administration of the carcinogen MNNG followed by intrarectal treatment with the secondary bile acids lithocholic acid and taurodeoxycholic acid gave more adenomas in the bile acid plus carcinogen group than in the group given carcinogen alone (Narisawa et al. 1974). In addition, lithocholic acid produced an increase in colonic adenocarcinomas in rats treated with MNNG (Reddy and Watanabe 1979). The bile acids given intrarectally without chemical carcinogen show no tumor-promoting properties (Reddy and Watanabe 1979). In another study, tumor promotion was observed in germ-free rats treated with MNNG and the primary bile acids sodium cholate or sodium chenodeoxycholate, suggesting the bile acids themselves promote tumors in the presence or absence of the fecal flora (Reddy and Watanabe 1979).

Rats treated with the direct-acting carcinogen MNU and fed either cholic acid or chenodeoxycholic acid showed an increase in colon neoplasms compared with animals treated only with carcinogen (Sarwal et al. 1979; Cohen et al. 1980). Thus, bile acids appear active as promoters either admixed with feces or administered intrarectally. Although the mechanism of action of bile acids has not been fully elucidated, cellular kinetic studies have given us leads as to their possible mode of action. Dietary cholic acid supplementation in rats has been shown, by virtue of the damaging detergent action of the bile acid, to stimulate colonic epithelial cell proliferation, widen the proliferative compartment and accelerate cell migration up the crypt walls (Deschner et al. 1981). The enhanced proliferative activity effectively shortens the turnover or replacement time of the mucosa as well as increasing the likelihood that a malignantly transformed cell will emerge and be expressed as a colonic tumor.

Other studies lend support to the role of bile acid in colon carcinogenesis. Using the carcinogen AOM, rats in which the bile duct had been surgically diverted to the middle of the small intestine produced an increase in colonic neoplasms (Chomchai et al. 1974). Similarly, rats which had undergone ileal resection or bypass followed by treatment with the carcinogen DMH also showed an enhanced tumor development (Nigro et al. 1973; Bull et al. 1979). This study suggests that total fecal bile acids may be more important in tumor formation than individual secondary bile acids (Nigro et al. 1973; Bull et al. 1979). Bile acid binding agents have given variable results in terms of their effect on tumor formation and development. Nigro et al. (1973) report that cholestyramine, a bile acid binding resin, enhances colon tumors induced by the carcinogen AOM. However, Cruse et al. (1981a), employing the carcinogen DMH and cholestyramine, failed to observe an increase in tumors. It appears that differences in experimental design may be important in tumor promotion models of carcinogenesis (Cruse et al. 1981b).

Bile Acids and Cancer in Animals – New Directions. The availability of bile acids to the colonic mucosa has been suggested as a mode of action for promotion of colon cancer. This effect may be inhibited by the presence of binding ions, particularly ionized calcium (Newmark et al. 1984). The hypothesis seems to be supported by an animal study which shows that deoxycholic acid has a reduced toxic effect on the colonic epithelium when administered in conjunction with dietary oral calcium (Wargovich et al. 1983). Studies using dietary calcium and bile acid in a rat colon cancer model will show whether calcium reduces bile acid availability and alters tumor incidence in vivo.

Bile Acids in Colon Tissue

A novel finding by Nair et al. (1977, 1978) has suggested that the secondary bile acid lithocholic acid is covalently bound to tissues via the epsilon amino group of lysine. Significant amounts of tissue-bound lithocholic acid have been reported in human liver (Nair et al. 1977); high concentrations of the tissue-bound lithocholic acid have been found in livers of rats treated with AOM (Nair et al. 1978). More important is the finding that tissue-bound lithocholic acid was isolated from a polyp of a patient with carcinoma in situ (Turjman and Nair 1981). To confirm these studies, tissue from patients with colonic neoplasms was examined; however, significant amounts of tissue-bound bile acids could not be detected nor could a relationship between tissue bile acids and colorectal disease be established (Gelb et al. 1982). These findings, however, cannot rule out a direct relationship between bile acids and cancer.

Studies in Man

Bile Acids and Colonic Disorders

Fecal bile acid profiles have been examined to determine if they are predictive of colon disease. For example, an elevation in fecal bile acids is found in patients with adenomas compared to controls (Reddy and Wynder 1977). A correlation between bile acid excretion and adenoma size has been postulated (Hill et al. 1978, 1983). Colorectal cancer is believed to progress through the adenoma-carcinoma sequence (Hill et al. 1978). Patients with colon cancer are reported to excrete more total fecal bile acids than other groups (Reddy and Wynder 1977). However, the fecal bile acid profile does not differ in patients with adenomas, cancer, or controls. Although there is some evidence that the ratio of lithocholic acid to deoxycholic acid is high in certain patients (Owen et al. 1983), the fecal bile acid profile may not be an indicator of colon cancer.

Fecal bile acid patterns have been examined in patients with other large bowel disorders. Analyses of fecal bile acid excretion in ulcerative colitis (UC) patients have given variable results. In an early study, it was reported that fecal bile acid excretion was similar in UC patients vs. controls (Hill et al. 1983); recently, patients with UC have been found to have significantly less bile acids than controls (Albert and Fromm 1987). The rapid intestinal transit time for UC patients would suggest an increase rather than a decrease in bile acid excretion. Patients with familial polyposis also have an increased risk for developing early large bowel cancer (Reddy et al. 1976a). These patients do not have altered bile acid metabolism but do have altered fecal cholesterol degradation (Bone et al. 1975). Whereas normal individuals are able to metabolize cholesterol to coprostanol, patients with familial polyposis cannot; consequently, cholesterol predominates in the feces. Whether this condition predisposes this group to early cancer is unknown. In summary, bile acid analyses per se are not correlated to colonic disorders. They appear to be important insofar as their presence stimulates cell proliferation thereby promoting the expression of any neoplastically transformed colonic epithelial stem cell.

Bile Acid and Nutrition

The role of diet on fecal bile acids and colon cancer has been explored in great detail. Two epidemiological studies include the role of fat and fiber on bile acid composition and concentration.

Bile Acids and Dietary Fat. Dietary fat has been implicated as a potential promoter of large bowel cancer in man (Reddy 1981a). The quantity of fat ingested appears to determine amounts of bile acids which reach the intestine as well as the composition of the intestinal microflora responsible for the degradation of the bile acids (Aries et al. 1969). In addition, individuals on high-fat diets appear to have increased concentrations of secondary bile acids in the feces, presumably because of the increased activity of the bacterial flora responsible for the formation of these compounds (Cummings et al. 1978; Talbot 1980; Reddy 1981b). Thus, the association of dietary fat with bile acid excretion and composition has suggested that there might be a relationship between fat, bile acids, and cancer risk. Recent studies have shown that *total* fat rather than the *type* of fat (saturated vs. unsaturated) is the important factor for the colon cancer–fat relationship (Connor et al. 1969; Brussard et al. 1983). From the data available, it can be postulated that a reduction in fat intake will lower the excretion of fecal bile acids; the hypothetical deleterious effects of the bile acids (if any) on the colonic mucosa over the life span of the individual will subsequently be reduced.

Bile Acids and Dietary Fiber. In contrast to fat, increased amounts of dietary fiber have been suggested as having beneficial effects, either by diluting the luminal contents or by binding compounds such as bile acids or carcinogens. For example, rural third world populations have a low colon cancer incidence; these populations consume high-fiber, low-fat diets and excrete less bile acids compared to populations consuming the typical Western-style diet. Rural Finnish populations, also having low colorectal cancer rates, have a high intake of high-fiber cereal products compared to subjects in New York consuming a Western diet; the Finnish population also has a reduced fecal bile acid excretion (Reddy et al. 1978). Further, Seventh Day Adventists, who consume vegetarian diets, also reportedly have a low rate for colon cancer (Phillips 1975). The mode of action of fiber on lowering colon cancer incidence remains unknown; however, dietary fiber may be beneficial to the Western population in general if indeed it reduces the incidence of colon cancer over time.

Bile Acids and Cholecystectomy. Factors which increase fecal bile acid excretion are believed to increase the risk of colon cancer. Removal of the gallbladder by cholecystectomy results in increased enterohepatic recycling and increased secretion of total and secondary bile acids; in other words, cholecystectomy increases the exposure of the intestinal lumen and intestinal bacteria to bile acids (Almond et al. 1973; Malagelada et al. 1973; Hepner et al. 1974). Studies have been performed to evaluate whether cholecystectomy increases the risk for colorectal cancer. Cholecystectomy did not increase the incidence of DMH-induced colon cancer in mice or alter the type of cancer or benign tumor which arose (Schattenkerk et al. 1980). Several case control studies showed an increased risk of colonic cancer after cholecystectomy (Vernick et al. 1980; Vernick and Kuller 1981; Turunen and Kivilaakso 1981; Alley and Lee 1983), especially in the proximal colon. However, other studies could not support these findings (Abrams et al. 1983; Narisawa et al. 1983; Blanco et al. 1984). To date, the available data do not support a firm conclusion on the relationship of cholecystectomy to colon cancer. It is possible that a relationship between cholecystectomy and colonic cancer exists due to some common factors such as increased exposure of the primary bile acid pool to the bacterial flora as well as increased formation of secondary bile acids (Lowenfels 1980).

Conclusions and Future Directions

Epidemiology has shown a significant correlation between colon cancer risk and fecal bile acid excretion, yet a clear, definitive relationship between the two has not yet emerged. It is difficult to transfer results of animal studies to the human situation. Nevertheless, most studies show that the tumor-promoting effects of bile acids are related to their effects on cell turnover. Factors which reduce turnover are beneficial, those which increase it appear harmful. Whether bile acids definitely alter the course of colonic neoplasia must await further study.

Acknowledgements. The authors wish to thank Dr. Erwin H. Mosbach for critically reviewing the chapter. This work was supported in part by USPHS grants CA 08748 from the National Cancer Institute and CA 26674 from the National Cancer Institute through the National Large Bowel Cancer Project (E. E. Deschner), and grant HL 24061 from the National Heart, Lung, and Blood Institute (E. H. Mosbach).

References

Abrams JS, Anton JR, Dreyfuss DC (1983) The absence of a relationship between cholecystectomy and the subsequent occurrence of cancer of the proximal colon. Dis Colon Rectum 26:141–144

Albert MB, Fromm H (1987) Inflammatory bowel disease and bile acids: what are the connections? Gastroenterology 93: 207–208

Alley PG, Lee SP (1983) The increased risk of proximal colonic cancer after cholecystectomy. Dis Colon Rectum 26: 522–524

Almond HR, Vlahcevic ZR, Bell CC, Gregory DH, Swell L (1973) Bile acid pools, kinetics and biliary lipid composition before and after cholecystectomy. N Engl J Med 289: 1213–1216

Ames BN, McCann J, Yamaski E (1975) Methods for detecting carcinogens and mutagens with the Salmonella mammalian microsome mutagenicity test. Mutat Res 31: 347–364

Aries V, Crowther JS, Drasar BS, Hill MJ, Williams REO (1969) Bacteria and etiology of cancer of the large bowel. Gut 10: 334–335

Armstrong B, Doll R (1975) Environmental factors and cancer incidence and mortality in different countries, with special reference to dietary practices. Int J Cancer 15: 617–631

Armstrong MJ, Carey MC (1982) The hydrophobic-hydrophilic balance of bile salts. Inverse correlation between reverse-phase high performance liquid chromatographic mobilities and micellar cholesterol-solubilizing capacities. J Lipid Res 23: 70–80

Autrup H, Stoner GD, Jackson F, Shamsuddin AKM, Barrett LA, Trump BF (1978) Explant culture of rat colons: a model system for studying metabolism of chemical carcinogens. In Vitro 14: 868–877

Bauer HG, Asp NG, Dahlquist A, Fredlund PE, Wyman M, Oste R (1981) Effect of two kinds of pectin and guar gum on 1,2-dimethylhydrazine initiation of colon tumors and on fecal β-glucuronidase activity in the rat. Cancer Res 41: 2518–2523

Bell GD, Whitney B, Dowling RH (1972) Gallstone dissolution in man using chenodeoxycholic acid. Lancet 2: 1213–1216

Bergstrom S, Danielsson H (1968) Formation and metabolism of bile acids. In: Code CF (ed) Handbook of physiology, sec 6, vol V. American Physiological Society, Washington, pp 2391–2407

Bird RP, Mercer NJH, Draper HH (1985) Animal models for the study of nutrition and human disease: colon cancer, atherosclerosis and osteoporosis. Adv Nutr Res 7: 155–186

Blanco D, Ross RK, Paganini-Hill A, Henderson BE (1984) Cholecystectomy and colonic cancer. Dis Colon Rectum 27: 290–292

Bone E, Drasar BS, Hill MJ (1975) Gut bacteria and their metabolic activities in familial polyposis. Lancet 1: 1117–1120

Brussard JH, Katan MB, Hautvast JGAJ (1983) Fecal excretion of bile acids and neutral steroid on diets differing in type and amount of dietary fat in young healthy persons. Eur J Clin Invest 13: 115–122

Bull AW, Soullier BK, Wilson PS, Hayden MT, Nigro ND (1979) Promotion of azoxymethane-induced intestinal cancer by high fat diets in rats. Cancer Res 39: 4956–4959

Carey MC (1982) The enterohepatic circulation. In: Arias I, Popper H, Schachter D, Shafritz DA (eds) The liver: biology and pathobiology. Raven, New York, pp 429–465

Carroll KK, Khor HT (1975) Dietary fat in relation to tumorigenesis. Prog Biochem Pharmacol 10: 308–353

Chomchai C, Bhadrachari N, Nigro ND (1974) The effect of bile on the induction of experimental intestinal tumors in rats. Dis Colon Rectum 17: 310–312

Cohen BI, Mosbach EH (1985) The role of bile acids in colon cancer. In: Vahouny G, Kritchevsky D (eds) Basic and clinical aspects of dietary fiber. Plenum, New York, pp 487–496

Cohen BI, Raicht RF, Deschner EE, Takahashi M, Sarwal AN, Fazzini E (1980) Effect of cholic acid feeding on N-methyl-N-nitrosourea-induced colon tumors and cell kinetics in rats. J Natl Cancer Inst 64: 573–578

Connor WE, Witiak DT, Stone DB, Armstrong ML (1969) Cholesterol balance and fecal neutral steroid and bile acid excretion in normal men fed dietary fats of different fatty acid composition. J Clin Invest 48: 1363–1375

Correa P, Haenszel W (1978) The epidemiology of large-bowel cancer. Adv Cancer Res 26: 1–141

Cruse JP, Lewin MR, Clark CG (1981a) The effects of cholic acid and bile salt binding agents on 1,2-dimethylhydrazine-induced colon carcinogenesis in the rat. Carcinogenesis 2: 439–443

Cruse JP, Lewin MR, Ferulano GP, Clark CG (1981b) Experimental evidence against the bile salt theory of colon carcinogenesis. Eur Surg Res 13: 117–124

Cummings JH, Wiggins HS, Jenkins DJA, Houston H, Jivraj T, Drasar BS, Hill MJ (1978) Influence of diets high and low in animal fat on bowel habit, gastrointestinal transit time, fecal microflora, bile acid and fat excretion. J Clin Invest 61:953–963

Cummings JH, Hill MJ, Jivraj T, Houston H, Branch WJ, Jenkins DJA (1979) The effect of meat protein and dietary fiber on colonic function and metabolism. I. Changes in bowel habit, bile acid excretion and calcium absorption. Am J Clin Nutr 32:2086–2093

Dales LG, Friedman GD, Ury HK, Thistle JL (1979) A case-control study of relationships of diet and other traits to colorectal cancer in American Blacks. Am J Epidemiol 109:132–144

Danzinger RG, Hofmann AF, Schoenfield LJ, Thistle JL (1972) Dissolution of cholesterol gallstones by chenodeoxycholic acid. N Engl J Med 286:1–8

Deschner EE, Cohen BI, Raicht RF (1981) The acute and chronic effect of dietary cholic acid on colonic epithelial cell proliferation. Digestion 21:290–296

Dowling RH (1977) Chenodeoxycholic acid therapy of gallstones. Clin Gastroenterol 6: 141–163

Fath RB, Deschner EE, Winawer SJ, Dworkin B (1984) Degraded carrageenan-induced colitis in CF1 mice: a clinical, histopathological and kinetic analysis. Digestion 29:197–203

Gelb AM, McSherry CK, Sadowsky JR, Mosbach EH (1982) Tissue bile acids in patients with colon cancer and colonic polyps. Am J Gastroenterol 77:314–317

Glauert HP, Bennink MR, Sander CH (1981) Enhancement of 1,2-dimethylhydrazine induced colon carcinogenesis in mice by dietary agar. Food Cosmet Toxicol 19:281–286

Gustafsson BE (1982) The physiological importance of the colonic microflora. Scand J Gastroenterol [Suppl] 77:117–131

Haenszel W, Locke FB, Segi M (1980) A case-control study of large bowel cancer in Japan. J Natl Cancer Inst 64:17–22

Hepner GW, Hofmann AF, Malagelada JR, Szczepanik PA, Klein PD (1974) Increased bacterial degradation of bile in acids in cholecystectomized patients. Gastroenterology 66:556–564

Hill MJ (1975) Metabolic epidemiology of dietary factors in large bowel cancer. Cancer Res 35:3398–3402

Hill MJ (1981) Metabolic epidemiology of large bowel cancer. In: De Cosse J, Sherlock P (eds) Gastrointestinal cancer. Nijhoff, The Hague, pp 187–226

Hill MJ, Morson BC, Bussey HJR (1978) Etiology of adenoma-carcinoma sequence in large bowel. Lancet 1:245–247

Hill MJ, Morson BC, Thompson MH (1983) The role of fecal bile acids (FBA) in large bowel carcinogenesis. Br J Cancer 48:143

Hofmann AF (1977) The enterohepatic circulation of bile acids in man. Clin Gastroenterol 6:3–24

Hofmann AF (1984) Chemistry and enterohepatic circulation of bile acids. Hepatology 4:4S–15S

Hofmann AF, Roda A (1984) Physicochemical properties of bile acids and their relationship to biological properties: an overview of the problem. J Lipid Res 25:1477–1489

Hofmann AF, Molino G, Milanese M, Belforte G (1983) Description and simulation of a physiological pharmacokinetic model for the metabolism and enterohepatic circulation of bile acids in man. Cholic acid in healthy man. J Clin Invest 71:1003–1022

Hylemon PB, Glass TL (1983) Biotransformation of bile acids and cholesterol by the intestinal microflora. In: Hentzes DJ (ed) Human intestinal microflora in health and disease. Academic New York, pp 189–213

Iser JH, Sali A (1981) Chenodeoxycholic acid: a review of its pharmacological properties and therapeutic use. Drugs 21:90–119

Jacobs LR (1983) Enhancement of rat colon carcinogenesis by wheat bran consumption during the stage of 1,2-dimethylhydrazine administration. Cancer Res 43:4057–4061

Jacobs LR, Lupton JR (1986) Relationship between colonic luminal pH, cell proliferation, and colon carcinogenesis in 1,2-dimethylhydrazine treated rats fed high fat diets. Cancer Res 46:1727–1734

Jain M, Cook GM, Davis FG, Grace MG, Howe GR, Miller AB (1980) A case-control study of diet and colo-rectal cancer. Int J Cancer 26:757–768

Jensen OM, MacLennan R, Wahrendorf J (1982) Diet, bowel function, faecal characteristics and large bowel cancer in Denmark and Finland. Nutr Cancer 4:5–19

Kaur AP, Bhat CM, Grewal RS (1985) Effect of cellulose incorporation in a low fiber diet on fecal excretion and digestability of nutrients in adolescent girls. Nutr Rep Int 32:383–388

Kelsey MI (1983) In vitro effects of bile acids. In: Autrup H, Williams GM (eds) Experimental colon carcinogenesis. CRC, Boca Raton, pp 241–253

Kern F, Birkner HJ, Ostrower VS (1979) Binding of the bile acids by dietary fiber. Am J Clin Nutr 31:S175–S179

Kirby RW, Anderson JW, Sieling B, Rees ED, Chen WJL, Miller RE, Kay RM (1981) Oat bran intake selectively lowers serum low density lipoprotein concentrations of hypercholestero-lemic men. J Clin Nutr 34:824–829

Kritchevsky D, Nair PP (1971) Chemistry of the bile acids. In: Nair PP, Kritchevsky D (eds) The bile acids. Plenum, New York, pp 1–10

Lack L, Weiner IM (1963) Intestinal absorption of bile salts and some biological implications. Gastroenterology 22:1334–1338

LaMont JF, O'Gorman TA (1978) Experimental colon cancer. Gastroenterology 75:1157–1196

Lingeman CH, Garner FM, Colonel VC (1972) Comparative study of intestinal adenocarci-nomas of animals and man. J Natl Cancer Inst 48:325–346

Lowenfels AB (1980) Epidemiology: gallstones and the risk of cancer. Gut 21:1090–1092

Macdonald IA, Bokkenheuser VD, Winter J, McLernon AM, Mosbach EH (1983) Degradation of sterols in the human gut. J Lipid Res 24:675–700

Mak KM, Chang WW (1978) Inhibition of DNA synthesis by 1,2-dimethylhydrazine and methylazoxymethanol acetate in rabbit colon mucosa in organ culture. J Natl Cancer Inst 61:799–805

Malagelada JR, Go VLW, Summerkill WHJ, Gamble WS (1973) Bile acid secretion and biliary bile acid composition altered by cholecystectomy. Dig Dis Sci 18:455–459

Mastromarino AJ, Reddy BS, Wynder EL (1978) Fecal profiles of anaerobic microflora of large bowel cancer patients and patients with nonhereditary large bowel polyps. Cancer Res 38:4459–4462

McCay PB (1983) Dietary fat and cancer – an overview. In: Roe D (ed) Diet, nutrition and cancer: from basic research to policy implications. Liss, New York, pp 7–17

McKillip CA, Owens RW, Bilton RF, Haslan EA (1983) Mutagenicity testing of steroids obtained from bile acid and cholesterol. Carcinogenesis 4:1179–1183

Moskovitz M, White C, Barnett RN, Stevens S, Russell E, Vargo D, Flock MH (1979) Diet, fecal bile acids, and neutral sterols in carcinoma of the colon. Dig Dis Sci 24:746–751

Mudd DG, McKelvey STD, Norwood W, Elmore DT, Roy AD (1980) Fecal bile acid concen-trations of patients with carcinoma or increased risk of carcinoma in the large bowel. Gut 21:587–590

Nair PP, Mendeloff AI, Vocci M, Bankoski J, Gorelik M, Herman G, Plapinger R (1977) Lithocholic acid in human liver: identification of ε-lithocholyl lysine in tissue protein. Lipids 12:922–929

Nair PP, Solomon R, Bankoski J, Plapinger R (1978) Bile acids in tissues: binding of lithocholic acid to protein. Lipids 13:966–970

Narisawa T, Magadia NE, Weisburger JH, Wynder EL (1974) Promoting effect of bile acid on colon carcinogenesis after intrarectal instillation of MNNG in rat. J Natl Cancer Inst 53:1093–1097

Narisawa T, Sano M, Sato M, Takahashi T, Arakawa H (1983) Relationship between chole-cystectomy and colonic cancer in low-risk Japanese population. A preliminary study. Dis Colon Rectum 26:512–515

NCI (1985) Diet and colon cancer: integration of the descriptive analytic, and metabolic epi-demiology. NCI Monogr 69:223–228

Newmark RL, Wargovich MJ, Bruce WR (1984) Colon cancer and dietary fat, phosphate, and calcium: a hypothesis. J Natl Cancer Inst 72:1323–1325

Nigro ND, Bull AW (1983) The two-step concept of intestinal carcinogenesis. In: Autrup H, Williams GM (eds) Experimental colon carcinogenesis. CRC, Boca Raton, pp 215–224

Nigro ND, Bhadrachari N, Chomchai C (1973) A rat model for studying colonic cancer: effect of cholestyramine on induced tumors. Dis Colon Rectum 16:438–443

Owen RW, Dodo M, Thompson MH, Hill MJ (1983) The fecal ratio of lithocholic acid to deoxycholic acid may be an important etiological factor in colorectal cancer. Eur J Cancer Clin Oncol 19:1307

Phillips R (1975) Role of life-style and dietary habits in risk of cancer among Seventh-Day Adventists. Cancer Res 35: 3513–3522

Pitot HC (1983) Contribution to our understanding of the natural history of neoplastic development in lower animals to the cause and control of human cancer. Cancer Surv 2: 519–537

Potter JD, McMichael AJ (1986) Diet and cancer of the colon and rectum. A case control study. J Natl Cancer Inst 76: 557–569

Reddy BS (1981a) Dietary fat and its relationship to large bowel cancer. Cancer Res 41: 3700–3705

Reddy BS (1981b) Diet and excretion of bile acids. Cancer Res 41: 3766–3768

Reddy BS (1983) Dietary fat and colon cancer. In: Autrup H, William GM (eds) Experimental colon carcinogenesis. CRC, Boca Raton, pp 225–239

Reddy BS, Ohmori T (1981) Effect of intestinal microflora and dietary fat on 3,2′-dimethyl-4-aminobiphenyl-induced colon carcinogenesis in F344 rats. Cancer Res 41: 1363–1367

Reddy BS, Watanabe K (1979) Effect of cholesterol metabolites and promoting effect of lithocholic acid in colon carcinogenesis in germfree and conventional F344 rats. Cancer Res 39: 1521–1524

Reddy BS, Wynder EL (1977) Metabolic epidemiology of colon cancer: fecal bile acids and neutral sterols in colon cancer patients and patients with adenomatous polyps. Cancer 39: 2533–2539

Reddy BS, Narisawa T, Maronpot R, Weisburger JH, Wynder EL (1975a) Animal models for the study of dietary factors and cancer of the large bowel. Cancer Res 35: 3421–3426

Reddy BS, Weisburger JH, Wynder EL (1975b) Effects of high risk and low risk diets for colon carcinogenesis on fecal microflora and steroids in man. J Nutr 105: 878–884

Reddy BS, Mastromarino A, Gustafson C, Lipkin M, Wynder EL (1976a) Fecal bile acids and neutral sterols in patients with familial polyposis. Cancer 38: 1694–1698

Reddy BS, Narisawa T, Weisburger JH, Wynder EL (1976b) Promoting effect of sodium deoxycholate on colonic adenocarcinomas in germfree rats. J Natl Cancer Inst 56: 441–442

Reddy BS, Mangat S, Weisburger JH, Wynder EL (1977a) Effect of high-risk diets for colon carcinogenesis or intestinal mucosal and bacterial β-glucuronidase activity in F344 rats. Cancer Res 37: 3533–3536

Reddy BS, Martin CW, Wynder EL (1977b) Fecal bile acids and cholesterol metabolites of patients with ulcerative colitis, a high risk group for development of colon cancer. Cancer Res 37: 1697–1701

Reddy BS, Watanabe K, Weisburger JH, Wynder EL (1977c) Promoting effect of bile acids in colon carcinogenesis in germfree and conventional F344 rats. Cancer Res 37: 3238–3242

Reddy BS, Hedges AR, Laakso K, Wynder EL (1978) Metabolic epidemiology of large bowel cancer, fecal bulk and constituents of high-risk North American and low-risk Finnish populations. Cancer 42: 2832–2838

Reddy BS, Cohen L, McCoy GD, Hill P, Weisburger JH, Wynder EL (1980a) Nutrition and its relationship to cancer. In: Klein G, Weinhouse S (eds) Advances in cancer research. Academic, New York, pp 237–345

Reddy BS, Sharma C, Darby L, Laakso K, Wynder EL (1980b) Metabolic epidemiology of large bowel cancer: fecal mutagens in high- and low-risk populations for colon cancer. A preliminary report. Mutat Res 72: 511–522

Reddy BS, Maeura Y, Wayman M (1983) Effect of dietary corn bran and autohydrolyzed lignin on 3,2-dimethyl-4-aminobiphenyl-induced intestinal carcinogenesis in male F344 rats. J Natl Cancer Inst 71: 419–423

Reiss B, Williams GM (1979) Conditions affecting prolonged maintenance of mouse and rat colon in organ culture. In Vitro 15: 877–890

Reiss B, Telang NT, Williams GM (1982) The application of organ culture to the study of colon carcinogenesis. In: Autrup H, Williams GM (eds) Experimental colon carcinogenesis. CRC, Boca Raton, pp 83–94

Reiss B, Weiss CJ, Tanaka T, Reddy B, Williams GM (1987) Effects of bile acids on carcinogen-exposed rat colon in organ culture and as subsequent long-term transplants. J Natl Cancer Inst 78: 107–113

Sarwal AN, Cohen BI, Raicht RF, Takahashi M, Fazzini E (1979) Effects of dietary administration of chenodeoxycholic acid on N-methyl-N-nitrosourea-induced colon cancer in rats. Biochim Biophys Acta 574: 423–432

Schattenkerk ME, Li AC, Jeppsson BW, Eggink WF, Jamieson CG, Ross JS, Matt RA (1980) Cholecystectomy has no influence on frequency of chemically induced colon cancer in mice. Br J Cancer 42:791–793

Shamsuddin AKM (1983) In vivo induction of colon cancer, dose and animal species. In: Autrup H, Williams GM (eds) Experimental colon carcinogenesis. CRC, Boca Raton, pp 51–62

Talbot JM (1980) The role of dietary fiber in diverticular disease. Fed Am Soc Exp Biol, Bethesda, MD

Turjman N, Nair PP (1981) Nature of tissue-bound lithocholic acid and its implications on the role of bile acids in carcinogenesis. Cancer Res 41:3761–3763

Turunen MJ, Kivilaakso EO (1981) Increased risk of colorectal cancer after cholecystectomy. Ann Surg 194:639–641

Vernick LJ, Kuller LH (1981) Cholecystectomy and right-sided colon cancer: an epidemiological study. Lancet 2:381–383

Vernick LJ, Kuller LH, Lohsoonthorn P, Rycheck RR, Redmond CK (1980) Relationship between cholecystectomy and ascending colon cancer. Cancer 45:392–395

Wargovich MJ, Eng VW, Newmark HL, Bruce WR (1983) Calcium ameliorates the toxic effect in deoxycholic acid on colonic epithelium. Carcinogenesis 4:1205–1207

Watabe J, Bernstein H (1985) The mutagenicity of bile acids using a fluctuation test. Mutat Res 158:45–51

Weisburger JH (1971) Colon carcinogens: their metabolism and mode of action. Cancer 28:60–70

Weisburger JH, Fiala ES (1983) Experimental colon carcinogens and their mode of action. In: Autrup H, Williams GM (eds) Experimental colon carcinogenesis. CRC, Boca Raton, pp 27–50

Weisburger JH, Reddy BS, Springarn NE, Wynder EL (1980) Current views on the mechanisms involved in the etiology of colorectal cancer. In: Winawer S, Schottenfeld D, Sherlock P (eds) Colorectal cancer: prevention, epidemiology and screening. Raven, New York, pp 19–42

Wilpart M, Mainguet P, Maskens A, Roberfroid M (1983) Mutagenicity of 1,2-dimethylhydrazine towards *Salmonella typhimurium,* co-mutagenic effect of secondary biliary acids. Carcinogenesis 4:45–58

Zaridze DG (1983) Environmental etiology of large bowel cancer (Guest editorial). J Natl Cancer Inst 70:389–400

Dietary Fiber, Fiber-Containing Foods, and Colon Cancer Risk

L. R. Jacobs

Section of Nutrition, Division of Gastroenterology, Cedars-Sinai Medical Center, 8700 Beverly
Boulevard, Los Angeles, California 90048, USA

Contents

Diet and Cancer Risk

A number of national agencies, many of which are involved in formulating public
health policy, have recommended major increases in the consumption of dietary fiber.
Among the justifications used for such recommendations is that this will help inhibit
the development of colorectal cancer. Some agencies have even attempted to "identify" the type and level of fiber that is anticarcinogenic. However, such health claims
are, in the opinion of this author, premature since the human data on dietary fiber
and cancer is at best circumstantial and certainly not consistent. There are many
studies in both humans and experimental animals that show no protective effect with
fiber, while several reports even indicate an enhancing effect. It is therefore important
to evaluate critically the scientific evidence both for and against the dietary fiber
hypothesis. For some investigators working in this area of cancer control, the fiber
question has almost become a religious issue with believers and skeptics. Unfortunately, this has led to a politicization of the issues and a certain lack of objectivity

in interpretation of the data. This situation has been further complicated by commercial pressures to eat more fiber, the supplementation of prepared foods with fibers, and by aggressive advertising of fiber supplements to the medical profession and general public.

The Fiber Hypothesis

The perception that dietary fiber is important in maintaining intestinal health goes back many years. Hippocrates noted that "wholemeal bread cleans out the gut and passes through as excrement, while white bread is more nutritious, as it makes less feces." Curiously much of the recent research in dietary fiber has been devoted to confirming these early observations. The work of Cleave (1956) rekindled interest in the relationships between dietary fiber, human health, and disease. Subsequently Burkitt (1971) and Trowell (1976) proposed a more specific role for dietary fiber in the prevention of various modern-day diseases, including colorectal cancer. Much of the early fiber research was confounded by the lack of a widely accepted definition of what constitutes dietary fiber and by a lack of simple, reproducible analytic methods to measure total dietary fiber.

Definitions of Dietary Fiber

A recent definition used by the United States Expert Panel on Dietary Fiber (Pilch 1987) is that dietary fibers are the endogenous components of plant materials in the diet which are resistant to digestion by enzymes produced by humans. Analytically dietary fiber is predominantly nonstarch polysaccharide and lignin. This analytical definition encompasses a variety of isolated polysaccharide-rich, plant-derived products, which may or may not be chemically modified, including brans, pectins, and gums. This definition excludes other substances in the plant wall such as phytates, cutins, saponins, lectins, proteins, waxes, silicon, and other organic constituents. Nonstarch polysaccharides include cellulosic and noncellulosic polysaccharides (hemicellulose, pectin, and other polysaccharides). Furthermore, it has been helpful, when studying the effects of dietary fibers on the upper gastrointestinal tract, to classify fibers as being either water soluble or insoluble. However, when considering the influence of fibers on the large bowel, the classification of "fermentable" (metabolized by colonic bacteria) and "nonfermentable" will probably be more useful.

Human Studies

The ideal way to prove that dietary fiber prevents colon cancer is to perform a prospective, randomized, controlled clinical trial. Ideally such a study should measure the effect of the intervention (a high-fiber diet) on disease outcome (development of colonic cancer). Such a study has at this time not been reported. Short of this, the next best design would be to measure the effect of high-fiber diets on predictors of colon carcinogenesis. Unfortunately, there are currently no available biological markers that can accurately predict colon risk. However, metabolic epidemiology studies provide a suggestion of what the outcomes of a dietary intervention are likely to be (see Metabolic Epidemiology).

Ecological (Correlational) Studies

Tables 1 and 2 summarize the results from 21 publications of which 13 (61.9%) show evidence consistent with a protective effect of fiber-containing foods. However, it should be pointed out that many of these reports use the same data set, i.e., Food and Agriculture Organization (FAO) food availability data and international cancer mortality rates. The older international studies are based on intake of crude fiber, which greatly underestimates total dietary fiber levels. However, crude and dietary fiber are highly correlated (Pilch 1987). It is nevertheless scientifically unsound to draw causal inferences from ecological studies, leading to the "ecological fallacy," in which an unmeasured confounding factor may be responsible for the association observed. For example, total caloric intake or the amount and type of dietary fat may be key determinants of cancer risk and could therefore confound the relationship between colon cancer and dietary fiber. Dietary fat is strongly inversely correlated with dietary fiber. Needless to say, the ecological correlation studies do not control for other dietary variables or for any of the other known risk factors associated with colon cancer.

Table 1. Ecological studies of dietary fiber, fiber-containing foods, and colon cancer risk (1973–1979)

Reference	Geographic location	Groups compared	Measure of dietary fiber	Association
Drasar and Irving (1973)	International	37 Countries	Crude fiber	None
Irving and Drasar (1973)	International	37 Countries	Cereals	Protective
Howell (1975)	International	37 Countries	Cereals, pulses	Protective
Armstrong and Doll (1975)	International	32 Countries	Cereals	Protective
Schrauzer (1976)	International	17 Countries	Cereals	Protective
International Agency for Research on Cancer, Intestinal Microecology Group (1977)	Finland, Denmark	Two Countries	Dietary fiber	Protective
Knox (1977)	International	20 Countries	Fruits, vegetables, wheat	Protective
Lyon and Sorenson (1978)	Utah, USA	One state vs. USA	Crude fiber	None
Hill et al. (1979)	Hong Kong	Three socio-economic groups	Fiber-rich foods	Risk-enhancing
Bingham et al. (1979)	United Kingdom	Nine regions	Dietary fiber Pentoses Vegetables	None Protective Protective
Liu et al. (1979)	International	20 Countries	Sum of fruits, vegetables, legumes, grains	Protective

Table 2. Ecological studies of dietary fiber, fiber-containing foods, and colon cancer risk (1980–1987)

Reference	Geographic location	Groups compared	Measure of dietary fiber	Association
Enstrom (1980)	California, Washington (Mormons)	Two states vs. USA	Fruits, vegetables	Protective Protective
Rozen et al. (1981)	Israel	Two regions	Crude fiber	Protective
Englyst et al. (1982)	Finland, Denmark	Four regions	Nonstarch polysaccharides	Protective
Helms et al. (1982)	Denmark	Two regions	Dietary fiber	None
Minowa et al. (1983)	Japan, Britain	Two countries	Dietary fiber	None
McKeown-Eyssen and Bright-See (1984)	International	38 countries	Fruit, vegetables Legumes, cereals	None Protective
Bingham et al. (1985)	United Kingdom	Nine regions	Pentoses Nonstarch polysaccharides	None Protective
Walker et al. (1986)	South Africa	Five racial-ethnic groups	Dietary fiber	None
Kuratsune et al. (1986)	Japan, England, Denmark	Three countries	Nonstarch polysaccharides	None
Rozen et al. (1987)	Israel	Three regions	Dietary fiber	None

For a detailed discussion of the numerous sources of error in such studies, the reader is referred elsewhere (Byers and Graham 1984; Morgenstern 1982; Lyon et al. 1983; Pilch 1987). Correlation studies use mortality rates to assess disease frequency, an insensitive measure since many subjects with this disease are cured and do not die from the cancer. The mortality from colorectal cancer in the United States is approximately 1 in 37 or 2.6% of all cancer deaths (Doll and Peto 1981). Similarly, the dietary data are obtained from populations the majority of which do not have and will not develop large bowel cancer. It is estimated that about 5% of the population in the United States will develop colorectal cancer. Another approach that attempts to circumvent some of these problems is the case-control study.

Case-Control Studies

As with the ecological studies, the case-control design is also retrospective. In general, the approach has been to determine the diet of colon cancer cases and to compare this with an appropriate control population. This assumes that recent dietary patterns are similar to those in the past and that recall is accurate. Although colorectal cancer occurs more frequently in the elderly, there is no data indicating that this is the result of environmental changes occurring late in life. In fact, it is likely that there is a long latency period between initiation, promotion, and the ultimate clinical expression of a tumor. This suggests that dietary patterns in childhood, adolescence, and early adulthood may be relevant to cancer risk. Certainly, once patients develop cancer, their dietary habits can change dramatically.

Nevertheless, these and other criticisms notwithstanding, there have been numerous case-control studies which are summarized in Tables 3 and 4. Of the 23 studies listed, 11 (48%) provide evidence for protection, nine (39%) show no effect, and four studies demonstrate evidence of risk enhancement. Compared with the ecological (correlation) studies, the case-control studies demonstrate no evidence of protection in the majority of cases and in 17% of reports there is evidence of risk enhancement. Frequently cited criticisms of case-control studies are that there are large errors in the measurements of nutrient intake and that the variability of fiber consumption in a given population is too small to demonstrate the fiber–colon cancer relationships observed in the international correlation studies. These criticisms are inherently weak since individual nutrient intake histories and measurements have been validated, are reproducible, and demonstrate differences in the intake of calories, fats, and other components.

All of these studies deal with the intake of fiber-containing foods since this is the usual source of dietary fiber. Thus, even in those studies showing a "protective" effect, it cannot be concluded that this is due exclusively to the fiber content of these foods, or whether the "protective factor" is some other component of fiber-containing foods. Eight studies associate vegetable intake with lower cancer risk. The cruciferous group of vegetables including cabbage, spinach, broccoli, and Brussels sprouts, as well as lettuce, have all been specifically identified with reduced colon cancer risk. This had led to the suggestion that a nonfiber component of vegetables, e.g., indoles, are antineoplastic. However, in animal studies, such compounds appear to be co-carcinogenic (Pence et al. 1986), while the feeding of cabbage actually enhances experimental colon carcinogenesis (Temple and El-Khatib 1987).

Table 3. Case-control studies of dietary fiber, fiber-containing foods, and colon cancer risk (1933–1979)

Reference	Geographic location	Size of study cases:controls	Measured of dietary fiber	Association
Stocks and Karn (1933)	United Kingdom	450:450	Whole-grain breads, vegetables	Protective
Higginson (1966)	Kansas, USA	340:1020	Fruits, cereals	None
Wynder and Shigematsu (1967)	New York City	791:309	Fruits, cereals, vegetables	None
Wynder et al. (1969)	Japan	69:307	Fruits, vegetables	None
Haenszel et al. (1973)	Hawaii	179:357	Vegetables, cereals	Risk-enhancing
Bjelke (1974a)	Norway	278:1394	Vegetables	Protective
Bjelke (1974b)	Minnesota, USA	373:1657	Vegetables	Protective
Modan et al. (1975)	Israel	198:396	Vegetables, fruit	Protective
Phillips (1975)	California, USA	41:123	High-fiber foods	None
Graham et al. (1978)	New York, USA	330:783	Vegetables	None
Dales et al. (1979)	San Francisco, USA (Blacks)	72:202	High-fiber foods	None
Martinez et al. (1979)	Puerto Rico	461:461	Cereals, crude fiber	Protective

Table 4. Case-control studies of dietary fiber, fiber-containing foods, and colon cancer risk (1980–1987)

Reference	Geographic location	Size of study cases:controls	Measures of dietary fiber	Association
Haenszel et al. (1980)	Japan	588:1176	Vegetables, cereals	Protective Risk-enhancing
Jain et al. (1980)	Canada	348:542	Crude fiber	None
Manousos et al. (1983)	Greece	100:100	Vegetables, cereals, fruits	Protective
Pickle et al. (1984)	Nebraska, USA	86:176	High-fiber foods	None
Bristol et al. (1985)	England	50:50	Dietary fiber	None
Tajima and Tominaga (1985)	Japan	93:186	Vegetables	Risk-enhancing
Potter and McMichael (1986)	Australia	419:732	Dietary fiber	Risk-enhancing
Tuyns (1986)	Belgium	1207:3521	High-fiber foods	Protective
Macquart-Moulin et al. (1986)	France	399:399	Fruits, cereals Vegetables	None Protective
Lyon et al. (1987)	Utah, USA	246:484	Dietary fiber	Weakly protective
Kune et al. (1987)	Australia	715:727	Dietary fiber Vegetables Cereals	Protective Protective None

Table 5. Case-control studies of dietary fiber, fiber-containing foods, and colorectal polyps

Reference	Geographic location	Size of study cases:controls	Measure of dietary fiber	Association
Hoff et al. (1986)	Norway	78:77	Cruciferous vegetables, cereals	Protective None
Macquart-Moulin et al. (1987)	France	252:238	Vegetables, cereals Fruits	None Protective

Colonic adenomatous polyps are premalignant tumors that are known to develop into adenocarcinoma. Two case-control studies (Table 5) of colorectal polyps found that cruciferous vegetables and fruits were protective whereas cereals and vegetables were not.

Cohort (Prospective) Studies

Three prospective studies are summarized in Table 6. Although prospective studies require large numbers of subjects and take a long time, dietary intake may be measured more accurately. Two of the studies in Table 6 showed no protective effect of fiber-containing foods, while the third demonstrated protection with rice and wheat. Without any completed prospective intervention studies, the cohort studies come the

Table 6. Prospective cohort studies of dietary fiber, fiber-containing foods, and colon cancer

Reference	Geographic location	Size of study (n)	Measure of dietary fiber	Association
Hirayama (1981)	Japan	265,118	Vegetables	None
			Rice and wheat	Protective
Kromhout et al. (1982)	The Netherlands	871	Dietary fiber	None
Phillips and Snowdon (1985)	California, USA Seventh Day Adventists	25,493	Vegetables, cereals, fruits	None

closest to being able to answer the question of whether dietary fiber may inhibit colon carcinogenesis. To date the results are inconsistent and cast doubt on the validity of the original fiber hypothesis. However, it does seem possible that certain, but not all, fiber-containing foods have antineoplastic properties, which may well be independent of their fiber content.

Metabolic Epidemiology

It is widely believed that colorectal cancer is the end result of a multistep process (Farber 1984) in which abnormal colonic metabolism plays a major role. The initiating event, or the factor that damages colonic cell DNA in humans, has not been identified. However, mutagenic activity is present in human feces and can easily be measured using salmonella tester strains. Bruce (1987) and co-workers have identified the major fecal mutagens as fecapentaenes, ethers of glycerol, and unsaturated alcohols. These are produced by Bacteroides and may be reduced with the feeding of supplemental dietary fiber in the form of whole grain bread (Reddy et al. 1987). In a recent review of this topic, Bruce (1987) concluded, however, that the weight of evidence no longer supports an important role for the fecapentaenes in colon cancer causation.

Although the identity of the carcinogen that causes human colon cancer may still be in doubt, a number of potentially important promoters of colonic cancer have been identified. Bile acids have been shown to promote tumor development in animals (Weisburger et al. 1983). Bile acids that are not reabsorbed in the terminal ileum spill over into the large intestine where they are degraded into secondary bile acids by the colonic microflora. When present in high concentrations, secondary bile acids may damage the surface epithelium of the colon and increase epithelial cell proliferation and turnover. This stimulation of colonic cell proliferation is thought to promote tumor development by increasing the population of cells in DNA synthesis (Cohen et al. 1980). Cells that are actively synthesizing new DNA are more susceptible to mutation and subsequent malignant transformation. More recent studies demonstrate that bile acids may directly stimulate cell replication and DNA synthesis, possibly by increasing ornithine decarboxylase activity and the activation of protein kinase C (Craven et al. 1987).

In general, those fibers that increase fecal bulk will decrease fecal bile acid concentration (Reddy et al. 1987). A greater fecal bulk will frequently speed up transit rate, especially if it is already delayed. Thus, by increasing bulk and transit rate, certain fibers can reduce the concentration of and mucosal contact time with any carcinogens and tumor promoters present in the colonic contents. By the same rationale, any antineoplastic factors present in the colonic lumen would also be effectively diminished by fibers that increase fecal bulk and transit rate.

Animal Studies

The only controlled prospective studies on dietary fiber and colon cancer have been performed with animal models. Although questions have been raised about the relevance of such models to human colon cancer, the animal data have provided considerable new information which has raised important new questions regarding mechanisms of actions that are relevant to humans. The carcinogen that has been the most widely used is 1,2-dimethylhydrazine dihydrochloride (DMH). This is usually administered systematically, but can be given orally, following which it is metabolized to a DNA-methylating agent. Administration of this compound to rodents produces both benign adenomas and malignant carcinomas of the large bowel. Because of the large number of animal studies using defined fiber sources, it is now possible to analyze results according to the type of fiber fed. Wheat bran has been the most widely studied fiber supplement. Animal experiments using DMH are summarized in Table 7. Two out of three experiments using mice showed tumor enhancement with wheat bran (Clapp 1984), whereas in the studies with rats eight out of 13 experiments (61.5%)

Table 7. Dietary wheat bran and dimethylhydrazine-induced colon cancer

Animal	Strain	Sex	Bran (%)	Effect	Reference
Mice	CF$_1$	F	40	P	Chen et al. (1978)
	Balb/c	M	20 SWW	E	Clapp et al. (1984)
		M	20 HSW	E	Clapp et al. (1984)
Rats	Wistar	F	20	N	Cruse et al. (1978)
		M	3.8[a]	P	Kroes et al. (1986)
	Sprague-Dawley	F	20	N	Barbolt and Abraham (1980)
		M	20	P	Barbolt and Abraham (1980)
		M	20	P	Wilson et al. (1977)
		M	20	P	Barbolt and Abraham (1978)
		M	20	N	Bauer et al. (1979)[b]
		M	20	P	Abraham et al. (1980)
		M	20	E	Jacobs (1983)[b]
		M	20	P	Jacobs (1983)[c]
	Chester Beatty	M	28	P	Fleiszer et al. (1978)
	Fischer 344	M	20	P	Barnes et al. (1983)
	Fischer 344	M	15	E	Pence et al. (1986)

[a] g/100 kcal.
[b] Fiber fed before and during carcinogen teatment (initiation).
[c] Fiber fed after carcinogen treatment (promotion).
E, enhancement; P, protective; N, no effect; SWW, soft winter wheat; HSW, hard spring wheat.

Table 8. Dietary wheat bran and experimental colon cancer

Carcinogen	Animal	Strain	Sex	Bran (%)	Effect	Reference
Azoxymethane	Rats	Sprague-Dawley	M	10	N	Nigro et al. (1979)
			M	20	P	Nigro et al. (1979)
			M	30	P	Nigro et al. (1979)
		Fischer 344	F	15	P	Watanabe et al. (1979)
		Fischer 344	M	15	P	Reddy et al. (1981)
N-Methyl-N-nitrosourea	Rats	Fischer 344	F	15	N	Watanabe et al. (1979)
3,2'-Dimethyl-4-aminobiphenyl	Rats	Fischer 344	M	15	P	Reddy and Mori (1981)
N-Methyl-N'-nitro-N-nitrosoguanidine	Rats	Wistar	M	3.8 g/ 100 kcal	P	Kroes et al. (1986)

P, protective; N, no effect.

Table 9. Dietary brans and experimental colon cancer

Carcinogen	Animal	Strain	Sex	Bran	%	Effect	Reference
3,2'-Dimethyl-4-aminobiphenyl	Rats	Fischer 344	M	Corn	15	E	Reddy et al. (1983)
1,2-Dimethylhydrazine	Rats	Fischer 344	M	Corn	20	E	Barnes et al. (1983)
	Rats	Wistar	M	Corn	4.5	P	Freeman et al. (1984)
	Mice	Balb/c	M	Corn	20	E	Clapp et al. (1984)
	Rats	Fischer 344	M	Rice	20	N	Barnes et al. (1983)
	Rats	Fischer 344	M	Soybean	20	N	Barnes et al. (1983)
	Mice	Balb/c	M	Soybean	20	E	Clapp et al. (1984)
	Rats	Sprague-Dawley	M	Oat	20	E	Jacobs and Lupton (1986)

E, enhancement; P, protective; N, no effect.

showed evidence of protection against tumor induction. The effect of wheat bran on tumor induction using four other carcinogens are summarized in Table 8. With the carcinogen azoxymethane (AOM), a metabolite of DMH, four out of five experiments demonstrated evidence of protection against tumor development. On the other hand, using N-methyl-N-nitrosourea (MNU), a direct-acting carcinogen, no protective effect was seen, whereas with 3,2'-dimethyl-4-aminobiphenyl (DMAB) and N-methyl-N'-nitro-N-nitrosoguanidine (MNNG) there was evidence of protection. With MNNG, protection was only observed when fat intake was high (Kroes et al. 1986). In summary, it appears that in nearly two-thirds of experiments in which wheat bran was fed to rodents there was evidence of decreased tumor development.

It is of interest, however, that other forms of bran do not exhibit the same protective effect. As shown in Table 9, there are four published studies using corn bran, of which three-quarters show evidence of tumor enhancement when corn bran was fed at a 15%–20% level. On the other hand, rice and soybean bran had no effect in two rat experiments, whereas soybean bran enhanced tumor development in mice. In one study, a 20% oat bran diet enhanced tumor development in rats. The mechanisms by which certain types of cereal bran inhibit while others enhance tumorigenesis has been examined. Clapp et al. (1984) found a positive correlation between tumor incidence and the percentage of neutral detergent fiber in the brans, but not between the individual components of cellulose, hemicellulose, or lignin. Jacobs (1984) showed that dietary wheat bran stimulates colonic epithelial cell growth and, when fed only during the stage of carcinogen exposure, enhances tumor development (Jacobs 1983). Paradoxically, a wheat bran supplement was found to inhibit tumor development when fed only during the post-carcinogen exposure stage (Jacobs 1983). Tumor enhancement with oat bran was found to correlate with its pH-lowering effect, a measure of its fermentability, and not with any other cellular measurement (Jacobs and Lupton 1986).

Results using dietary cellulose are summarized in Table 10. When the carcinogen AOM was used, three out of six experiments (50%) showed evidence of protection while the remainder showed no effect. This was a slightly lower level of protection than that found with DMH, where five out of eight experiments (62.5%) showed evidence of protection. The experiments with wheat bran and cellulose suggest that the type of carcinogen used may determine whether a particular fiber inhibits tumorigenesis. Compared with wheat bran, cellulose appeared to be about equally protective.

The studies examining the effects of pectin on experimental colon cancer are summarized in Table 11. The one study in which the carcinogen AOM was used showed evidence of tumor protection, in contrast to those studies using DMH, where four out of six experiments showed evidence of tumor enhancement. When the

Table 10. Dietary cellulose and experimental colon cancer

Carcinogen	Animal	Strain	Sex	Fiber (%)	Effect	Reference
Azoxymethane	Rats	Fischer	M	20	N	Ward et al. (1973)
		Fischer	M	40	N	Ward et al. (1973)
		Sprague-Dawley	M	10	N	Nigro et al. (1979)
		Sprague-Dawley	M	20	P	Nigro et al. (1979)
		Sprague-Dawley	M	30	P	Nigro et al. (1979)
	Mice	Albino Swiss	M	26	P	Galloway et al. (1986)
1,2-Dimethyl-hydrazine	Rats	Wistar	M	4.5	P	Freeman et al. (1978)
		Wistar	M	4.5	P	Freeman et al. (1980)
		Wistar	M	9.0	P	Freeman et al. (1980)
		Wistar	M	5.0	N	Wilpart and Roberfroid (1987)
		Wistar	M	15	N	Wilpart and Roberfroid (1987)
		Sprague-Dawley	M	22	P	Trudel et al. (1983)
		Sprague-Dawley	M	10	N	Jacobs and Lupton (1986)
		Sprague-Dawley	M	10	P	Roberts-Andersen et al. (1987)

P, protective; N, no effect.

Table 11. Dietary pectin and experimental colon cancer

Carcinogen	Animal	Strain	Sex	Fiber (%)	Effect	Reference
Azoxymethane	Rats	Fischer 344	F	15	P	Watanabe et al. (1979)
1,2-Dimethyl-hydrazine	Rats	Sprague-Dawley	M	6.5	E	Bauer et al. (1979)
		Wistar	M	4.5	N	Freeman et al. (1980)
		Wistar	M	9.0	N	Freeman et al. (1980)
		Sprague-Dawley	M	5.0 HM	E	Bauer et al. (1981)
		Sprague-Dawley	M	5.0 LM	E	Bauer et al. (1981)
		Sprague-Dawley	M	10	E	Jacobs and Lupton (1986)
N-Methyl-N-nitrosourea	Rats	Fischer 344	F	15	N	Watanabe et al. (1979)

E, enhancement; P, protective; N, no effect; HM, high methoxylated; LM, low methoxylated.

Table 12. Miscellaneous dietary fibers and dimethylhydrazine-induced colon cancer

Animal	Strain	Sex	Fiber	%	Effect	Reference
Rats	Wistar	M	Fybogel	15	P	Wilpart and Roberfroid (1987)
	Sprague-Dawley	M	Carrot	20	N	Bauer et al. (1979)
	Sprague-Dawley	M	Seaweeds	0.05 −2	P	Yamamoto and Maruyama (1985)
	Sprague-Dawley	M	Psyllium husk	10	P	Roberts-Andersen et al. (1987)
	Sprague-Dawley	M	Guar gum	5	N	Bauer et al. (1981)
	Sprague-Dawley	M	Guar gum	10	E	Jacobs and Lupton (1986)
	Fischer 344	M	Konjac mannan	20	P	Mizutani and Mitsuoka (1983)
	Fischer 344	M	Carageenan	6	P	Arakawa et al. (1986)
Mice	CF$_1$	M	Agar	7	E	Glauert et al. (1981)
	CF$_1$	M	Agar	9	E	Glauert et al. (1981)
	Swiss, albino	M	Metamucil	20	E	Toth (1984)
	Swiss, albino	F	Metamucil	20	N	Toth (1984)
	Swiss	M	Cabbage	13	N	Temple and El-Khatib (1987)
	Swiss	F	Cabbage	13	E	Temple and El-Khatib (1987)

E, enhancement; P, protective; N, no effect; Metamucil, psyllium hydrophilic mucilloid; Fybogel, Mucillage from seed of *Ispaghula husk ex Plantago ovata Forsk*.

direct-acting carcinogen MNU was used, there was no modulation of tumor development.

The effect of miscellaneous fibers on DMH-induced colon cancer are summarized in Table 12. In rats, protective effects were reported with Fybogel, edible seaweeds, psyllium husk, Konjac mannan, and carageenan, but enhancement with 10% guar gum. In mice, tumor enhancement was observed with agar and cabbage. In a study by Toth (1984), Metamucil (psyllium hydrophilic mucilloid) decreased the tumor yield

Table 13. Miscellaneous dietary fibers and experimental colon cancer

Carcinogen	Strain of rat	Sex	Fiber	%	Effect	Reference
Azoxymethane	Fischer 344	F	Carageenan	15	E	Watanabe et al. (1978)
	Sprague-Dawley	M	Alfalfa	10	N	Nigro et al. (1979)
	Sprague-Dawley	M	Alfalfa	20	N	Nigro et al. (1979)
	Sprague-Dawley	M	Alfalfa	30	P	Nigro et al. (1979)
	Fischer 344	F	Alfalfa	15	N	Watanabe et al. (1979)
N-Methyl-N-nitrosourea	Fischer 344	F	Alfalfa	15	E	Watanabe et al. (1979)
3,2'-Dimethyl-4-aminobiphenyl	Fischer 344	M	Lignin	7.5	P	Reddy et al. (1983)

E, enhancement; P, protective; N, no effect.

in mice by more than 50% compared with controls, but this was greater than the expected number of tumors and therefore interpreted as tumor enhancement.

The effect of miscellaneous fibers on tumor induction, using carcinogens other than DMH, are summarized in Table 13. With AOM, undegraded carageenan produced tumor enhancement, whereas a high level of alfalfa showed protection. Using the direct-acting carcinogen MNU, alfalfa was found to enhance tumor development. With the carcinogen DMAB, a lignin supplement inhibited tumor development.

Based on these studies we begin to see that the effect of a specific dietary fiber on tumor development is related to its physiochemical properties. In general, those fibers that are more insoluble and less fermentable, such as cellulose and wheat bran, are the most successful (in about 60% of studies) at inhibiting tumor development. This is in contrast to the viscous and more fermentable fibers such as the pectins and gums which have been associated with increased tumor production. Corn bran (high in hemicellulose) would appear to be an exception to this, since it is not very soluble or fermentable but does enhance tumor development. For these reasons it is important to study the metabolic and physiological effects of dietary fibers on the intestine in order to gain further insight into the mechanisms by which high-fiber diets modify tumor development.

Mechanisms of Action

The earlier work of Burkitt (1971) and Walker (1978) indicated that high-fiber diets were associated with increased fecal bulk and faster rates of intestinal transit. These observations prompted the hypothesis (Burkitt 1971) that these changes would dilute out any carcinogens or tumor promoters present within the intestinal lumen while also reducing the time available for their interaction with the intestinal epithelium. However, human and animal studies do not support the concept that transit times are important in the prevention of colon cancer, whereas fecal bulk does show an inverse correlation (International Agency for Research on Cancer Intestinal Microecology Group 1977; Cummings et al. 1982). A number of in vitro studies have demonstrated that different fibers are able to bind carcinogens (Smith-Barbaro et al. 1981; Gulliver et al. 1983) and potential tumor promoters (Kritchevsky and Story 1974); however, the relative importance of these effects in vivo either in humans or animals has not been determined.

Metabolic Activity of the Intestinal Microflora

The effects of different dietary fibers on the colonic microflora have been studied extensively. Earlier investigations attempted to measure the effects of high-fiber diets on individual bacterial species. However, more recently the emphasis has shifted toward studying the functional impact by measuring the activity of microbial enzymes considered to be important in carcinogen activation (Goldin and Gorbach 1976). Enzymes measured include β-glucuronidase (Lindop et al. 1985) which appears to be important in activating AOM in the rodent colon cancer model, possibly by hydrolyzing the conjugate of methylazoxymethanol in the intestinal lumen (Takada et al. 1982). Similarly, β-glucosidase appears to convert glucosides to toxic aglycones. Azoreductase and nitroreductase both form nitroso and N-hydroxy compounds from azo and aromatic nitro compounds, respectively. 7-α-Dehydroxylase is important in the degradation of primary to secondary bile acids. These degraded bile acids are considered by some to be the main promoters of colon cancer (Weisburger et al. 1983). Bile acids may also be converted from dihydroxy bile acids to carcinogenic polynuclear hydrocarbons. Although dietary fibers clearly modulate cecal and fecal bacterial enzyme activity (Mallett et al. 1983, 1984, 1986; Rowland et al. 1983), the relationship between bacterial enzyme activity and tumor development still requires further delineation.

Mineral Bioavailability

Dietary fibers can chelate chemicals present in the bowel lumen. If these are tumor promoters or carcinogens, then this may decrease their toxic effects. The cation exchange capacity of fibers leads to binding of minerals such as calcium, magnesium, iron, and zinc. Mineral binding may be further increased by the phytic and oxalic acids which are frequently present in fiber-containing foods. However, the fermentation of soluble fibers within the large bowel liberates fiber-bound minerals, which are then free to be absorbed by the colon. Raising the concentration of intraluminal calcium has been shown to bind fatty acids and free bile acids, thereby reducing their mitogenic activity (Wargovich et al. 1984). Phytic acid, which is present in cereals, has been shown to complex with iron, preventing hydroxyl radical formation and lipid peroxidation, events thought to be important in the process of tumor development (Graf and Eaton 1985).

Fermentation and Short Chain Fatty Acids

When dietary fiber or any other nonabsorbed polysaccharide enters the large bowel, it is fermented by anaerobic microorganisms, resulting in the production of short chain fatty acids (SCFA) (Cummings 1983; Nyman and Asp 1982). Studies have shown that in vivo infusions of SCFA will stimulate colonic cell growth (Sakata and Yajima 1984) and that butyrate is an important substrate for the colonic epithelial cell (Roediger 1982). In vitro studies, using human colon cancer cell lines, have also shown that butyrate is antineoplastic, inhibiting tumor cell growth and producing a less malignant phenotype (Kruh 1982; Kim et al. 1982). During fermentation pH falls (Cummings 1983; Jacobs and Lupton 1986), the greater acidity inhibiting bile acid and carcinogen metabolism (Thornton 1981). When pH drops, the solubility of free fatty acids and free bile acids is diminished, thereby decreasing their potential promoter activity (Wargovich et al. 1984). The colonic fermentation of fiber and the resultant changes in luminal metabolism and cell physiology appear to play a major role in determining the ultimate action of individual fibers on colon carcinogenesis.

Bile Acid Excretion and Fiber Fermentability

According to the bile acid hypothesis, there is a direct correlation between fecal bile concentration and colon carcinogenesis. While cellulose and wheat bran reduce both fecal bile acid concentration and tumor development, corn bran and oat bran increase fecal bile acid excretion and enhance tumorigenesis. However, pectin, agar, guar gum, and alfalfa enhance experimental colon carcinogenesis without increasing rat fecal bile acids and may even lower bile acid concentrations (Story 1986).

This is in contrast to the relationship between fiber fermentability and colonic tumorigenesis. Fibers that tend to inhibit tumorigenesis, such as cellulose and wheat bran, are poorly fermented. However, those fibers reported to enhance experimental colon carcinogenesis, including pectin, guar gum, oat bran, agar, and carageenan, are all highly fermentable. Thus, while the effect of fibers on bile acid metabolism and excretion is a significant factor, the fermentability of fibers would appear to be an equally important determinant of which fibers inhibit and which enhance colon tumor development.

Lignans

Lignans are a group of estrogen-like compounds that have antineoplastic properties and can inhibit DNA synthesis (Adlercreutz 1984). Lignans are constituents of certain higher plants and may also be synthesized by the colonic bacteria from fiber-rich foods. The role of lignans in colon carcinogenesis has not been adequately explored and requires further investigation.

Intestinal Cell Proliferation

Specific dietary fibers can modify intestinal epithelial cell morphology and proliferation. In the large bowel, wheat bran, pectin, and guar produce the greatest mucosal growth effect (Jacobs and White 1983; Jacobs and Lupton 1984). Maximal stimulation of growth occurs in the cecum and proximal colon, the major sites for SCFA production (Mitchell et al. 1985), while in the distal colon, where SCFA are metabolized and absorbed, growth effects are less but still present (Jacobs and White 1983; Jacobs and Lupton 1984). Similarly, in carcinogen-exposed rats, dietary wheat bran, pectin, and guar have each been found to stimulate colonic cell proliferation, whereas cellulose and oat bran produce no significant response (Jacobs 1984; Jacobs and Lupton 1986). The mechanism by which specific fibers stimulate colonic cell proliferation appears to be mediated, at least in part, through large bowel fermentation. Passage of dietary fiber into the large intestine results in fermentation by anaerobic microflora and the production of SCFA and a lower luminal pH (Cummings 1983). Both SCFA (Sakata and Yajima 1984) and an acidic luminal pH (Lupton et al. 1985) stimulate colonic cell proliferation. These trophic effects of dietary fibers and colonic fermentation products appear to play an important role in the enhancement of colon carcinogenesis. Growth factors in general have been shown to promote tumor development (Farber 1984). This growth effect may explain why a substantial number of experimental and human studies have failed to demonstrate any protective effect with fiber supplements or fiber-containing foods.

pH of Intestinal Contents

In a recent study designed to examine the relationship between colonic cell proliferation, large bowel fermentation, and experimental colon carcinogenesis, Jacobs and Lupton (1986) found that fermentation of dietary fiber was associated with a reduction in the pH of large bowel luminal contents. Furthermore, the level of luminal acidity was inversely correlated with tumor frequency. Thus, as luminal contents became more acid, the frequency and yield of tumors increased. Although fermentable fibers such as pectin and guar stimulated cell proliferation, no consistent relationship between cell proliferation and colon cancer frequency could be shown. Having demonstrated an inverse relationship between pH and colon tumorigenesis in animals fed high-fiber diets, subsequent studies examined the effect of lowering colonic pH using dietary sorbitol and lactulose. In an earlier study it was demonstrated that the addition of either 10% sorbitol or lactulose to the diet reduced the pH of large bowel contents and stimulated mucosal cell proliferation (Lupton et al. 1985). In a series of experiments completed recently it was demonstrated that chronic acidification of colonic luminal contents with either sorbitol (Jacobs 1986 a) or lactulose (Jacobs 1986 b) was associated with increased distal colon tumors. This is in contrast to the tumor enhancement seen with fermentable fibers, where increased colon carcinogenesis occurred primarily in the proximal colon (Jacobs and Lupton 1986). Ingram and Castleden (1980) also studied lactulose but found no effect on DMH-induced colon cancer, whereas Samelson et al. (1985) reported that lactulose or sodium sulphate decreased the number DMH-induced tumors per rat but not the incidence of animals with tumor.

These data do not strongly support the hypothesis that an acid pH in the colonic lumen inhibits colon carcinogenesis (Thornton 1981). Human epidemiological studies have shown an association between a reduced colon cancer risk and a low fecal pH (Walker et al. 1986). However, in these populations (Walker et al. 1986) the fecal pH values could not be explained by differences in fiber intake alone. A recently proposed mechanism to explain this is that there may be a greater degree of carbohydrate malabsorption (leading to greater colonic fermentation) in those individuals at lower cancer risk (Thornton et al. 1987). Thus, the relationships between colonic epithelial cell proliferation, large bowel fermentation, luminal pH, SCFAs, fecal bile acid levels, and colon carcinogenesis are of a highly complex nature and require further investigation in both animals and, most importantly, in humans.

Summary

Human studies have in general been retrospective and uncontrolled and as a result cannot be used as convincing evidence in support of the fiber hypothesis. It is of concern that some human studies report that certain fiber-containing foods may even be associated with tumor enhancement. While this falls far short of implicating dietary fiber as a promoter of human colon cancer, it does perhaps argue for a more considered and cautious approach to recommending high-fiber diets as a means of cancer prevention. The animal data show that different sources of dietary fiber produce markedly different effects on colon carcinogenesis. While some fibers exhibit protective properties, others clearly promote tumor development. The mechanisms behind these opposing actions require further investigation. However, it is clear that dietary fibers do modulate the carcinogenic process and as such provide a valuable tool for probing the mechanisms and stages of colon tumor development.

Dietary fiber appears to play a major role in the regulation of normal intestinal function and in the maintenance of a healthy intestinal mucosa. Whether a fiber-deficient diet predisposes to colon carcinogenesis seems to be a very different issue from the role of supplemental fiber in cancer prevention. This is further complicated by not knowing what constitutes a normal level of fiber intake. In the interim it would perhaps be best to advise the general public to consume a moderate diet that contains vegetables, fruits, and whole grains. This will provide a varied source of fiber-containing foods and, if consumed in sufficient quantity, will optimize intestinal transit and bulk according to individual needs. Fiber supplements appear at present to have no place in colon cancer prevention. To be any more specific about what type of fiber to recommend seems premature at this time, whereas for quantity a range of 20–35 g of dietary fiber per day has recently been suggested (Pilch 1987).

References

Abraham R, Barbolt TA, Rodgers JB (1980) Inhibition by bran of the colonic cocarcinogenicity of bile salts in rats given dimethylhydrazine. Exp Mol Pathol 33:133–143

Adlercreutz H (1984) Does fiber-rich food containing animal lignan precursors protect against both colon and breast cancer? An extension of the "fiber hypothesis." Gastroenterology 86:761–766

Arakawa S, Okumura M, Yamada S, Ito M, Tejima S (1986) Enhancing effect of carageenan on the induction of rat colonic tumors by 1,2-dimethylhydrazine and its relation to β-glucuronidase activities in feces and other tissues. J Nutr Sci Vitaminol (Tokyo) 32:481–485

Armstrong B, Doll R (1975) Environmental factors and cancer incidence and mortality in different countries, with special reference to dietary practices. Int J Cancer 15:617–631

Barbolt TA, Abraham R (1978) The effect of bran on dimethyl-hydrazine-induced colon carcinogenesis in the rat. Proc Soc Exp Biol 157:656–659

Barbolt TA, Abraham R (1980) Dose-response, sex difference, and the effect of bran in dimethylhydrazine-induced intestinal tumorigenesis in rats. Toxicol Appl Pharmacol 55:417–422

Barnes DS, Clapp NK, Scott SA, Oberst DL, Berry SG (1983) Effects of wheat, rice, corn and soybean bran on 1,2-dimethylhydrazine-induced large bowel tumorigenesis in F344 rats. Nutr Cancer 5:1–9

Bauer HG, Asp N-G, Oste R, Dahlqvist A, Fredlund PE (1979) Effect of dietary fiber on the induction of colorectal tumors and fecal β-glucuronidase activity in the rat. Cancer Res 39:3752–3756

Bauer HG, Asp N-G, Dahlqvist A, Fredlund PE, Nyman M, Oste R (1981) Effect of two kinds of pectin and guar gum on 1,2-dimethylhydrazine initiation of colon tumors and on fecal β-glucuronidase activity in the rat. Cancer Res 41:2518–2523

Bingham SA, Williams DRR, Cole TJ, James WPT (1979) Dietary fiber and regional large-bowel cancer mortality in Britain. Br J Cancer 40:456–463

Bingham SA, Williams DRR, Cummings JH (1985) Dietary fibre consumption in Britain: new estimates and their relation to large bowel cancer mortality. Br J Cancer 52:399–402

Bjelke E (1974a) Case-control study in Norway. Scand J Gastroenterol 9 (Suppl 31):42–48

Bjelke E (1974b) Case-control study in Minnesota. Scand J Gastroenterol 9 (Suppl 31):49–53

Bristol JB, Emmett PM, Heaton KW, Williamson RCN (1985) Sugar, fat, and the risk of colorectal cancer. Br Med J 291:1467–1470

Bruce WR (1987) Recent hypotheses for the origin of colon cancer. Cancer Res 47:4237–4242

Burkitt DP (1971) Epidemiology of cancer of the colon and rectum. Cancer 28:3–13

Byers T, Graham S (1984) The epidemiology of diet and cancer. Adv Cancer Res 41:1–69

Chen W-F, Patchefsky AS, Goldsmith HS (1978) Colonic protection from dimethylhydrazine by a high fiber diet. Surg Gynecol Obstet 147:503–506

Clapp NK, Henke MA, London JF, Shock TL (1984) Enhancement of 1,2-dimethylhydrazine-induced large bowel tumorigenesis in Balb/c mice by corn, soybean, and wheat brans. Nutr Cancer 6:77–85

Cleave TL (1956) The neglect of natural principles in current medical practice. J Roy Nav Med Serv 42:55–82

Cohen BI, Raicht RF, Deschner EE, Takahashi M, Sarwal AN, Fazzini E (1980) Effect of cholic acid feeding on N-methyl-N-nitrosourea-induced colon tumors and cell kinetics in rats. J Natl Cancer Inst 64:573–578

Craven PA, Pfanstiel J, DeRubertis FR (1987) Role of activation of protein kinase C in the stimulation of colonic epithelial proliferation and reactive oxygen formation by bile acids. J Clin Invest 79:532–541

Cruse JP, Lewin MR, Clark CG (1978) Failure of bran to protect against experimental colon cancer in rats. Lancet ii:1278–1280

Cummings JH (1983) Fermentation in the human large intestine: evidence and implications for health. Lancet i:1206–1209

Cummings JH, Branch WJ, Bjerrum L, Paerregaard A, Helms P, Burton R (1982) Colon cancer and large bowel function in Denmark and Finland. Nutr Cancer 4:61–66

Dales LG, Friedman GD, Ury HK, Grossman S, Williams SR (1979) A case-control study of relationships of diet and other traits to colorectal cancer in American Blacks. Am J Epidemiol 109:132–144

Doll R, Peto R (1981) The causes of cancer. Quantitative estimates of avoidable risks of cancer in the United States today. J Natl Cancer Inst 66:1191–1308

Drasar BS, Irving D (1973) Environmental factors and cancer of the colon and breast. Br J Cancer 27:167–172

Englyst HN, Bingham SA, Wiggins HS, Southgate DAT, Seppanen R, Helms P, Anderson V, Day KC, Choolun R, Collinson E, Cummings JH (1982) Nonstarch polysaccharide consumption in four Scandinavian populations. Nutr Cancer 4:50–60

Enstrom JE (1980) Health and dietary practices and cancer mortality among California Mormons. In: Chairns J, Lyon JL, Skolnick M (eds) Cancer incidence in defined populations. Banbury report no 4. Cold Spring Harbor, New York, pp 69–92

Farber E (1984) The multistep nature of cancer development. Cancer Res 44:4217–4223

Fleiszer D, Murray D, MacFarlane J, Brown RA (1978) Protective effect of dietary fiber against chemically induced bowel tumors in rats. Lancet ii:552–553

Freeman HJ, Spiller GA, Kim YS (1978) A double-blind study on the effect of purified cellulose dietary fiber on 1,2-dimethylhydrazine-induced rat colonic neoplasia. Cancer Res 38:2912–2917

Freeman HJ, Spiller GA, Kim YS (1980) A double-blind study on the effects of different purified cellulose and pectin fiber diets on 1,2-dimethylhydrazine-induced rat colonic neoplasia. Cancer Res 40:2661–2665

Freeman HJ, Spiller GA, Kim YS (1984) Effect of high hemicellulose corn bran in 1,2-dimethylhydrazine-induced rat intestinal neoplasia. Carcinogenesis 5:261–264

Galloway DJ, Owen RW, Jarrett F, Boyle P, Hill MJ, George WD (1986) Experimental colorectal cancer: the relationship of diet and faecal bile acid concentration to tumour induction. Br J Surg 73:233–237

Glauert HP, Bennick MR, Sander CH (1981) Enhancement of 1,2-dimethylhydrazine-induced colon carcinogenesis in mice by dietary agar. Food Cosmet Toxicol 19:281–286

Goldin BR, Gorbach SL (1976) The relationship between diet and rat fecal bacterial enzymes implicated in colon cancer. J Natl Cancer Inst 57:371–375

Graf E, Eaton JW (1985) Dietary suppression of colon cancer. Fiber or phytate. Cancer 56:717–718

Graham S, Dayal H, Swanson M, Mittelman A, Wilkinson G (1978) Diet in the epidemiology of cancer of the colon and rectum. J Natl Cancer Inst 61:709–714

Gulliver WP, Kutty KP, Laher JM, Barrowman JA (1983) In vitro interaction of 7,12-dimethylbenz[a]anthracene and its biliary metabolites with dietary fibers. J Natl Cancer Inst 71:207–210

Haenszel W, Berg JW, Segi M, Kurihara M, Locke FB (1973) Large-bowel cancer in Haiwaiian Japanese. J Natl Cancer Inst 51:1765–1779

Haenszel W, Locke FB, Segi M (1980) A case-control study of large bowel cancer in Japan. J Natl Cancer Inst 64:17–22

Helms P, Jorgensen IM, Paerregaard A, Bjerrum L, Poulsen L, Mosbech J (1982) Dietary patterns in Them and Copenhagen, Denmark. Nutr Cancer 4:34–40

Higginson J (1966) Etiological factors in gastrointestinal cancer in man. J Natl Cancer Inst 37:527–545

Hill M, MacLennan R, Newcombe K (1979) Diet and large bowel cancer in three socioeconomic groups in Hong Kong. Lancet i:436

Hirayama T (1981) A large-scale cohort study on the relationship between diet and selected cancers of digestive organs. In: Bruce WR, Correa P, Lipkin M, Tannenbaum SR, Wilkins TD (eds) Gastrointestinal cancer: endogenous factors. Banbury report no 7. Cold Spring Harbor, New York, pp 409–429

Hoff G, Moen IE, Trygg K, Frølich W, Sauar J, Vatn M, Gjone E, Larsen S (1986) Epidemiology of polyps in the rectum and sigmoid colon. Evaluation of nutritional factors. Scand J Gastroenterol 21:199–204

Howell MA (1985) Diet as an etiological factor in the development of cancers of the colon and rectum. J Chronic Dis 28:67–80

Ingram DM, Castleden WM (1980) The effect of dietary lactulose on experimental large bowel cancer. Carcinogenesis 1:893–895

International Agency for Research on Cancer Intestinal Microecology Group (1977) Dietary fiber, transit-time, faecal bacteria, steroids and colon cancer in two Scandinavian populations. Lancet ii:207–211

Irving D, Drassar BS (1973) Fibre and cancer of the colon. Br J Cancer 28:462–463

Jacobs LR (1983) Enhancement of rat colon carcinogenesis by wheat bran consumption during the stage of 1,2-dimethylhydrazine administration. Cancer Res 43:4057–4061

Jacobs LR (1984) Stimulation of rat colonic crypt cell proliferative activity by wheat bran consumption during the stage of 1,2-dimethylhydrazine administration. Cancer Res 44:2458–2463

Jacobs LR (1986a) Enhancement of experimental colon cancer and production of colitis in rats fed sorbitol. Clin Res 35:441A

Jacobs LR (1986b) Enhancement of experimental rat colon cancer with dietary lactulose. Gastroenterology 90:1473

Jacobs LR, Lupton JR (1984) Effect of dietary fibers on rat large bowel mucosal growth and cell proliferation. Am J Physiol 246:G378–G385

Jacobs LR, Lupton JR (1986) Relationship between colonic luminal pH, cell proliferation, and colon carcinogenesis in 1,2-dimethylhydrazine treated rats fed high fiber diets. Cancer Res 46:1727–1734

Jacobs LR, White FA (1983) Modulation of mucosal cell proliferation in the intestine of rats fed a wheat bran diet. Am J Clin Nutr 37:945–953

Jain M, Cook GM, Davis FG, Grace MG, Howe GR, Miller AB (1980) A case-control study of diet and colo-rectal cancer. Int J Cancer 26:757–768

Kim YS, Tsao D, Marita A, Bella A (1982) Effect of sodium butyrate on three human colorectal adenocarcinoma cell lines in culture. In: Malt RA, Williamson RCN (eds) Colonic carcinogenesis. MTP Press, Lancaster, pp 317–323

Knox EG (1977) Foods and diseases. Br J Prev Soc Med 31:71–80

Kritchevsky D, Story JA (1974) Binding of bile salts in vitro by non-nutritive fiber. J Nutr 104:458–462

Kroes R, Beems RB, Bosland MC, Bunnik GSJ, Sinkeldam EJ (1986) Nutritional factors in lung, colon, and prostate carcinogenesis in animal models. Fed Proc Fed Am Soc Exp Biol 45:136–141

Kromhout D, Bosschieter EB, de Lezenne Coulander C (1982) Dietary fiber and 10-year mortality from coronary heart disease, cancer and all causes. The Zutphen study. Lancet ii:518–522

Kruh J (1982) Effect of sodium butyrate, a new pharmacological agent, on cells in culture. Mol Cell Biochem 42:65–82

Kune S, Kune GA, Watson LF (1987) Case-control study of dietary etiological factors: the Melbourne colorectal cancer study. Nutr Cancer 9:21–42

Kuratsune M, Honda T, Englyst HN, Cummings JH (1986) Dietary fiber in the Japanese diet as investigated in connection with colon cancer risk. Jpn J Cancer Res 77:736–738

Lindop R, Tasman-Jones C, Thomsen LL, Lee SP (1985) Cellulose and pectin alter intestinal β-glucuronidase (EC 3.2.1.31) in the rat. Br J Nutr 54:21–26

Liu K, Stamler J, Moss D, Garside D, Persky V, Soltero I (1979) Dietary cholesterol, fat and fibre, and colon-cancer mortality. Lancet ii:782–785

Lupton JR, Coder DM, Jacobs LR (1985) Influence of luminal pH on rat large bowel epithelial cell cycle. Am J Physiol 249:G382–G388

Lyon JL, Sorenson AW (1978) Colon cancer in a low-risk population. Am J Clin Nutr 31:S227–S230

Lyon JL, Gardner JW, West DW, Mahoney AM (1983) Methodological issues in epidemiological studies in diet and cancer. Cancer Res (Suppl) 43:2392s–2396s

Lyon JL, Mahoney AW, West DW, Gardner JW, Smith KR, Sorensen AW, Stanish W (1987) Energy intake: its relationship to colon cancer risk. J Natl Cancer Inst 78:853–861

Macquart-Moulin G, Riboli E, Cornée J, Charnay B, Berthezène P, Day N (1986) Case-control study on colorectal cancer and diet in Marseilles. Int J Cancer 38:183–191

Macquart-Moulin G, Riboli E, Cornée J, Kaaks R, Berthezène P (1987) Colorectal polyps and diet: a case-control study in Marseilles. Int J Cancer 40:179–188

Mallett AK, Wise A, Rowland IR (1983) Effect of dietary cellulose on the metabolic activity of the rat cecal microflora. Arch Toxicol 52:311–317

Mallett AK, Wise A, Rowland IR (1984) Hydrocolloid food additives rat caecal microbial enzyme activities. Food Chem Toxicol 22:415–418

Mallett AK, Rowland IR, Bearne CA (1986) Influence of wheat bran on some reductive and hydrolytic activities of the rat cecal flora. Nutr Cancer 8:125–131

Manousos O, Day NE, Trichopoulos D, Gerovassilis F, Tzonou A, Polychronopoulou A (1983) Diet and colorectal cancer: a case-control study in Greece. Int J Cancer 32:1–5

Martinez I, Torres R, Frias Z, Colon JR, Fernandez N (1979) Factors associated with adenocarcinomas of the large bowel in Puerto Rico. In: Birch JM (ed) Epidemiology. Advances in medical oncology, research and education, vol 3. Pergamon, New York, pp 45–52

McKeown-Eyssen GE, Bright-See E (1984) Dietary factors in colon cancer: international relationships. Nutr Cancer 6:160–170

Minowa M, Bingham S, Cummings JH (1983) Dietary fiber intake in Japan. Hum Nutr Appl Nutr 37 A:113–119

Mitchell BL, Lawson MJ, Davies M, Grant MK, Roediger WEW, Illman RJ, Topping DL (1985) Volatile fatty acids in the human intestine: studies in surgical patients. Nutr Res 5:1089–1092

Mizutani I, Mitsuoka T (1983) Effect of Konjac mannan on 1,2-dimethylhydrazine-induced intestinal carcinogenesis in Fischer F344 rats. Cancer Lett 19:1–6

Modan B, Barell V, Lubin F, Modan M, Greenberg RA, Graham S (1975) Low-fiber intake as an etiological factor in cancer of the colon. J Natl Cancer 55:15–18

Morgenstern H (1982) Uses of ecological analysis in epidemiological research. Am J Public Health 72:1336–1344

Nigro ND, Bull AW, Klopfer BA, Pak MS, Campbell RL (1979) Effect of dietary fiber on azoxymethane-induced intestinal carcinogenesis in rats. J Natl Cancer Inst 62:1097–1102

Nyman M, Asp N-G (1982) Fermentation of dietary fiber components in the rat intestinal tract. Br J Nutr 47:357–366

Pence BC, Buddingh F, Yang SP (1986) Multiple dietary factors in the enhancement of dimethylhydrazine carcinogenesis: main effect of indole-3-carbinol. J Natl Cancer Inst 77:269–276

Phillips RL (1975) Role of life-style and dietary habits in risk of cancer among Seventh-Day Adventists. Cancer Res 35:3513–3522

Phillips RL, Snowdon DA (1985) Dietary relationships with fatal colorectal cancer among Seventh-Day Adventists. J Natl Cancer Inst 74:307–317

Pickle LW, Greene MH, Ziegler RG, Toledo A, Hoover R, Lynch HT, Fraumeni JF (1984) Colorectal cancer in rural Nebraska. Cancer Res 44:363–369

Pilch SM (ed) (1987) Physiological effects and health consequences of dietary fiber. Life Sciences Research Office, Federation of American Societies for Experimental Biology, Bethesda, Maryland

Potter JD, McMichael AJ (1986) Diet and cancer of the colon and rectum: a case-control study. J Natl Cancer Inst 76:557–569

Reddy BS, Mori H (1981) Effect of dietary wheat bran and dehydrated citrus fiber on 3,2-dimethyl-4-aminobiphenyl-induced intestinal carcinogenesis in F344 rats. Carcinogenesis 2:21–25

Reddy BS, Mori H, Nicolais M (1981) Effect of dietary wheat bran and dehydrated citrus fiber on azoxymethane-induced intestinal carcinogenesis in Fischer 344 rats. J Natl Cancer Inst 66:553–557

Reddy BS, Maeura Y, Wayman M (1983) Effect of dietary corn bran and autohydrolyzed lignin on 3,2-dimethyl-4-aminobiphenyl-induced intestinal carcinogenesis in male F344 rats. J Natl Cancer Inst 71:419–423

Reddy BS, Sharma C, Simi B, Engle A, Laakso K, Puska P, Korpela R (1987) Metabolic epidemiology of colon cancer: effect of dietary fiber on fecal mutagens and bile acids in healthy subjects. Cancer Res 47:644–648

Roberts-Andersen J, Mehta T, Wilson RB (1987) Reduction of DMH-induced colon tumors in rats fed psyllium husk or cellulose. Nutr Cancer 10:129–136

Roediger WEW (1982) Utilization of nutrients by isolated epithelial cells of the rat colon. Gastroenterology 83:424–429

Rowland IR, Wise A, Mallett AK (1983) Metabolic profile of caecal micro-organisms from rats fed indigestible plant cell-wall components. Food Chem Toxicol 21:25–29

Rozen P, Hellerstein SM, Horwitz C (1981) The low incidence of colorectal cancer in a "high risk" population: its correlation with dietary habits. Cancer 48:2692–2695

Rozen P, Horwitz C, Tabenkin C, Ron E, Katz L (1987) Dietary habits and colorectal cancer incidence in a second-defined kibbutz population. Nutr Cancer 9 (2–3):177–184

Sakata T, Yajima T (1984) Influence of short chain fatty acids on the epithelial cell division of digestive tract. Q J Exp Physiol 69:639–648

Samelson SL, Nelson RL, Nyhus LM (1985) Protective role of fecal pH in experimental colon carcinogenesis. J R Soc Med 78:230–233

Schrauzer GN (1976) Cancer mortality correlation studies. II. Regional association of mortalities with the consumptions of foods and other commodities. Med Hypotheses 2:39–49

Smith-Barbaro P, Hanson D, Reddy BS (1981) Carcinogen binding to various types of dietary fiber. J Natl Cancer Inst 67:495–497

Stocks P, Karn MN (1933) A cooperative study of the habits, home life, dietary and family histories of 450 cancer patients and of an equal number of control patients. Ann Eugen (London) 5:237–280

Story JA (1986) Modification of steroid excretion in response to dietary fiber. In: Vahouny GV, Kritchevsky D (eds) Dietary fiber. Basic and clinical aspects. Plenum, New York, pp 253–264

Tajima K, Tominaga S (1985) Dietary habits and gastrointestinal cancer: A comparative case-control study of stomach and large intestinal cancers in Nagoya, Japan. Jpn J Cancer Res 76:705–716

Takada H, Hirooka T, Hiramatsu Y, Yamamoto M (1982) Effect of β-glucuronidase inhibitor on azoxymethane-induced colonic carcinogenesis in rats. Cancer Res 42:331–334

Temple NJ, El-Khatib S (1987) Cabbage and vitamin E: their effect on colon tumor formation in mice. Cancer Lett 35:71–77

Thornton JR (1981) High colonic pH promotes colorectal cancer. Lancet i:1081–1083

Thornton JR, Dryden A, Kelleher J, Losowsky MS (1987) Super-efficient starch absorption. A risk factor for colonic neoplasia? Dig Dis Sci 32:1088–1091

Toth B (1984) Effect of Metamucil on tumour formation by 1,2-dimethylhydrazine dihydrochloride in mice. Food Chem Toxicol 22:573–578

Trowell H (1976) Definition of dietary fiber and hypotheses that it is a protective factor in certain diseases. Am J Clin Nutr 29:417–427

Trudel JL, Senterman MK, Brown RA (1983) The fat/fiber antagonism in experimental colon carcinogenesis. Surgery 94:691–696

Tuyns AJ (1986) A case-control study on colorectal cancer in Belgium. Preliminary results. Soz Praventivmed 31:81–82

Walker ARP (1978) The relationship between bowel cancer and fiber content in the diet. Am J Clin Nutr 31:S248–S251

Walker ARP, Walker BF, Walker AJ (1986) Fecal pH, dietary fibre intake, and proneness to colon cancer in four South African populations. Br J Cancer 53:489–495

Ward JM, Yamamoto RS, Weisburger JH (1973) Cellulose dietary bulk and azoxymethane-induced intestinal cancer. J Natl Cancer Inst 51:713–715

Wargovich MJ, Eng VWS, Newmark HL (1984) Calcium inhibits the damaging and compensatory proliferative effects of fatty acids on mouse colon epithelium. Cancer Lett 23:253–258

Watanabe K, Reddy BS, Wong CQ, Weisburger JH (1978) Effect of dietary undegraded carageenan on colon carcinogenesis in F344 rats treated with azoxymethane or methylnitrosourea. Cancer Res 38:4427–4430

Watanabe K, Reddy BS, Weisburger JH, Kritchevsky D (1979) Effect of dietary alfalfa, pectin and wheat bran on azoxymethane- or methylnitrosourea-induced colon carcinogenesis in F344 rats. J Natl Cancer Inst 63:141–145

Weisburger JH, Reddy BS, Barnes MS, Wynder EL (1983) Bile acids but not neutral sterols, are tumor promoters in the colon in man and in rodents. Environ Health Perspect 50:101–107

Wilpart M, Roberfroid M (1987) Intestinal carcinogenesis and dietary fibers: the influence of cellulose on Fybogel chronically given after exposure to DMH. Nutr Cancer 10:39–51

Wilson RB, Hutcheson DP, Wideman L (1977) Dimethylhydrazine-induced colon tumors in rats fed diets containing beef fat or corn oil with and without wheat bran. Am J Clin Nutr 30:176–181

Wynder EL, Shigematsu T (1967) Environmental factors of cancer of the colon and rectum. Cancer 20:1520–1561

Wynder EL, Kajitani T, Ishikawa S, Dodo H, Takano A (1969) Environmental factors of cancer of the colon and rectum. II. Japanese epidemiological data. Cancer 23:1210–1220

Yamamoto I, Marugama H (1985) Effect of dietary seaweed preparations on 1,2-dimethylhydrazine-induced intestinal carcinogenesis in rats. Cancer Lett 26:241–251

Colorectal Bacteria in Colorectal Carcinogenesis

M.J. Hill

Public Health Laboratory Service – Centre for Applied Microbiology and Research,
Porton Down, Salisbury, Wiltshire, SP4 0JG, UK

Contents

Introduction

Although the importance of the gut bacterial flora to the general well-being of the host was recognised in the last century by Metchnikoff, detailed studies were hampered by the lack of equipment and techniques for cultivating the oxygen-sensitive components of the flora. Interest waned in the early decades of this century, and only the role of bacteria as intestinal pathogens was considered, the beneficial effects of the gut flora being ignored. The subject was revived in the 1960s with the development of anaerobic cabinet techniques for the culture of the vast majority of intestinal organisms, and our knowledge of the composition and the function of the gut bacterial flora has grown steadily since then.

In this chapter I will summarise the current state of knowledge of the composition of the gut bacterial flora, the factors controlling the flora and, in particular, its relation to diet. I will then describe the metabolic activity of the flora as it relates to studies of colorectal carcinogenesis. I will conclude by discussing the gut flora in relation to the prevention of colorectal carcinogenesis.

Gut Bacterial Flora in Adult Humans

In the normal healthy adult human, the flora of the upper gastrointestinal tract is very sparse except during the early stages of a meal. Gastric acid secretion maintains the stomach as a bactericidal environment; during a meal the acid is buffered allowing the survival of salivary organisms and those present in the food, and consequently a bolus of organism enters the small intestine with the food. Pancreatic secretions and bile are bactericidal to most organisms and only those resistant to such controlling factors survive. In addition, the volume of such secretions greatly dilutes the flora of the small bowel. The rapid transit of small bowel contents and the efficient flushing of the mucosal crypts which controls surface growth ensures that bacterial multiplication in the small bowel is minimised.

In consequence, it is clear that the "inoculum" for the flora of the human colon does not come from above, with the nutrients, but must be maintained locally. In contrast to the small bowel, the large intestine maintains a rich profuse bacterial flora dominated by the strictly anaerobic non-spring rods (*Bacteroides* spp, *Eubacterium* spp, *Bifidobacterium* spp and *Propionibacterium* spp). The composition of the faecal flora is summarised in Table 1. In terms of genera, the flora is similar to that of the mouth; the major distinguishing characteristic of the faecal bacteria flora, other than that the vast majority are anaerobic organisms, is that the dominant organism are all

Table 1. Bacterial flora of faeces and of the colonic mucosa

Bacterial group	Presence in the flora		Bacterial group	Presence in the flora	
	Faeces	Mucosa		Faeces	Mucosa
Anaerobic non-sporing rods			Microaerophilic		
Gram negative			organisms		
Bacteroides spp	10^{11}	+++	*Lactobacillus* spp	10^8	++
Fusobacterium spp	10^9	++	*Streptococcus* spp	10^8	+++
Gram positive			Facultative rods		
Bifidobacterium spp	10^{10}	++	Gram negative		
Eubacterium spp	10^{10}	+	*Escherichia* spp	10^7	++
Propioni-			*Klebsiella* spp	++	+
bacterium spp	10^{10}		*Proteus* spp	++	+
Anaerobic cocci			Gram positive		
Gram negative			*Corynebacterium* spp	++	±
Veillonella spp	10^5	++	Facultative cocci		
Megasphaera spp	+	+	Gram negative		
Gram positive			*Neisseria* spp	10^7	±
Peptococcus spp	++	+	Gram positive		
Peptostrepto-			*Staphylococcus* spp	+	±
coccus spp	++	+	*Micrococcus* spp	++	±
Spiral organisms			Spore-forming organisms		
Spirochaetes	±	±	Anaerobic –		
Brachyspira	±	±	*Clostridium* spp	10^5	++
			Aerobic – *Bacillus* spp	10^5	+

bile resistant. Thus, whereas the oral bacteroides are almost entirely bile sensitive (e.g. *B. melaninogenicus*, *B. oralis*, *B. gingivalis*), those in faeces belong mainly to the *B. fragilis* group of bile-resistant organisms (*B. fragilis*, *B. thetaiotaomicron*, *B. distasonis*, *B. vulgatus*); the bile-resistant enterobacteria are an important component of the facultative flora of faeces but are absent from the mouth; oral streptococci are bile sensitive (*S. sanguis*, *S. salivarius*, *S. milleri*), but in the colon the bile-resistant *S. faecalis* and *S. faecium* are present in large numbers.

There have been many detailed studies of the intestinal bacterial flora (e.g. Moore and Holdeman 1974; Finegold et al. 1975). These serve to accentuate the complexity of the flora (there are at least 400 different species) but do little to improve our understanding; for most practical purposes, the importance of the flora is related to its metabolic activity rather than to its taxonomic diversity.

Table 1 also illustrates the qualitative similarity between the faecal flora and the colonic mucosal flora in humans. The organisms that dominate the faecal flora are also present in large numbers in the mucosal flora, although their relative proportions are very different. Whereas in faeces the anaerobic organisms dominate the aerobes by a factor of 10^2-10^3, in the mucosal flora the dominance is by a factor of only 1 to 10.

Factors Controlling the Composition of the Flora

The major factors determining the composition of the colonic flora are nutrient availability, physico-chemical state, bacterial interactions and surface growth.

Nutrient Availability. The intestinal flora has a spartan existence since most of the readily available nutrients are removed from the intestine by the digestive process. The major nutrients available to the flora are (a) desquamated intestinal mucosal cells and digestive secretions; (b) those components of the diet which are not metabolised by mucosal or digestive enzymes; (c) those nutrients that would normally be digested but which are modified and rendered indigestible by the cooking process (e.g. resistant starch), or which are protected from digestion by resistant "shells" (e.g. of lignin in lignified plant material). A major feature of the colonic ecosystem is the very low concentration of glucose and the consequent absence of any glucose repression of inducible enzymes. The consequence of this is that, in contrast to the oral flora (where many inducible enzymes are repressed by the high glucose availability), the colonic flora is able to produce its full repertoire of enzymes in response to the presence of novel nutrients.

Physico-Chemical State. Organisms differ in their ability to grow under different conditions with respect to pH, Eh, oxygen tension, temperature, osmotic pressure, etc. Thus lactobacilli, streptococci and bifidobacteria are able to thrive at acidic pH values that would inhibit, for example, coliform bacteria or *Bacteroides* spp. At the other end of the pH range, *Proteus* spp are more tolerant to alkaline pH values than, for example, streptococci or lactobacilli. Whereas *Bacteroides* spp, *Bifidobacterium* spp, *Veillonella* spp, etc. are killed by even traces of oxygen in the environment (i.e. are obligate anaerobes), *Pseudomonas* spp and many *Bacillus* spp have an absolute requirement for oxygen (i.e. are obligate anaerobes). Between these two extremes we have the microaerophilic organisms (which can tolerate small amounts of oxygen but do not utilise it) such as lactobacilli and streptococci, and facultative organisms (which use oxygen when it is available but which utilise anaerobic pathways in its absence) such as *Escherichia coli*. The strictly anaerobic organisms grow much more readily than facultative species under anaerobic conditions; consequently the gut bacterial flora is dominated by the non-sporing, strictly anaerobic genera *Bacteroides* spp, *Bifidobacterium* spp, *Eubacterium* spp and *Propionibacterium* spp. The facultative organisms, in the context of the gut, may be considered as oxygen scavengers; they are the only organisms that utilise oxygen since the conditions are not sufficiently aerobic, even at the mucosal surface, to support strictly aerobic organisms. Since the oxygen tension at the mucosal surface is higher than in the lumen (as a result of diffusion from the mucosal cells), the dominance of the flora by strictly anaerobic genera is less pronounced at that site.

Most soil organisms grow optimally at 20°–30°C; skin organisms are able to grow rapidly at 30°C, but human intestinal organisms (and human pathogens) have an optimal growth temperature of 37°C. A consequence of this is that many environmental organisms that are able to survive passage through the stomach and small bowel nevertheless find it difficult to flourish in the human gut because of the adverse temperature.

Bacterial Interactions. In order to protect their ecological niche, bacteria produce a range of toxic substances active against competing bacterial species or genera. Examples are bacteriocines and bacteriophage (active against different strains of the same species) and antibiotics (normally active against organisms belonging to other genera). The consequence of this is that a balanced community of organisms is established in an ecosystem which then shows great colonisation resistance. In the human colon the serotype of the dominant *E. coli* strain is very stable for long periods despite being continually challenged by strains of other serotypes. Because the growth of potential competitors is suppressed by the toxic substances produced by the whole bacterial community, invasion of the gut by pathogens is greatly facilitated by any treatment which suppresses the normal bacterial flora such as antibiotic treatment (hence antibiotic-associated diarrhoea, pseudomembranous colitis, etc.).

Surface Growth. Bacteria tend to grow on surfaces in preference to the free fluid phase. The advantages of surface growth include nutrient availability (the surface often being a nutrient supply such as, in the gut, a food particle), a high local concentration of minerals (which tend to adsorb to surfaces) and the opportunity to produce a high local cell density and, consequently, a high concentration of antibacterial products for protecting the ecological niche. In the context of the gut, the surfaces of importance are the intestinal mucosa and, in the gut lumen, the undigested solid food particles.

Relation Between Diet and Gut Flora

Because of the relation between nutrient supply and the physico-chemical environment and the composition of the bacterial flora, it is reasonable to assume that the gut flora is related to diet. Nevertheless, until relatively recently there was little firm

Table 2. The relation between diet and the faecal bacterial flora

Dietary change	Effect on faecal flora
Increased fat	None
Increased protein	None
Fibre supplements	
Wheat bran	None
Bagasse	None
Pectin	None
Guar	None
Added lactulose	None

Table 3. The effect of a residue-free diet on the faecal bacterial flora (for details and references see Hudson et al. 1984)

Residue-free diet	Energy source	Time (days)	Persons (n)	Effect on the flora per gram of faeces
CDD6	Glucose	14	8	Marked decrease in all organisms
CDD7		14	8	Marked decrease in enterococci and lactobacilli
CDD6	Oligosaccharide	8–10	3	Decrease in enterococci and very oxygen-sensitive anaerobes
CDD6	Oligosaccharide	14	3	Decrease in enterococci and lactobacilli
3200AS	Oligosaccharide	12	14	Decrease in enterococci
Howard diet	Oligosaccharide	7	6	Decrease in enterococci, lactobacilli and veillonellae

evidence of such a relation. Table 2 lists some examples of dietary manipulations that have been studied in relation to the gut bacterial flora; in all of these examples the faecal flora was assumed to be representative of the intestinal flora. In none of the examples was the effect on the composition of the faecal bacterial flora notable except when a soluble defined diet with zero residue was used. Table 3 lists some studies of the relation between residue-free diets and the faecal bacterial flora. When a glucose-based diet was used, the effect on the composition of the flora was profound; when other energy sources were used, the effect was very much smaller and was largely limited to a few genera or species. It was necessary to carry out extremely detailed studies (e.g. Finegold et al. 1975; Maier et al. 1974) in order to detect statistically significant changes in the flora, and in no case was the change of any biological significance.

The clue to this conundrum was the realisation that the major site of gut bacterial metabolism is the proximal colon and that the distal colon makes little contribution to the overall metabolic activity of the flora. Some of the evidence for this is given in Table 4. In patients with a left hemicolectomy, the extent of bile acid and of neutral steroid metabolism (excreted in faeces) and the production of volatile phenols (excreted in urine) was similar to that in persons with a complete colon. In the case of all three substrates, the extent of metabolism was very low in patients with a total

Table 4. Evidence that the major site of gut bacterial metabolism is the proximal colon from the metabolism of various substrates in patients with total colectomy, hemicolectomy and no surgery

	Total colectomy	Hemicolectomy		Normal colon
		Right	Left	
Cholesterol degradation	±	+	+ + +	+ + +
Bile acid dehydroxylation	−	+	+ + +	+ + +
Urinary volatile phenol production	−	+	+ + +	+ + +
Tryptophan metabolism	−	ND	+ + +	+ + +

ND, not determined.

Table 5. The effect of diet on the bacterial flora of ileostomy fluid

Dietary change	Effect
Increased dietary fibre	General increase in all organisms
Increased dietary protein	Increase in total aerobes, coliforms and streptococci
Increased dietary fat	Increase in total anaerobes, bacteroides and clostridia

colectomy. When dietary manipulation was carried out on patients with a colectomy, a profound effect on the flora was observed (Table 5). Further, whereas a two-fold increase in dietary protein resulted in an increased amount of protein entering the colon (as determined from the analysis of ileostomy effluent), there was no change in the faecal protein concentration. Similarly, increased dietary fibre causes an increase in the amount of carbohydrate entering the colon but very little increase in faecal carbohydrate. The effect of diet on the faecal flora (and the absence of an effect on the faecal flora) can therefore be related to nutrient supply. Similarly, lactulose has a profound effect on the flora of the proximal colon (Florent et al. 1985) but little effect on the faecal flora (Vince et al. 1974). The concentration of lactulose in faeces is undetectable, and so the results can again be related to nutrient supply. They can also be related to pH since Bown et al. (1974) showed that lactulose caused a massive acidification of the caecum (to yield a pH of 4–5) but no change in faecal pH. Presumably, the fatty acids generated in the caecum (and responsible for the change in pH) are absorbed during colonic transit.

In summary, diet has a profound effect on the flora of the proximal colon but little effect on the faecal flora. This is significant because the proximal colon is the site of bacterial metabolism.

Metabolic Activity of the Gut Bacterial Flora

The metabolic activity of the gut bacterial flora has been studied using pure cultures in vitro, chemostat simulations of the gut flora and in vitro studies.

In Vitro Studies

The metabolic activity of the gut bacterial flora has been reviewed extensively by Smith (1966), Drasar and Hill (1974) and by Hill (1986). Table 6 lists some of the types of reaction carried out by the flora; these are principally hydrolytic and reductive in nature. The hydrolytic enzymes include the glycosidases, proteases and amidases, lipases, sulphatases, etc. Hawksworth et al. (1971) studied some important glycosidases of pure strains of gut bacteria and showed that, whereas *E. coli* produced the highest specific activity of β-glucuronidase, the numerical dominance of the non-sporing, strictly anaerobic bacteria means that *E. coli* contributed less than 0.1% of the caecal β-glucuronidase activity. Similarly, although streptococci are the producers of the highest specific activity of β-glucosidase, the intestinal activity of this enzyme is produced mainly by the non-sporing anaerobic bacteria.

Proteolysis has been studied using a range of substrates; in older studies the substrates tended to be meat, gelatin, casein, etc.; in recent years specific amide hydrolases have been studied and used taxonomically in the identification of gut bacteria. Regardless of the specific activity, numerical considerations make it certain that almost all of the protein digestion occurring in the colon is the result of the action of enzymes produced by the non-sporing anaerobic bacteria.

The major reductive reactions in the gut are oxoreductases, nitroreductases, hydrogenation of double bonds and dehydroxylations. Many of these reactions have been studied in less detail than the hydrolases and only nitrate reductase has been used extensively in the taxonomy of gut bacteria. The reductive reactions of bacteria are of metabolic value as a means to control the redox potential of the environment and as a source of terminal hydrogen acceptors.

Whole Animal Studies

Much of the information on the metabolic activities of the flora of the digestive tract stemmed from whole animal studies. The production of glycosidases by gut bacteria

Table 6. The types of reactions carried out by the gut bacterial flora, with some examples

Class of reaction	Examples	Function
Hydrolytic	Glycosidases (β-glucosidase, β-galactosidase, etc.)	Carbohydrate metabolism
	Proteinases, peptidases tryptophanase, tyrosinase	Protein metabolism
	lipases, esterases	Fat metabolism
Reductions	Azoreductase	Metabolism of food colours
	Nitrate reductase	
	Amino reductase	e.g. Chloramphenicol inactivation
	Cholesterol reductase	Cholesterol metabolism
Oxidations	Hydroxysteroid dehydrogenases	Bile acid metabolism
	Steroid nuclear dehydrogenases	Bile acid metabolism
Eliminations	Bile acid dehydroxylase	Bile acid metabolism
	Amino acid decarboxylases	

would be well known to bacteriologists because so many of the standard tests in bacterial identification are of "sugar fermentations". Salicin, amygdalin, aesculin, etc. are plant glucosides and tests of "fermentation" of these "sugars" are of the relative speed with which the β-glucosidase of the particular strain utilises the test compound as a substrate. However, in vitro results only give the capacity of individual organisms to carry out the reaction; whole animal studies are needed to determine which ones are carried out under the conditions prevailing in the gut. The metabolism of a range of substrates of possible relevance to human carcinogenesis has been investigated, involving some using the enzymes already described above. Examples of glycosidases, in this context, are β-glucuronidase in the enterohepatic circulation of polycyclic aromatic hydrocarbons (PAHs) and β-glucosidase in the metabolism of the plant glucoside cycasin (methylazoxymethanolglucoside). PAHs, ingested from environmental sources, are detoxified by hydroxylation then conjugation as glucuronides; these conjugates are hydrolysed by bacterial β-glucuronidase to yield the (non-carcinogenic) hydroxylated PAHs, which may be further dehydroxylated to yield the parent PAH (Renwick and Drasar 1976). Kinoshita and Gelboin (1978) showed that during hydrolysis of the conjugate by glucuronidase a short-lived highly active intermediate is formed which binds to DNA and hence is potentially carcinogenic. Cycasin is a plant glucoside which is metabolised by bacterial β-glucosidase to yield methylazoxymethanol; this is a potent colon carcinogen in rodents, but has still to be shown to be carcinogenic in humans. The gut mucosal β-glucosidase is highly substrate specific and is not active on cycasin; the bacterial enzyme is much less substrate specific and is able to hydrolyse cycasin readily. Until recent years it was debated whether cycasin was unique or was an example of a family of carcinogenic glucosides produced by plants. The recent studies of the mutagenicity of plant products suggest the latter; a large number of compounds are not mutagenic in their natural state but are highly active after treatment with β-glucosidase.

Nitrate reductase is widely used as a taxonomic test; the importance of the enzyme in human carcinogenesis derives from the role of bacteria as the source of nitrite (from nitrate) in the body. This is important because the N-nitroso compounds are a family of potent carcinogens in all animal species in which they have been tested and nitrite is an essential precursor of endogenous N-nitrosation. The dietary load of nitrite has been estimated by many groups (e.g. White 1975) and has been shown to be very low (less than 1 mg per day). However, the dietary load of nitrate is very much higher (White 1975) and a small fraction of the dietary nitrate is reduced to nitrite in the mouth (Bartholomew and Hill 1984). Dietary nitrate is absorbed rapidly from the upper small intestine and is secreted in saliva, sweat, tears, etc. before final excretion in urine (Bartholomew and Hill 1984). Of the nitrate secreted in saliva a proportion (usually 20% – 50%) is reduced to nitrite by the salivary flora; consequently the vast proportion of nitrite entering the stomach is the result of bacterial reduction of nitrate in the mouth and very little is of dietary origin.

Other sites of formation of nitrite by bacterial action in the human body are the stomach, the urinary bladder, large bowel and the uterine cervix. The normal stomach is highly acidic, has only a transient flora and so is not a site for local nitrite production. However, in the neutral stomach there is a rich bacterial flora and a high rate of local nitrite formation. The normal urinary bladder is free from bacteria, and there is no nitrate reduction; in the infected urinary bladder, in contrast, there is (numerically) a rich bacterial flora, long incubation times between micturations and consequently high amounts of nitrite are generated. Since we know that nitrate is secreted in saliva, sweat, tears and gastric juice, it is likely that it is secreted in all body secretions. The normal vaginal flora does not include large numbers of nitrate reducers, and the normal vaginal nitrite concentration is low; in vaginal infection the flora is greatly modified and includes nitrate reducers, and it is likely that the vaginal nitrite concentration is high. Finally, it is likely that some nitrate is secreted into the normal colon and very rapidly metabolised to nitrite and beyond; however, in patients with urine diversion into the sigmoid colon (ureterosigmoid anastomosis) urine rich in nitrate is conducted into the colon where it is reduced by the profuse local bacterial flora (Stewart et al. 1981).

A number of amino acids are metabolised in vivo to yield products known to be carcinogens, co-carcinogens, tumour promoters, mutagens or co-mutagens. Tyrosine is metabolised in the gut to yield volatile phenols which are absorbed from the gut, conjugated as sulphates or glucuronides, and excreted in the urine. The principal urinary volatile phenols (UVP) are phenol and p-cresol. The amount of UVP is decreased to very small levels by total colectomy, by colonic wash-out or by treatment with certain antibiotic cocktails (Table 7). It is related to diet and varies between populations. A number of volatile phenols, including the UVPs, have been shown to be promoters of skin carcinogenesis in rodents where the initiating carcinogen was PAH (Boutwell and Bosch 1959). Tryptophan is metabolised in the human to a wide range of products which are excreted in the urine. These are the products of both hepatic and bacterial metabolism; all of them *could* be produced by the gut bacterial flora (the pathways for their production were all demonstrated first in bacteria), and we have no information on the relative importance of the colonic flora and hepatic metabolism as contributors to the urinary pool of tryptophan metabolites. Many of the metabolites have been shown to be tumour promoters or initiators in rodent model systems and they have been claimed to be of importance in the causation of non-industrial bladder cancers (Bryan 1971). Methionine is metabolised in vitro to its

Table 7. The daily excretion of UVP in various populations and patient groups

	UVP	
	Total (mg/day)	Cresol/phenol (mg/day)
British living in London	68.1	5.0
Danes living in Copenhagen	93.9	6.9
Danes living in Them	63.4	2.7
Finns living in Helsinki	70.9	3.1
Finns living in Perrikala	68.4	5.5
British consuming 140 g protein per day	108.1	
60 g protein per day	74.1	
Patients with: Total colectomy	6.2	0.2
Left hemicolectomy	61.5	12.0
Small bowel overgrowth	140.2	2.0
Pre-operative bowel preparation	21.6	8.0

S-ethyl analogue ethionine by a range of bacterial species (Farber 1963). Ethionine is a potent carcinogen (Fisher and Mallette 1961), but it has not been studied in the context of the production of carcinogens by gut bacteria.

Bile acids are synthesised in the liver as cholic acid (CA) and chenodeoxycholic acid (CDC) and are secreted in bile as their glycine or taurine conjugates. They are absorbed from the terminal ileum by an active transport process and are returned to the liver via the portal vein for resection in the bile. The function of bile acids in fat digestion, and their enterohepatic circulation has been reviewed by Hoffmann (1977). Although the recovery of bile acids from the terminal ileum is very efficient, 1%–4% escape to the colon. In addition to the efficiency of recovery from the terminal ileum, various factors (mostly dietary) contribute in determining the amount of bile acid entering the colon and therefore, being exposed to the gut bacteria (Table 8). In the colon the bile acids are extensively metabolised, the principal reactions being deconjugation, hydroxysteroid oxido-reduction at the 3, 7 and 12 positions, 7α-dehydroxylation and nuclear dehydrogenation at the 4–5 position (reviewed by Hill 1975). Of the bile acid metabolites, the two major ones found in faeces are deoxycholic acid (DC) and lithocholic acid (LA) formed by the 7α-dehydroxylation of the hepatic bile acids CA and CDC, respectively. Both DC and LA have been shown to be tumour promoters in animal models and co-mutagens in bacterial mutagenesis assay systems (Table 9). They have also been implicated in human large bowel cancer, and this will be discussed in detail later.

The other bile acid metabolites of interest are the products of nuclear dehydrogenation. Certain clostridia, referred to as "nuclear dehydrogenating (NDH) clostridia" (Goddard et al. 1975), or simply as "NDC", are able to introduce double bonds into the steroid nucleus in conjugation with a 3-oxo group. The products of this reaction are structurally similar to families of known carcinogens, but the evidence that they may be of importance in colorectal cancer is derived almost entirely from epidemiological studies and will be discussed later in this chapter.

Table 8. Factors controlling the faecal loss of bile acids. (From Hill 1980.)

Dietary change	Faecal bile acids loss	
	Per day	Concentration
Increased protein	None	None
Increased digestible carbohydrate	None	None
Increased fat	Increase	Increase
Increased dietary fibre		
Wheat bran	None	Decrease
100 g wheat bran	Increase	Decrease
Oat bran	Increase	Increase
Bagasse	Increase	None
Pectin	Increase	Increase
Guar	Increase	None
Cellulose	None	Decrease
Added lactulose/mannitol	Increase	Decrease
Residue-free diet	Decrease	Decrease

Table 9. Evidence that the bile acids DCA and LA are tumour promoters, co-mutagens, mutagens, etc.

Bile acid	Test system	Observation
DC	Drosophila	Mutagenicity
	Ames test	Co-mutagenicity to a variety of mutagens
	Rodent colon	Promoter of colon carcinogenesis
	Human studies	Epidemiology relates DCA to colon cancer risk in populations
LA	Cell transformation	Mutagenicity
	Ames test	Co-mutagenicity to a variety of mutagens
	Rodent colon	Promoter of colon carcinogenesis
	Human studies	Epidemiology relates LA to colon cancer risk in individuals (LA/DC ratio)

Bacterial Metabolism in Various Colorectal Subsites

Bacterial metabolism has already been discussed briefly in the section on the relation between diet and the gut bacterial flora. There is a growing body of evidence that the major site of bacterial metabolism in the large intestine is the proximal region – the caecum and ascending colon. This has already been summarised in Table 4. In studies of persons at post mortem, the metabolism of cholesterol was as extensive in the ascending colon as in faeces in more than 80% of persons (Boyer et al. 1984). In cannulated pigs similar results were obtained to those seen in humans (Fadden et al. 1984). Clearly, this observation requires an explanation, and it is likely that this is to be found in (a) the high metabolic activity of the flora which results in the metabolism of a high proportion of the substrate in the proximal colon; (b) the relatively fluid conditions in the proximal colon which allow easy mixing of substrate and bacteria (in contrast to the situation in faeces where it is clear that the access of bacterial enzymes to substrates is limited by the viscosity of the matrix). For the reasons given above, it is clear that, in a study of the role of gut bacteria in colorectal carcinogenesis, it is the caecal and not the faecal flora that should be studied. Nevertheless, for reasons of accessibility, all studies to date have been carried out on faeces.

Sentinel Enzymes

Because the gut bacteria can produce metabolites with carcinogenic potential by a number of routes, some workers (led by Goldin and Gorbach 1977) have advocated the study of a set of "sentinel enzymes" instead of attempting to culture the total bacterial flora or of needing to opt for a particular metabolite or enzyme. The value of this approach is that enzyme activities can be assayed with reasonable accuracy whereas estimates of bacterial counts are extremely inaccurate. In consequence, subtle differences or alterations in the bacterial flora, which certainly could not be detected by classical bacteriological methods, might be detected by assaying the sentinel enzymes.

The enzymes chosen included β-glucuronidase, β-glucosidase, azoreductase, nitro-reductase and bile acid 7α-dehydroxylase. Users of the sentinel enzymes have had many successes in detecting changes in the faecal flora resulting from dietary change. However, the modifications have been small, and it has been impossible to determine whether the changes in enzyme activity have been due to changes in the relative proportions of enzyme producers and non-producers or to a change in the specific activity of enzyme produced by the enzyme producers with no change in relative numbers.

Although the major problem perceived with studies of sentinel enzymes is that of interpretation of the results, a much more serious problem is that the method has been applied to the analyses of faeces.

Colorectal Bacteria in Relation to Cancer Prevention

In a discussion of colorectal bacteria in relation to cancer prevention, it is first necessary to determine whether bacteria actually have a role in the disease. If so, the nature of the role needs to be determined, from which the best strategies for cancer prevention can be devised.

Evidence of a Role for Colorectal Bacteria in Human Cancer

A major source of evidence of a role for the colorectal bacterial flora in carcinogenesis is from animal studies. It was noticed by Bakke and Midtvedt (1970) that the rate of spontaneous hepatoma formation was very much lower in germ-free rats than in rats with a normal bacterial flora. In studies of colon carcinogenesis in which rats are given the closely related potent carcinogens dimethylhydrazine (DMH) or azoxymethane (AOM), the rate of tumour development was very much slower in germ-free than in conventional rats (Reddy et al. 1974). This was not, of course, seen when the direct-acting carcinogen N-methyl-N'-nitro-N-nitrosoguanidine (MNNG) was used.

Germ-free animals differ greatly from their conventional relatives because the lack of a bacterial flora has a profound effect on the development of the immune system and also on the functioning of the gut. For example, lack of a gut bacterial flora results in a massive accumulation of intestinal mucin and shed mucosal cells (which would normally be digested by the flora), and a consequence of this is that the germ-free rats have a massive caecum that can account for a high proportion of the total body weight of the animal. In order to try to avoid these problems, Goldin and Gorbach (1981) studied the effect of suppressing the gut bacterial flora using anti-biotic cocktails known to be effective in that respect. They confirmed that the rate of DMH-induced colorectal tumour formation was very much lower in the antibiotically treated than in the untreated rats.

There has been a host of studies of the effect of surgically diverting the faecal stream on the rate of tumour formation. For example Williamson et al. (1980) showed, using a range of surgical procedures to isolate different parts of the gut of rodents treated with colon carcinogens, that the rate of tumour formation in the isolated section was always much lower than that in the portions of the gut with a normal faecal stream. They concluded that the faecal stream was a major factor in the promotion of colorectal tumours in this animal model.

There is, of necessity, much less evidence of a role for the gut flora in human colorectal carcinogenesis. The delivery of germ-free babies is well documented, but in no case has the infant been preserved in that state for prolonged periods of time, and so there is no information on the effect of germ-free status. Patients are often maintained on antibiotic cocktails designed to suppress the gut flora for long periods of time. However, such patients are usually short-lived and are not a suitable study population for colorectal cancer risk. However, there have been reports that diversion of the faecal stream (in, for example, patients treated by colostomy and in whom a length of rectum is not removed) causes regression of rectal polyps in polyposis patients (Cole and Holden 1959).

Evidence for a Role for Colorectal Bacteria in Colorectal Cancer

The evidence that bacteria in general are important has been given above. Considerable amounts of effort have been expended in trying to identify specific bacterial activities that might be incriminated in colorectal carcinogenesis. These include the enterohepatic circulation of PAHs, the 7α-dehydroxylation of bile acids, the nuclear dehydrogenation of bile acids and the production of "faecal mutagens".

Enterohepatic Circulation of PAHs. PAHs are ingested with food or as pollutants and are conjugated by the liver as their glucuronides before secretion in the bile and elimination from the body. Because of their hydrophilicity, the glucuronides are not absorbed from the small bowel and so are exposed to the vast bacterial population of the large intestine where they are deconjugated (Renwick and Drasar 1976). The aglycone released is the hydroxy PAH which is not carcinogenic; however, Renwick and Drasar then demonstrated that gut bacterial isolates, particularly clostridia, dehydroxylated the aglycone to yield the parent (and carcinogenic) PAH. From this basis they postulated a role for bacterial β-glucuronidase and PAHs in colorectal carcinogenesis. Later studies by Kinoshita and Gelboin (1978) showed that during β-glucuronidase action a short-lived, high-energy intermediate was released which readily bound to DNA and so was potentially carcinogenic. On the basis of studies such as these, β-glucuronidase was included in the group of sentinel enzymes proposed by Goldin and Gorbach (1977) and described earlier.

A problem with this hypothesis is the very high activity of β-glucuronidase in the bacterial flora of the large bowel. Based on the data of Fernandez et al. (1985) on the flora of the terminal ileum and on the enzyme activities reported by Hawksworth et al. (1971), it can be calculated that the β-glucuronidase activity at that site would rapidly hydrolyse all of the biliary PAH in the proximal colon. Thus the highly active intermediate could only be incriminated in cancer of the proximal large bowel (the aetiology of which is known to be distinct from that of the distal colon; Jensen 1985).

7α-dehydroxylation of Bile Acids. There is a body of evidence suggesting a role for bile acid 7α-dehydroxylase in the causing of colorectal cancer. The key study was carried out by Mastromarino et al. (1976) who showed that the activity of the enzyme was

much higher in the faeces of persons with colorectal cancer than in faeces from healthy control persons. These results have been repeated by T. Jivraj and M. Hill (unpublished results).

The products of the action of the 7α-dehydroxylase on the primary bile acids synthesised by the liver (CA and CDC) are DC and LA, respectively. Studies by many groups have shown that DC and LA are potent tumour promoters in the rodent colon, whilst the parent primary bile acids are inactive. Similarly Wilpart et al. (1983) have shown that DC and LA are potent co-mutagens, whilst the primary bile acids are inactive. Table 9 lists the evidence implicating the products of 7α-dehydroxylation in colorectal carcinogenesis. Studies of the ability of gut bacteria to carry out this reaction show that the enzyme is only produced by the strictly anaerobic genera together with some strains of faecal streptococci (Hill 1975). The enzyme has been studied in detail by Aries and Hill (1970) and by Hylemon and Stellwag 1976. Because it has been so strongly implicated in colorectal carcinogenesis, the bile acid 7α-dehydroxylase was included in the list of sentinel enzymes proposed by Goldin and Gorbach (1977) and described earlier.

Nuclear Dehydrogenation of Bile Acids. The evidence of a role for NDC in colorectal cancer comes from studies of populations, case-control studies and studies of high-risk patient goups, all of which show that an increased risk of colorectal cancer is associated with an increased risk of carrying NDC. The evidence is summarised in Table 10. Unfortunately, in a study of the minor faecal bile acids, the number and amount of unsaturated bile acid found was disappointing (Wait et al. 1985). However, there was copious evidence of the formation of such compounds since they are intermediates in the formation of allo bile acids, a number of which were found consistently by Wait et al., Wilpart et al. (1983) demonstrated that the allo bile acids (with 5α configuration) were more potent co-mutagens than the 5β-analogues synthesised by the liver.

Faecal Mutagen. A faecal mutagen was reported by Bruce et al. (1977) in faeces. Further studies of this mutagen revealed it to be a family of icosapentenoyl glycerol ethers (Gupta et al. 1983). Reports of the mutagen and of the assay methods resulted in a spate of epidemiological studies relating faecal mutagen activity to the risk of malignancy, but all of these studies were heavily criticised by Vennitt (1982) who

Table 10. Evidence that clostridia capable of producing unsaturated bile acids are associated with an increased risk of colorectal cancer

Type of study	Observation
Comparison of populations	NDC carriage correlated with incidence of CRC
Case-control studies	Carriage of NDC much higher in cases than in controls
Adenoma patients	NDC carriage correlated with adenoma size (a major risk factor in CRC)
Patients with partial colitis of more than 10 years' duration	Carriage of NDC related to severity of dysplasia

CRC, colorectal cancer.

pointed out the very great fluctuations in activity within a stool and between stools in an individual. Until better assay methods have been applied, the role of the faecal mutagen in human colorectal cancer remains controversial.

Possible Strategies for Cancer Prevention

If colorectal bacteria have a role in colorectal carcinogenesis, then various strategies for cancer prevention might be possible including (a) removing or decreasing the numbers of key bacteria; (b) decreasing the substrate concentration; or (c) changing the physico-chemical environment in the colon to one less favourable to the production of harmful metabolites.

The first of these possibilities can be dismissed rapidly because no safe method is available for modifying the faecal flora, and too little is known about the caecal flora to be able to permit recommendations.

Changing the substrate concentration is likely to be more fruitful and this may be achieved by dietary manipulation. Table 8 lists the effects of various dietary modifications on the faecal bile acid concentration. In recent years it has been suggested that a high intake of dietary calcium results in a high colonic concentration of the cation which then forms insoluble soaps with the colonic bile acids (Newmark et al. 1984). This inactivates or ameliorates the toxic effects of bile acids on the colonic mucosa (Wargowich et al. 1983; Rafter et al. 1986) and provides a possibly simple and effective method of countering the effects of bile acids; this is being studied in a number of centres.

The optimal conditions for the production and activity of many of the bacterial enzymes of interest in colorectal carcinogenesis include a neutral pH and highly reducing and anoxic environment. Although the conditions are difficult to modify in general, the pH can be manipulated by dietary means. It has been established that the caecal pH can be acidified by administration of lactulose (Bown et al. 1974; Florent et al. 1985), and it has been suggested that acidification of the colon would be of value in decreasing the risk of colorectal cancer (Hill 1974; Thornton 1981; Berge Henegouwan et al. 1987). In this respect any "non-fermentable" sugar (i.e. non-fermentable by intestinal enzymes) will have a similar effect, but the extent of acidification will depend on the rate of fermentation of the sugar bacterial enzymes. Alternatives to lactulose therefore include some sugar alcohol such as mannitol, lactitol, xylitol.

References

Aries VC, Hill MJ (1970) Degradation of steroids by intestinal bacteria. II. Enzymes catalysing the oxidoreduction of the 3α-, 7α- and 12α-hydroxyl group. Biochim Biophys Acta 202: 535–544

Bakke OM, Midtvedt T (1970) Influence of germ-free status on the excretion of simple phenols of possible significance in tumour promotion. Experientia 26: 519

Bartholomew B, Hill MJ (1984) The pharmacology of dietary nitrate and the origin of urinary nitrate. Food Chem Toxicol 22: 789–795

Berge Henegouwen GP, Van Der Werf S, Ruben A (1987) Effect of long-term lactulose ingestion on secondary bile salt metabolism in man: potential protective effect of lactulose in colonic carcinogenesis. Gut 28: 675–680

Boutwell RK, Bosch DK (1959) The tumour promoting effect of phenol and related compounds on the mouse skin. Cancer Res 19:413–427

Bown RL, Gibson JA, Sladen GE, Hicks B, Dawson AM (1974) Effects of lactulose and other laxatives on ileal and colonic pH as measured by a radiotelemetry device. Gut 15:999–1004

Boyer J, Day DW, Hill MJ (1984) Site of cholesterol metabolism in the human gut. Trans Biochem Soc 12:1104–1105

Bruce WR, Varghese AJ, Furrer R, Land PC (1977) A mutagen in the feces of normal humans. In: Hiatt H, Watson J, Winsten J (eds) Origins of human cancer. Cold Spring Harbor, New York, p 1641–1646

Bryan GT (1971) The role of urinary tryptophan metabolites in the etiology of bladder cancer. Am J Clin Nutr 24:841–847

Cole JW, Holden WD (1959) Post-colectomy regression of adenomatous polyps in the human colon. Arch Surg 79:385–392

Drasar BS, Hill MJ (1974) Human intestinal flora. Academic, London

Fadden K, Owen R, Hill MJ et al. (1984) Steroid degradation along the gastrointestinal tract: the use of the cannulated pig as a model system. Trans Biochem Soc 12:1105–1106

Farber E (1963) Ethionine carcinogenesis. Adv Cancer Res 7:383

Fernandez F, Kennedy H, Hill MJ, Truelove S (1985) The effect of diet on the bacterial flora of ileostomy fluid. Microb Aliments Nutr 3:47–52

Finegold SM, Flora DJ, Attebury HR, Sutter VL (1975) Fecal bacteriology of colonic polyp patients and control patients. Cancer Res 35:3407–3417

Fisher JF, Mallette MF (1961) The natural occurrence of ethionine in bacteria. J Gen Physiol 45:1–13

Florent C, Fluorie B, Leblond A et al. (1985) Influence of chronic lactulose ingestion on the colonic metabolism of lactulose in man (an in vivo study). J Clin Invest 75:608–613

Goddard P, Fernandez F, West B et al. (1975) The nuclear dehydrogenation of steroids by intestinal bacteria. J Med Microbiol 8:429–435

Goldin B, Gorbach SL (1977) Alterations in fecal microflora enzymes related to diet, age, lactobacillus supplements and dimethylhydrazine. Cancer 40:2421–2426

Goldin B, Gorbach SL (1981) Effects of antibiotics on incidence of rat intestinal tumors induced by 1,2-dimethylhydrazine. J Natl Cancer Inst 67:877–880

Gupta I, Baptista J, Bruce WR et al. (1983) Structures of fecal pentaenes, the mutagens of bacterial origin from human feces. Biochemistry 22:241–245

Hawksworth GM, Drasar BS, Hill MJ (1971) Gut bacteria and the hydrolysis of glycosidic bonds. J Med Microbiol 4:451–457

Hill MJ (1974) Steroid nuclear dehydrogenation and colon cancer. Am J Clin Nutr 27:1475–1480

Hill MJ (1975) The role of colon anaerobes in the metabolism of bile acids and steroids and its relation to colon cancer. Cancer 36:2387–2400

Hill MJ (1980) Conservation of bile acids. In: Fumigalli R, Kritchevsky D, Paoletti R (eds) Drugs affecting lipid metabolism. Elsevier, Amsterdam, pp 89–96

Hill MJ (1986) Microbial metabolism in the digestive tract. CRC, Boca Raton

Hofmann AF (1977) The enterohepatic circulation of bile acids in man. Clin Gastroineterol 6:3–24

Hudson MJ, Borriello SP, Hill MJ (1984) Elemental diets and the bacterial flora of the gastrointestinal tract. In: Russell R (ed) Elemental diets. CRC, Boca Raton, pp 105–126

Hylemon PB, Stellwag EJ (1976) Bile acid biotransformation rates of selected gram-positive and gram-negative intestinal anaerobic bacteria. Biochem Biophys Res Commun 69:1088–1094

Jensen OM (1985) The role of diet in colorectal cancer. In: Joossens J, Hill M, Geboers J (eds) Diet and human carcinogenesis. Elsevier, Amsterdam, pp 137–147

Kinoshita N, Gelboin H (1978) β-Glucuronidase catalysed hydrolysis of benzy-α-pyrene-3-glucuronide and binding to DNA. Science 199:307–310

Maier B, Flynn M, Burton G et al. (1974) Effects of a high beef diet on the bowel flora: a preliminary report. Am J Clin Nutr 27:1470–1474

Mastromarino A, Reddy BS, Wynder EL (1976) Metabolic epidemiology of colon cancer: enzymic activity of the fecal flora. Am J Clin Nutr 29:1455–1460

Metchnikoff E (1903) In: Chalmers M (ed) The nature of man: studies in optimisting philosophy. Putram, New York, p 254

Moore WEC, Holdeman LV (1974) Human fecal flora: the normal flora of 20 Japanese Hawaiians. Appl Microbiol 27:961–979

Newmark HL, Wargovich MJ, Bruce WR (1984) Colon cancer, dietary fat, phosphate and calcium: a hypothesis. JNCI 72:1323–1325

Rafter J, Eng V, Furrer R, Medline A, Bruce WR (1986) Effects of calcium and pH on the mucosal damage produced by deoxycholic acid in the rat colon. Gut 27:1320–1329

Reddy BS, Weisburger JH, Narisawa T, Wynder EL (1974) Colon carcinogenesis in germ-free rats with dimethylhydrazine and N-methyl-N-nitro-N-nitroso-guanidine. Cancer Res 34:2368–2372

Renwick AG, Drasar BS (1976) Environmental carcinogens and large-bowel cancer. Nature 263:234–235

Smith RL (1966) The biliary secretion and enterohepatic circulation of drugs and other organic compounds. Prog Drug Res 9:300–360

Stewart M, Hill MJ, Pugh RC, Williams JP (1981) The role of N-nitrosamines in carcinogenesis at the ureterocolic anastomosis. Br J Urol 53:115–118

Thornton JR (1981) High colonic pH promotes colorectal cancer. Lancet i:1081–1082

Vennitt S (1982) Faecal mutagens in the aetiology of colonic cancer. In: Malt R, Williamson R (eds) Colonic carcinogenesis. MTP Press, Lancaster, pp 59–72

Vince A, Zeegen R, Drinkwater JE, O'Grady FW, Dawson AM (1974) The effect of lactulose on the faecal flora of patients with hepatic encephalopathy. J Med Microbiol 7:163

Wait R, Thompson MH, Hill MJ (1985) Faecal steroids and colorectal cander: allo bile acids. Br J Cancer 52:445

Wargovich MJ, Eng V, Newmark HL, Bruce WR (1983) Calcium ameliorates the toxic effect of deoxycholic acid on colonic epithelism. Carcinogenesis 4:1205–1207

White JW (1975) Relative significance of dietary sources of nitrate and nitrite. J Agric Food Chem 23:886–894

Williamson RCN, Bauer F, Terpstra O, Ross JS, Malt RA (1980) Contrasting effects of subtotal enteric bypass, enterectomy and colectomy on azoxymethane-induced intestinal carcinogenesis. Cancer Res 40:538–543

Wilpart M, Mainguet P, Maskens A, Roberfroid M (1983) Structure – activity relationship amongst biliary acids showing co-mutagenicity towards 1,2-dimethylhydrazine. Carcinogenesis 4:1239–1241

Ethanol and Colorectal Carcinogenesis

H. K. Seitz and U. A. Simanowski

Department of Internal Medicine, University of Heidelberg, Bergheimerstr. 58,
D-6900 Heidelberg, FRG

Contents

Introduction

Ethanol has to be considered as one of the most important toxins consumed regularly and in high quantities by humans. Throughout history, alcoholic beverages have been widely used for their pleasant taste and their mood-altering effects. However, during the last few decades alcohol consumption has steadily increased worldwide, and alcoholism has become one of the major health problems. Haevy alcohol ingestion exerts a deleterious effect on almost every organ and tissue of the human body. The most important ethanol-related diseases are hepatic cirrhosis, pancreatitis, cardio-myopathy, hematological and neurological disorders, infections such as tuberculosis, and tumor development.

Epidemologic studies and animal experiments have identified ethanol as a cocar-cinogen and tumor promoter for various organs including the upper alimentary and respiratory tract (Seitz and Simanowski 1986), the liver (Lieber et al. 1986), the breast (Schatzkin et al. 1987; Willett et al. 1987), and the rectum (Seitz and Simanowski 1988). This chapter will focus on epidemiologic studies and animal experiments with respect to ethanol and colorectal carcinogenesis. The main emphasis, however, will be on possible mechanisms by which alcohol may influence tumor occurrence in the large intestine.

Epidemiology

In 1974 Breslow and Enstrom were the first to raise the possibility of an association between beer consumption and the occurrence of rectal cancer. In a retrospective study, average annual age-adjusted cancer mortality rates for 1950–1967 were correlated with per capita consumption of spirits, wine, and beer as estimated from tax receipts in 41 states of the United States and in 24 other countries. The strongest single association found was between rectal but not colon cancer and beer consumption (Enstrom 1977). Other retrospective cohort studies followed confirming these data. McMichael et al. (1979) analyzed time trends in cancer mortality from 1921 in the United States, England and Wales, Australia, and New Zealand in relation to changes in per capita consumption of alcohol. For rectal cancer, and to a lesser extent for colon cancer, the most consistent correlate in comparison across time, and between place, sex and age-group was again beer intake. Similar observations have been made by Knox (1977) who analyzed alcohol intake and chief causes of mortality in 20 different countries including European countries, the Unites States, Canada, and Japan; by Kono and Ikeda (1979) who found, in a retrospective study based on geographic correlations between standardized mortality ratios and alcohol consumption, a significant correlation between cancer of the rectum and wine ingestion in Japanese males; and by Potter et al. (1982) who found that changes in beer consumption over time correlate with subsequent changes in rectal cancer, particularly among younger age groups.

At an individual level, various case-control studies have collected data on alcohol consumption and large bowel cancer. In 1979–1981, 419 patients with colon and rectal cancer and 732 controls were questioned regarding diet and alcohol (Potter and McMichael 1986). Cancer cases were a population-based series reported in the South Australian Central Cancer Registry, were 30–74 years of age, and were resident in metropolitan Adelaide. Total alcohol intake (but not specifically beer) was associated with increased risk of both colon and rectal cancer in women. In addition, in both sexes there was an increased risk of large intestinal cancer associated with spirit consumption. Two further case-control studies also reported an increased risk for cancer of both colon and rectum in relation to beer intake (Bielke 1973; Wynder and Shigematsu 1967), whereas one study failed to show such an association (Graham et al. 1978). Another study was conducted in Japan and also failed to detect a relationship between beer consumption and rectal cancer (Wynder et al. 1969). However, in Japan beer consumption is low (International Statistics on Alcoholic Beverages 1977) and rectal cancer might therefore be more related to exposure variables of greater inter-individual heterogeneity. Unfortunately some case-control studies have treated large bowel cancer as a single entity without differentiation between colon and rectum (Potter et al. 1982; Pernu 1960; Higginson 1966). In these studies only Higginson (1966) observed a higher risk of rectal cancer for beer drinkers. Furthermore, two follow-up studies in Norway, one of over 12000 middle-aged men, the other of approximately 1700 male alcoholics have also observed such an increased risk for beer consumers (Sundby 1967; Bjelke 1973).

In two recent studies of brewery workers, no excess risk of bowel cancer was inferred in the Copenhagen study (Jensen 1979), whereas in Dublin a two-fold excess of rectal cancer was observed with beer consumption (Dean et al. 1979). However, re-examination of the Danish data suggests that there may have been some increased risk for this group of brewery workers relative to that of social class peers (Potter et al. 1982). Another explanation for the controversial results between the Copenhagen and

Dublin studies was attributed to the fact that Danish beers have a significantly lower dimethylnitrosamine content than Irish beers (Lieber et al. 1986).

Subsequently, two prospective studies have been performed with respect to alcohol consumption and large bowel cancer in the United States. In Hawaii 8006 subjects were followed for an average of approximately 14 years. The study showed an approximate three-fold risk of developing rectal but not colon cancer when 1 liter beer or more was ingested regularly every day (Pollack et al. 1984). Similar results were published from southern California where 11 888 residents of a retirement community were followed up for 4½ years. Here daily alcohol drinkers experienced a nearly two-fold increase in risk for rectal cancer (Wu et al. 1987).

Taking all these data from retrospective, prospective, and case-control studies together, chronic alcohol consumption seems to be associated with a small but significant increase of cancer risk for the rectum, but far less for the colon. This increased risk seems mainly due to beer consumption, although alcohol itself may also affect rectal carcinogenesis. In this context it should be noted that small amounts of nitrosamines have been found in beers (Spiegelhalder et al. 1979).

Animal Experiments

Ethanol per se is not a carcinogen (Ketcham et al. 1963). However, when administered to animals in combination with a chemical carcinogen, ethanol may be cocarcinogenic for some organs under certain experimental conditions, especially when given before or together with the carcinogen, or it may act as a tumor promoter when administered after tumor initiation (Seitz and Simanowski 1988). Thus, chronic ethanol consumption enhances chemically induced carcinogenesis in the upper alimentary (Giebel 1967; Gabrial et al. 1982) and respiratory tract (McCoy et al. 1981; Castonguay et al. 1984) and in the liver (Porta et al. 1985; Takada et al. 1986; Driver and McLean 1986). Factors which influence the effect of ethanol on carcinogenesis in animals include the type of carcinogen used, as well as the dose, duration, and means of carcinogen- and ethanol administration (Seitz 1985a). One of the most important factors seems to be the means of alcohol application. If alcohol is added to the drinking water, ethanol intake may be extremely low, but nutritional deficiencies may occur which can influence carcinogenesis (Seitz and Simanowski 1986, 1987, 1988). Thus, only the administration of ethanol as a liquid diet, first introduced by Lieber and DeCarli (1970), guarantees an adequate ethanol intake and takes care of nutritional factors.

Table 1 summarizes the results of chronic ethanol ingestion on chemically induced colorectal carcinogenesis in rats. In two of the eight studies ethanol was given in the drinking water, and the results of these experiments have, therefore, to be questioned (Howarth and Pihl 1985; Nelson and Samelson 1985). When the two procarcinogens dimethylhydrazine (DMH) and azoxymethane (AM) have been used to induce colorectal tumors, different results have been reported, mainly depending on the experimental conditions. In these studies it is important to note that both compounds need metabolic activation by cytochrome P-540-dependent microsomal enzymes to become carcinogenic (Fig. 1). The results of these studies depend on the ethanol dose used and on the timing of ethanol administration (Hamilton et al. 1987a, 1987b; Seitz et al.

Table 1. Effect of ethanol on chemically induced colorectal carcinogenesis in rats

References	Carcinogen	Ethanol administration	Ethanol effect
Seitz et al. (1984)	DMH, s.c.	6% l.d. (36% total calories), preinduction	Increased rectal but not colonic tumors
Howarth and Pihl (1985)	DMH, s.c.	5% d.w., induction	No effect
Nelson and Samelson (1985)	DMH, s.c.	5% d.w., preinduction/induction	No effect
McGarrity et al. (1986)	DMH, s.c.	6% l.d. (36% total calories), preinduction	No effect
Garzon et al. (1987)	AMMN, i.r.	6% l.d. (36% total calories), preinduction/induction	Increased rectal tumors
Hamilton et al. (1987b)	AOM, s.c.	l.d. (11%, 22%, 33% total calories), preinduction/induction, postinduction	Inhibition of tumor development in the left but less in the right colon. Higher ethanol intake has a stronger inhibitory effect. No effect when ethanol is given in the postinduction phase.
Hamilton et al. (1987a)	AOM, s.c.	l.d. (9%, 18% total calories ethanol), (12%, 23% total calories beer), preinduction/induction	High ethanol inhibits tumors in the right but not in the left colon, while low ethanol enhances tumors in the left colon but not in the right colon. No effect of beer
Seitz et al. (1987b)	AMMN, i.r.	i.g. (4.8 g/kg body weight per day), preinduction/induction	Increased rectal tumors. Carcinogenesis was further stimulated when cyanamide, an acetaldehyde dehydrogenase inhibitor was administered additionally

DMH, 1,2-dimethylhydrazine; AMMN, Azetoxymethyl-methylnitrosamine; AOM, Azoxymethane; s.c., subcutaneously; i.r., intrarectally; l.d., liquid diets; d.w., drinking water; i.g., intragastrically.

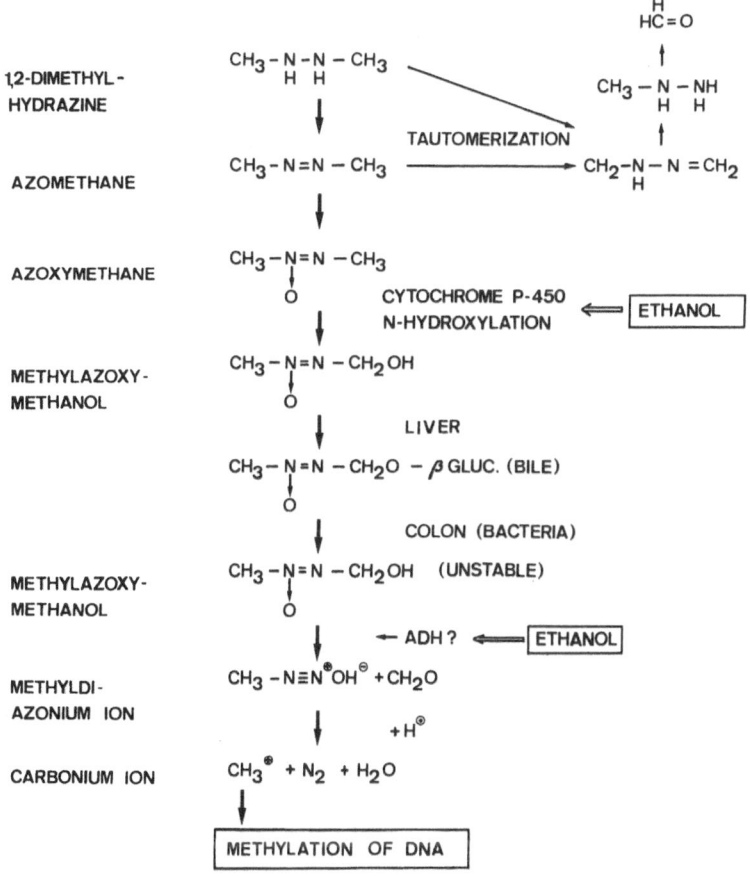

Fig. 1. Metabolism of 1,2-dimethylhydrazine (DMH) and possible effect of ethanol

1984). The conclusions derived from those experiments are as follows:

- The modulation of experimental colonic tumorigenesis by chronic dietary beer and ethanol consumption is due to alcohol rather than to other beverage constituents.
- The tumorigenesis in the right and left colorectum is affected differently by alcohol and may depend on the levels of alcohol consumption. Thus, high alcohol intake (18%–33% of total calories) inhibits carcinogenesis in the right colon and has no effect on the left colon, while lower ethanol consumption (9%–12% of total calories) enhances tumor development in the left colon without effect on the right colon.
- Ethanol affects carcinogenesis during the preinduction and/or induction phase, including carcinogen metabolism, but not during the postinduction phase (promotion).
- An interaction between ethanol and procarcinogen metabolism does occur and this may influence tumor incidences.

It must be emphasized that in one experiment with DMH, ethanol ingestion only enhanced tumor development in the rectum (last 5 cm), but not in the remaining large intestine (Seitz et al. 1984). In this study ethanol was given during acclimatization and initiation, but at the time of procarcinogen application ethanol was not present in the body. In a similar study by McGarrity et al. (1986), these results could not be confirmed.

In addition, in two more recent animal experiments, the primary carcinogen acetoxymethyl-methylnitrosamine (AMMN) was used to induce rectal tumors. This carcinogen does not need metabolic activation to exert its carcinogenic power and is applied locally to the rectal mucosa of rats (Wiessler 1975). The animals were endoscopied regularly (Narisawa et al. 1975; Merz et al. 1981), and tumor occurrence was registered. Alcohol was given continuously before (preinduction) and during tumor initiation and during tumor promotion. Since chronic ethanol administration given either as a liquid diet (Garzon et al. 1987) or intragastrically (Seitz et al. 1987b) accelerates the appearance of rectal tumors induced by AMMN, it seems most likely that alcohol enhances carcinogenesis, at least in part, by local mechanisms in the rectal mucosa and not only by increasing the activation of procarcinogens.

Possible Mechanisms by which Ethanol May Affect Colorectal Carcinogenesis

Ethanol may increase the susceptibility of various tissues to chemical carcinogenesis by a variety of mechanisms such as activation of chemical procarcinogens, altering the metabolism and/or distribution of carcinogens, interference with the repair of carcinogen-mediated DNA alkylation and the immune response, stimulating cellular regeneration, and exacerbation of dietary deficiencies (Lieber et al. 1986; Seitz and Simanowski 1986, 1988) (Fig. 2). With respect to the effect of ethanol on colorectal carcinogenesis, two factors may be of particular interest, namely increased activation of procarcinogens and local ethanol-mediated effects in the rectal mucosa leading to tissue injury and hyperregeneration which favors carcinogenesis.

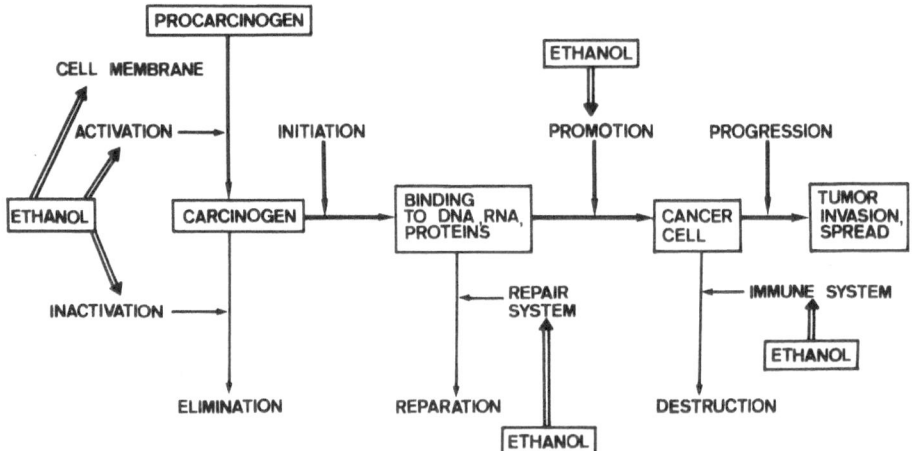

Fig. 2. Simplified scheme of two-step carcinogenesis and possible effects of ethanol

Effect of Ethanol on the Activation of Procarcinogens

Many environmental carcinogens exist in their procarcinogenic form and require metabolic activation by microsomal cytochrome P-450-dependent enzymes (Lieber et al. 1979). The activated procarcinogens exhibit a high capacity to bind to macromolecules such as DNA, RNA, or proteins and thus lead to initiation of the carcinogenic process. Induction of microsomal enzyme activities increases the mutagenic effect of many compounds in the Ames salmonella mutagenesis assay (Ames et al. 1975). Since the extent of metabolic activation of various secondary carcinogens can be correlated with microsomal enzyme activities (Felton and Nebert 1975; Conney 1982), factors such as environmental pollutants, drugs, and diet which can influence the activity of this enzyme system are also expected to affect tumor formation in animals exposed to carcinogens. In the light of this fact it seems important that ethanol is a well-known microsomal enzyme "inducer" in the liver and in other tissues (Lieber 1985; Seitz et al. 1978, 1981a, b; Seitz and Simanowski 1987), but not in the colon (Seitz et al. 1982). Both ethanol and procarcinogens are metabolized via cytochrome P-450-dependent microsomal pathways, and therefore interactions between the two compounds occur as demonstrated in Fig. 3.

If ethanol and a procarcinogen are present at the same time, ethanol inhibits the activation of the procarcinogen (Fig. 3B), and carcinogenesis may also be inhibited. During chronic ethanol consumption, microsomal enzyme activity increases, and microsomal ethanol oxidation is enhanced. Under these conditions the activation of the procarcinogen is still inhibited (Fig. 3C). However, when ethanol is withdrawn from the organism at this stage of microsomal enzyme induction, an increased activation of the procarcinogen occurs (Fig. 3D) possibly resulting in an enhancement of carcinogenesis. Thus, it has been shown that ethanol inhibits the hepatic microsomal activation of azoxymethan (AM) (Sohn et al. 1987) and of dimethylnitrosamine

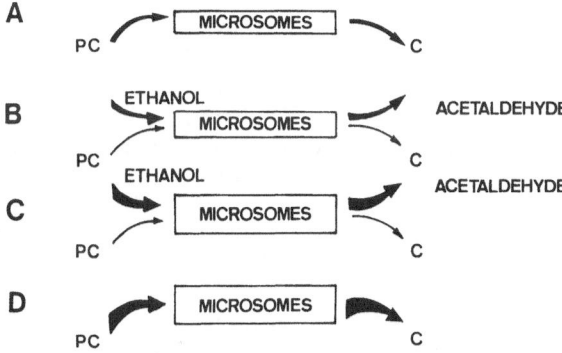

Fig. 3A–D. Interaction between microsomal metabolism of ethanol and procarcinogens. In the presence of ethanol the microsomal activation of procarcinogens (*PC*) to ultimative carcinogens (*C*) is inhibited (**B**), while ethanol is metabolized to acetaldehyde. Chronic ethanol ingestion increases microsomal cytochrome P-450 and microsomal enzyme activity. Thus, in the presence of ethanol, microsomal ethanol oxidation is enhanced and procarcinogen activation is still inhibited (**C**). Following withdrawal of ethanol, procarcinogen activation is enhanced (depending on the time interval between the last drink and procarcinogen exposure) due to microsomal enzyme induction (**D**)

(DMN) (Sohn et al. 1987; Peng et al. 1982), while the activation of these two procarcinogens was strikingly enhanced following chronic ethanol consumption when ethanol was withdrawn (Sohn et al. 1987; Garro et al. 1981).

The conversion of AOM to methylazoxymethanol (MAM) is catalyzed by a microsomal cytochrome P-450-dependent N-hydroxylase in the liver (Fiala 1977) and in the colon (Wargovich and Felkner 1982; Glauert and Bennink 1983). Pretreatment of animals with microsomal enzyme inducers such as phenobarbital, chrysene (Fiala 1977), or ethanol (Sohn et al. 1987) leads to an increased metabolism of AOM to carbon monoxide, probably through an induction of the microsomal enzyme. On the other hand, agents which inhibit DMH metabolism (Fiala et al. 1977) also inhibit DMH-induced colorectal carcinogenesis in vivo (Wattenberg 1975). It therefore seems possible that the effect of ethanol observed in the animal experiment with DMH and AOM can be attributed, at least in part, to the alcohol-related changes in the metabolism of the procarcinogen. In the light of these facts, it is understandable why high ethanol intake leading to high ethanol blood concentrations results in an inhibition of colorectal carcinogenesis and low alcohol intake does not. The presence of ethanol during tumor initiation also inhibits tumor development (Hamilton et al. 1987b), while its absence at a stage of enzyme induction enhances the carcinogenic process (Seitz et al. 1984). However, it is not clear why ethanol under certain experimental conditions stimulates tumor occurrence in the left colon and rectum but not in the right colon (Hamilton et al. 1987a; Seitz et al. 1984).

Another enzyme possibly involved in DMH metabolism is alcohol dehydrogenase (ADH) (Fig. 1). It has been suggested by Schoenthal (1973) that the conversion of MAM to the diazonium ion is enzymatically catalyzed by ADH. This concept is supported by the observation that the incidence of DMH- or MAM-induced intestinal tumors is paralleled by the activity of intestinal mucosal ADH (Grab and Zedeck 1977). Both tumor yield and ADH activity are highest in the large intestine and in the duodenum but low in the jejunum or ileum (Grab and Zedeck 1977; Mezey 1975). Furthermore, ADH inhibitors such as pyrazole (Zedeck and Tan 1978; Zedeck 1980) or butylated hydroxyanisole (BHA) inhibit both colonic carcinogenesis and colonic ADH activity (Wattenberg and Sparnens 1979). However, it was shown recently by Fiala et al. (1984) in the ADH-lacking deer mouse that MAM can also be metabolized by a non-ADH pathway. Thus, the inhibitory effect of BHA and pyrazole on chemically induced colonic carcinogenesis was possibly due to an inhibition of microsomal cytochrome P-450-dependent enzyme activities (Stohs and Wu 1982; Fiala et al. 1978) and not to their effect on ADH.

Local Mechanisms

The fact that chronic ethanol ingestion enhances rectal carcinogenesis induced by the local application of the primary carcinogen AMMN, which does not require metabolic activation, suggests that alcohol also acts by local mechanisms in the rectal mucosa and not by enhancing the activation of procarcinogens alone (Garzon et al. 1987).

Bile acids, which may be involved as tumor promoters in colorectal carcinogenesis as discussed by Cohen and Deschner in another chapter of this book, do not play an important role in ethanol-associated colorectal cancer since chronic ethanol consumption, although increasing biliary bile acid output (Sieg and Seitz 1987), does not change fecal bile acid excretion and pattern (Seitz et al. 1984; Cohen and Raicht 1981).

However, one important feature in intestinal carcinogenesis is the change in mucosal cell renewal modulating response to chemical carcinogens as discussed by Simanowski and Wright elsewehre in this book. Utilizing the metaphase arrest technique with vincristine, cell proliferation was selectively increased in the rectal mucosa of chronically ethanol-fed rats when compared to controls (Simanowski et al. 1986). A similar stimulatory effect of alcohol on cell regeneration has already been reported for the esophagus where ethanol also acts as a cocarcinogen (Mak et al. 1987). A concomitant increase in the proliferative compartment size of the rectal crypt due to ethanol ingestion was also found. Such hyperproliferation and expansion of the proliferative compartment of the crypt toward the intestinal lumen appears to be predictive of increased susceptibility to chemical carcinogens as pointed out in the chapter by Lipkin. Cell regeneration is triggered by polyamines, and their synthesis is regulated by the activity of ornithine decarboxylase (ODC). ODC activity was found to be significantly enhanced after chronic ethanol consumption, but falls rapidly in the colonic mucosa after cessation of ethanol intake (Hamilton and Luk 1987; Seitz, unpublished observation).

The rectal hyperproliferation observed after alcohol ingestion may be of secondary compensatory nature, since light microscopy of rectal mucosa from alcoholics reveals superficial cell damage, which returns to normal following alcohol abstinence for 2 weeks (Brozinski et al. 1979), and since the life span of functional epithelial cells in the rectal crypt is reduced (Simanowski et al. 1986).

Some gastrointestinal hormones such as gastrin, enteroglucagon (EG), and peptide YY may cause hyperregeneration in the intestinal mucosa. Acute and chronic ethanol consumption increase serum concentrations of EG (Simanowski et al. 1989) which could lead to an additional stimulation of cell regeneration in the colon without explaining the difference in cell turnover between the right and the left colon following ethanol ingestion.

It has been suspected that acetaldehyde (AA), a rather toxic metabolite of ethanol, may cause the rectal tissue injury observed in the alcoholic. Significantly high concentrations of AA have been found in the distal colon after alcohol application (Seitz et al. 1987a). These AA concentrations were significantly elevated compared to the proximal colon and to the liver when calculated per gram of tissue. In addition, increased ADH activity has been found in the mucosa derived from the distal colon when compared to the proximal large intestine (Seitz et al. 1984) which may favor AA accumulation through ethanol oxidation. However, it seems impossible that the colonic ADH with its low activity is capable of producing the striking accumulation of AA in the rectum. It is therefore hypothesized that bacterial production of AA especially in the distal colon (where the highest bacteria counts occur) may be responsible for the AA formation and that the observed ADH activity in the mucosal cytoplasm may be due, at least in part, to a contamination by bacterial ADH. This theory is supported by the fact that various aldehydes, including AA, can be detected in vitro following incubation of feces with ethanol (Levitt et al. 1982).

Most recent data on the effect of ethanol on AMMN-induced rectal cancer further support the concept that AA is involved in ethanol-associated rectal carcinogenesis.

Animals which received ethanol and cyanamide, a potent AA-dehydrogenase inhibitor, exhibited an earlier occurrence of rectal tumors compared to animals which received ethanol alone (Seitz et al. 1987b). In these experiments AA concentrations were significantly elevated in the serum and in the colonic mucosa following the application of cyanamide.

Conclusion

Although conflicting results have been reported, ethanol may have a cocarcinogenic effect on the distal colon or rectum in animal experiments. Ethanol may enhance colorectal carcinogenesis (a) by enhancing the activation of the procarcinogens; and (b) by local mechanisms possibly mediated by AA.

Acknowledgements. Original studies have been supported by the Deutsche Forschungsgemeinschaft (Se 333/1, 2, 4-1, 6-1, 2) and by the Gerhardt Katsch Studienfond der Deutschen Gesellschaft für Verdauungs- und Stoffwechselerkankungen.

References

Ames BN, McCann J, Yamasaki E (1975) Methods for detecting carcinogens and mutagens with the salmonella/mammalian-microsomes mutagenicity test. Mutat Res 31:347–364

Bjelke E (1973) Epidemiological studies of cancer of the stomach, colon and rectum. Thesis, Ann Arbor University Microfilms

Breslow NE, Enstrom JE (1974) Geographic correlations between mortality rates and alcohol, tobacco consumption in the United States. JNCI 53:631–639

Brozinski S, Fami K, Grosberg JJ (1979) Alcohol ingestion-induced changes in the human rectal mucosa: light and electron microscopic studies. Dis Colon Rectum 21:329–335

Castonguay A, Rivenson A, Trushin N, Reinhardt J, Spathopoulos S (1984) Effect of chronic ethanol consumption on the metabolism and carcinogenicity of N'-nitrosonornicotine in F 344 rats. Cancer Res 44:2285–2290

Cohen BI, Raicht RF (1981) Sterol metabolism in the rat: effect of alcohol on sterol metabolism in two strains of rats. Alcoholism 5:225–229

Conney AG (1982) Induction of microsomal enzymes by foreign chemicals and carcinogenesis by polycyclic hydrocarbons. Cancer Res 42:4875–4917

Dean G, MacLennan R, McLoughlin H, Shelley E (1979) The cause of death of blue collar workers at a Dublin brewery 1954–1973. Br J Cancer 40:581–598

Driver HE, McLean AEM (1986) Dose-response relationship for initiation of rat liver tumors by diethylnitrosamine and promotion by phenobarbitone or alcohol. Food Chem Toxic 24:241–245

Enstrom JE (1977) Colorectal cancer and beer drinking. Br J Cancer 35:674–683

Felton JS, Nebert DW (1975) Mutagenesis of certain activated carcinogens in vitro associated with genetically mediated increases in monooxygenase activity and cytochrome P-450. J Biol Chem 250:6769–6778

Fiala ES (1977) Investigations into the metabolism and mode of action of the colon carcinogen 1,2-dimethylhydrazine and azoxymethane. Cancer 40:2436–2445

Fiala ES, Bobota G, Kulakis C, Wattenberg W, Weisburger JH (1977) Effects of disulfiram and related compounds on the metabolism in vivo of the colon carcinogen 1,2-dimethylhydrazine. Biochem Pharmacol 26:1763–1768

Fiala ES, Kulakis C, Christiansen G, Weisburger JH (1978) Inhibition of the metabolism of the colon carcinogen azomethane by pyrazole. Cancer Res 38:4515–4521

Fiala ES, Caswell N, Sohn OS, Felder MR, McCoy GD, Weisburger JH (1984) Non-alcohol dehydrogenase-mediated metabolism of methylazoxymethanol in the deer mouse, *Peromyscus maniculatus*. Cancer Res 44:2885–2891

Gabrial GN, Schrager TF, Newberne PM (1982) Zinc deficiency, alcohol, and retinoid: association with esophageal cancer in rats. JNCI 68:785–789

Garro AJ, Seitz HK, Lieber CS (1981) Enhancement of dimethylnitrosamine metabolism and activation to a mutagen following chronic ethanol consumption in the rat. Cancer Res 41:120–124

Garzon FT, Simanowski UA, Berger MR, Schmähl D, Kommerell B, Seitz HK (1987) Acetoxymethyl-methylnitrosamine (AMMN)-induced colorectal carcinogenesis is stimulated by chronic alcohol consumption. Alcohol Alcohol (Suppl) 1:501–502

Giebel W (1967) Experimentelle Untersuchungen zur Synkarzinogenese beim Ösophaguskarzinom. Arch Geschwulstforsch 30:181–189

Glauert HP, Bennink MR (1983) Metabolism of 1,2-dimethylhydrazine by cultured rat colon epithelial cells. Nutr Cancer 5:78–86

Grab DJ, Zedeck MS (1977) Organ specific effects of the carcinogen methylazoxymethanol related to the metabolism by nicotinamide adenosine dinucleotide dependent dehydrogenases. Cancer Res 37:4182–4190

Graham S, Dayal H, Swanson M, Mittelman A, Wilkinson G (1978) Diet in the epidemiology of cancer of the colon and rectum. JNCI 61:709–714

Hamilton SR, Hyland J, McAvinchey D, Chaudhry Y, Hartka L, Kim HT, Cichon P, Floyd J, Turjman N, Kessie G, Nair PP, Dick J (1987a) Effects of chronic dietary beer and ethanol consumption on experimental colonic carcinogenesis by azoxymethane in rats. Cancer Res 47:1551–1559

Hamilton SR, Luk GD (1987) Induction of colonic mucosal ornithine decarboxylase activity by chronic dietary ethanol consumption in the rat (Abstract). Gastroenterology 92:1423

Hamilton SR, Sohn OS, Fiala ES (1987b) Effects of timing and quantity of chronic dietary ethanol consumption on azoxymethane-induced colonic carcinogenesis and azoxymethane metabolism in Fischer 344 rats. Cancer Res 47:4305–4311

Higginson J (1966) Etiological factors in gastrointestinal cancer in man. JNCI 37:527–545

Howarth AE, Pihl E (1985) High fat diet promotes and causes distal shift of experimental rat colonic cancer – beer and alcohol do not. Nutr Cancer 6:229–235

International Statistics on Alcoholic Beverages (1977) Finnish Foundation for Alcohol Studies, Helsinki, Vol 27

Jensen OM (1979) Cancer morbidity and cause of death among Danish brewery workers. Int J Cancer 23:454–463

Ketcham AS, Wexler H, Mantel N (1963) Affects of alcohol in mouse neoplasia. Cancer Res 23:667–670

Knox EG (1977) Foods and diseases. Br J Prevent Soc Med 31:71–80

Kono S, Ikeda M (1979) Correlation between cancer mortality and alcoholic beverages in Japan. Br J Cancer 40:449–455

Levitt MD, Doizaki W, Levine AS (1982) Hypothesis: metabolic activity of the colonic bacteria influences organ injury from ethanol. Hepatology 2:598–600

Lieber CS (1985) Ethanol metabolism and pathophysiology of alcoholic liver disease. In: Seitz HK, Kommerell B (eds) Alcohol related diseases in gastroenterology. Springer, Berlin Heidelberg New York Tokyo, pp 19–47

Lieber CS, DeCarli LM (1970) Quantitative relationship between the amount of dietary fat and the severity of the alcoholic fatty liver. Am J Clin Nutr 23:474–478

Lieber CS, Seitz HK, Garro AJ, Worner TM (1979) Alcohol related diseases and carcinogenesis. Cancer Res 39:2863–2886

Lieber CS, Garro AJ, Leo MA, Mak KM, Worner TM (1986) Alcohol and cancer. Hepatology 6:1005–1019

Loury DJ, Kado NY, Byard JL (1985) Enhancement of hepatocellular genotoxicity of several mutagens from amino acid pyrolysates and broiled foods following ethanol pretreatment. Food Chem Toxic 23:661–667

Mak KM, Leo MA, Lieber CS (1987) Effect of ethanol and vitamin A deficiency on epithelial cell proliferation and structure in the rat esophagus. Gastroenterology 93:362–370

McCoy GD, Chen CB, Hecht SS (1979) Enhanced metabolism and mutagenesis of nitrosopyrro-lidine in liver fractions isolated from chronic ethanol-consuming hamsters. Cancer Res 39: 793–796

McCoy GD, Hecht SS, Katayama S, Wynder EL (1981) Differential effect of chronic ethanol consumption on the carcinogenicity of *N*-nitrosopyrrolidine and *N'*-nitrosonornicotine in male Syrian hamsters. Cancer Res 41:2849–2854

McGarrity TJ, Via EA, Colony PC (1986) Changes in tissue sialic acid content and staining in dimethylhydrazine (DMH)-induced colorectal cancer: effects of ethanol (Abstract). Gastro-enterology 90:1543

McMichael AJ, Potter JD, Hetzel BS (1979) Time trends in colorectal cancer mortality in relation to food and alcohol consumption: USA, UK, Australia and New Zealand. Int J Epidemiol 8:295–303

Merz R, Wagner I, Habs M, Schmähl D (1981) Endoscopic diagnosis of chemically induced autochthonous colonic tumors in rats. Hepatogastroenteroloy 28:53–57

Mezey E (1975) Intestinal function in chronic alcoholism. Ann NY Acad Sci 252:215–227

Narisawa T, Wong CQ, Weisburger JH (1975) Evaluation of endoscopic examination of colon tumors in rats. Dig Dis 20:928–934

Nelson RL, Samalson SL (1985) Neither dietary ethanol nor beer augments experimental colon carcinogenesis in rats. Dis Colon Rectum 28:460–462

Peng R, Yong-Tu Y, Yang CS (1982) The induction and competitive inhibition of a high affinity microsomal nitrosodimethylamine demethylase by ethanol. Carcinogenesis 3:1457–1461

Pernu J (1960) An epidemiological study on cancer of the digestive organs and respiratory system. Ann Med Int Fenn 49 (Suppl) 33:1–117

Pollack ES, Nomura AMY, Heilbrun LK, Stemmermann GN, Green SB (1984) Prospective study of alcohol consumption and cancer. N Engl J Med 310:617–621

Porta EA, Markell N, Dorado RD (1985) Chronic alcoholism enhances hepatocarcinogenicity of diethylnitrosamine in rats fed a marginally methyl-deficient diet. Hepatology 5:1120–1125

Potter JD, McMichael AJ (1986) Diet and cancer of the colon and rectum: a case control study. JNCI 76:557–569

Potter JD, McMichael AJ, Hartshorne JM (1982) Alcohol and beer consumption in relation to cancers of bowel and lung: an extended correlation analysis. J Chronic Dis 35:833–842

Schatzkin A, Jones DY, Hoover RN, Taylor PR, Brinton LA, Ziegler RG, Harvey EB, Carter CL, Licitra LM, Dufour MC, Larson DB (1987) Alcohol consumption and breast cancer in the epidemiologic follow-up study of the first national health and nutrition examination survey. N Engl J Med 316:1169–1173

Schoenthal R (1973) The mechanism of cocarcinogenic nitro- and related compounds. Br J Cancer 28:436–439

Seitz HK (1985a) Ethanol and carcinogenesis. In: Seitz HK, Kommerell B (eds) Alcohol related diseases in gastroenterology. Springer, Berlin Heidelberg New York Tokyo, pp 192–212

Seitz HK (1985b) Alcohol effects on drug-nutrient interaction. Drug Nutr Interact 4:143–164

Seitz HK, Simanowski UA (1986) Ethanol and gastrointestinal carcinogenesis. Alcoholism 10:33–40

Seitz HK, Simanowski UA (1987) Metabolic and nutritional effects of alcohol. In: Hathcock JN (ed) Nutritional toxicology, vol II. Academic, New York, pp 63–104

Seitz HK, Simanowski UA (1988) Alcohol and carcinogenesis. Ann Rev Nutr 8:99–119

Seitz HK, Garro AJ, Lieber CS (1978) Effect of chronic ethanol ingestion on intestinal metabo-lism and mutagenicity of benzo[a]pyrene. Biochem Biophys Res Commun 85:1061–1066

Seitz HK, Garro AJ, Lieber CS (1981a) Sex dependent effect of chronic ethanol consumption in rats on hepatic microsome mediated mutagenicity of Benzo[a]pyrene. Cancer Lett 13:97–102

Seitz HK, Garro AJ, Lieber CS (1981b) Enhanced pulmonary and intestinal activation of procarcinogens and mutagens after chronic ethanol consumption in the rat. Eur J Clin Invest 11:33–38

Seitz HK, Bösche J, Czygan P, Veith S, Kommerell B (1982) Microsomal ethanol oxidation in the colonic mucosa of the rat: effect of chronic ethanol ingestion. Arch Pharmacol 310:81–84

Seitz HK, Czygan P, Waldherr R, Veith S, Raedsch R, Kässmodel H, Kommerell B (1984) Enhancement of 1,2-dimethylhydrazine induced rectal carcinogenesis following chronic ethanol consumption in the rat. Gastroenterology 86:886–891

Seitz HK, Simanowski UA, Garzon FT, Peters TJ (1987a) Alcohol and cancer (Letter to the editor). Hepatology 7:616

Seitz HK, Garzon FT, Simanowski UA, Schmähl D (1987b) Erhöhte Azetaldehydkonzentrationen als mögliche Ursache der tumorfördernden Wirkung von Alkohol im Rektum der Ratte (Abstract). Z. Gastroenterol 8:551

Sieg A, Seitz HK (1987) Increased production, hepatic conjugation, and biliary secretion of bilirubin in the rat following chronic ethanol consumption. Gastroenterology 93:261–266

Simanowski UA, Seitz HK, Baier B, Kommerell B, Schmidt-Gayk H, Wright NA (1986) Chronic ethanol consumption selectively stimulates rectal cell proliferation in the rat. Gut 27:278–282

Simanowski UA, Hubalek K, Ghatei MA, Bloom SR, Polak JM, Seitz HK (1989) Effects of acute and chronic ethanol administration on the gastrointestinal hormones gastrin, enteroglucagon, pancreatic glucagon and PYY in the rat. Digestion (in press)

Sohn OS, Fiala ES, Puz C, Hamilton SR, Williams GM (1987) Enhancement of rat liver microsomal metabolism of azoxymethane to methylazoxymethanol by chronic ethanol administration: similarity to the microsomal metabolism of N-nitrosomethylamine. Cancer Res 47:3123–3129

Spiegelhalder B, Eisenbrand G, Preussmann R (1979) Contamination of beer with trace quantities of N-nitrosodimethylamine. Food Cosmet Toxicol 17:29–31

Steele CM, Ioannides C (1986) Differential effects of chronic alcohol administration to rats on the activation of aromatic amines to mutagens in the Ames test. Carcinogenesis 7:825–829

Stohs SJ, Wu CLJ (1982) Effect of various xenobiotics and steroids on aryl hydrocarbon hydroxylase of intestinal and hepatic microsomes from male rats. Pharmacology 25:237–249

Sundby P (1967) Alcoholism and mortality. Rutgers Center on Alcohol Studies. New Brunswick, p 107

Takada A, Nei J, Takase S, Matsuda Y (1986) Effects of ethanol on experimental hepatocarcinogenesis. Hepatology 6:65–72

Wargovich MJ, Felkner IC (1982) Metabolic activation of DMH by colonic microsomes: a process influenced by dietary fat. Nutr Cancer 4:146–153

Wattenberg LW (1975) Inhibition of dimethylhydrazine-induced neoplasia of the large intestine by disulfiram. JNCI 54:1005–1006

Wattenberg LW, Sparnens VL (1979) Inhibitory effects of butylated hydroxyanisole on methylazoxymethanol acetate induced neoplasia of the large intestine and on nicotinamide adenine dinucleotide dependent alcohol dehydrogenase activity in mice. JNCI 63:219–222

Wiessler M (1975) Chemie der Nitrosamine. II. Synthese a-funktioneller Dimethylnitrosamine. Tetrahedron Lett 30:2575–2578

Willett WC, Stampfer MJ, Colditz GA, Rosner BA, Hennekens CH, Speizer FE (1987) Moderate alcohol consumption and the risk of breast cancer. N Engl J Med 316:1174–1180

Wright NA, Alison M (1984) The biology of epithelial cell populations. Clarendon, Oxford, pp 860–867

Wu AH, Paganini-Hill A, Ross RK, Henderson BE (1987) Alcohol, physical activity and other risk factors for colorectal cancer: a prospective study. Br J Cancer 55:687–694

Wynder EL, Shigematsu T (1967) Environmental factors of cancer of the colon and rectum. Cancer 20:1520–1561

Wynder EL, Kajitani T, Ishakawa S, Dodo H, Takano A (1969) Environmental factors of the colon and rectum. II. Japanese epidemiological data. Cancer 23:1210–1220

Zedeck MS (1980) Colon carcinogenesis and the role of dehydrogenase activity: inhibition of tumorigenesis by pyrazole. Prev Med 9:346–351

Zedeck MS, Tan QH (1978) Effect of pyrazole on tumor induction by methylazoxymethanol (MAM) acetate: relationship to metabolism of MAM. Pharmacologist 20:174–180

Pathophysiologic Mechanisms
in Colorectal Carcinogenesis

Environmental and Dietary Carcinogens Possibly Related to Colorectal Cancer

M. J. Wargovich and P. J. Hu

Section of Gastrointestinal Oncology and Digestive Diseases, Department of Medical Oncology, Division of Medicine, The University of Texas, M. D. Anderson Cancer Center, 1515 Holcombe Boulevard, Houston, Texas 77030, USA

Contents

Introduction

Since the early beginnings of research in the field of chemical carcinogenesis scientists have suspected that factors in the environment may contribute to the genesis of human cancers. Because the human diet is essentially a compilation of many and varied chemical nutrients, it has been logical to assume that some of the nutrients could be related to the carcinogenic process. We live, however, in a sea of environmental chemicals. Many of these agents, which may lack nutritional properties, can pass through the oral gateway and into the digestive tract where they may be involved figuring in some way in initiation and promotion, the two conceptual divisions of chemical carcinogenesis.

Among the neoplasms of the digestive tract, colorectal cancer has a high prevalence in industrialized Western countries. Epidemiological studies have often cited the similarity of life styles and dietary patterns as causal factors in the evolution of colorectal cancer in the populations of these countries. For example, at a macronutrient level, the diet of Britons compares with that of people in the United States, Canada, the Federal Republic of Germany, and Australia; these nations rank amongst the world's highest in terms of prevalence of colorectal cancer. Though as economically advanced, the people of Japan, where traditional dietary patterns largely prevail (though rapidly becoming westernized), are not at risk for the disease.

Table 1. Environmental agents possibly related to colon cancer

Exogenous sources	Endogenous sources
Polycyclic aromatic hydrocarbons	N-nitroso carcinogens
Hydrazines	Fecapentaenes
Cycasin	Lipid peroxides
Carrageenan	*Schistosoma japonicum*
Protein pyrolysates	

Thus the search for environmental or dietary carcinogens responsible for colorectal cancer has been a focus of intensive laboratory research. As yet, few naturally occurring dietary carcinogens can be directly implicated in the etiology of colon cancer. However, a number of carcinogenic agents either derived from the environment or created endogenously could have a role in the disease (Table 1).

Exogenous Sources of Dietary Carcinogens

Polycyclic Aromatic Hydrocarbons: Benzo[*a*]pyrene

Since man first used fire to cook food, carcinogens derived from the combustion of fats and oils or the use of hydrocarbons as fuels have been generated. Polycyclic aromatic hydrocarbons (PAHs) have been detected in cooked beef and the consumption of beef correlates strongly with the incidence of colon cancer in humans (Lijinsky and Ross 1967). Of the PAHs possibly linked to forms of human cancer, benzo[*a*]pyrene (BaP), first demonstrated as a carcinogen by Cook et al. in 1933, is found in significant amounts in the human diet (Lo and Sandi 1978). BaP is one of the most extensively studied procarcinogens in chemical carcinogenesis and induces a wide variety of tumors (Dipple 1976). In the gastrointestinal tract BaP is converted from the lipophilic, unreactive, polynuclear structures that characterize PAHs to highly electrophilic, carcinogenic, and soluble diol epoxides. This oxidative process is mediated by the cytochrome P450 enzymes found in many tissues (Levin et al. 1982). The gastrointestinal epithelium of rodents and man is capable of converting BaP to the carcinogenic metabolites (Gower and Wills 1986). In experiments by Autrup et al. (1982), cultured epithelial cells from the bronchus, esophagus, duodenum, and colon from each of 15 patients showed marked metabolism of BaP to DNA-binding conjugates for all four organs. Seven strains of mice were used in an experiment by Anderson et al. (1982) to examine the colonic metabolism and cytotoxicity of BaP. In their experiment, intrarectal administration of BaP caused significant cytotoxicity as measured by nuclear anomalies and elevated thymidine labeling. Evidence of BaP metabolism was also confirmed in two epithelial cells lines (duodenum and colon) of germ-free rats (Quaroni and Isselbacher 1981). One conundrum of significant biological interest is that BaP administered within the colon fails to induce cancer at that site, in spite of the evidence in favor of its rapid and complete metabolism in the organ (Anderson et al. 1983; Toth 1980) and overwhelming tumorigenicity in other organs (IARC 1973). Therefore, the risk to the human colon of BaP remains unclear.

Hydrazines

Edible mushrooms may contain hydrazines and substituted hydrazine derivatives. From the most commonly consumed species, *Agaricus bisporus, Cortinellus shiitake,* and *Gyomitra esculentra,* several hydrazines of tumorigenic potential have been isolated. *N*-Methyl-*N*-formylhydrazine and *N*-methylhydrazine isolated from mushrooms are tumorigenic in rodents (Toth 1979). Investigations by Toth et al. (1978, 1984) indicated tumorigenic activity of a metabolite of agaratine (also found in the common mushroom) in lungs and blood vessels of mice. In a subsequent study, Toth and Erickson (1986) found that feeding mice raw *Agaricus bisporus* induced tumors of the forestomach, bone, liver, and lungs. Colorectal cancer induction by naturally occurring hydrazines in mushrooms has not been shown, but methylated hydrazines (which do not occur in nature) are among the most powerful of the alkylating carcinogens used to induce experimental forms of gastrointestinal neoplasms, most notably, colorectal cancer in rodents.

Cycasin

Unlike the hydrazines in mushrooms, nuts of the trees belonging to the Cycas family (consumed for their starch content in parts of Guam, Kenya, and Japan) have yielded compounds of extraordinary carcinogenicity (Kobiyashi 1972). Cycasin, a substance derived from cycad nuts, and its aglycone methylazoxymethanol (MAM) are very potent in inducing colorectal cancer in rodents. Long-term feeding of cycasin frequently induced colon cancers in rats, but it also induced tumors of the liver, lungs, and ear canals (Laquer 1965). MAM is nearly unique among experimentally used carcinogens because of its high organospecificity for the large bowel (Zedeck and Sternberg 1974). As yet, the mechanism of its specificity for the colon is not understood. Recent evidence suggests that MAM, once having left the liver, is transported to the colonic mucosa via the blood stream (Matsubara et al. 1978). An earlier hypothesis suggesting that MAM was conjugated to glucuronic acid in the liver and subsequently cleaved in the colon by β-glucuronidase was questioned by the experiment of Rubio et al. (1980) who showed that removal of the colon from the bile stream did not protect the exteriorized segment from MAM tumorigenesis initiated by dimethylhydrazine, a precursor of MAM.

An appreciation for risk of colorectal cancer from consumption of cycad nuts has not been observed. In fact, the countries where cycads are consumed rank among the world's lowest in risk for colon cancer. Perhaps the carcinogenicity of cycasin and its derivatives is unique to the experimental conditions under which the compounds are used in animal tumorigenesis studies. No evidence of increased risk of cancer of the colon has been demonstrated for these compounds when the native nuts are consumed in man (Hirono et al. 1970).

Carrageenan

Carrageenan is an additive extracted from red seaweed that is used in a variety of foods as a thickening agent and emulsifier. Though the native substance is innocuous, the degraded form (which is acid hydrolyzed) was once used clinically as an antipeptic agent (Anderson 1961). Severe changes in the colonic mucosa have been reported in the rabbit colon following oral administration of degraded carrageenan. Squamous metaplasia and colonic polyps were observed by Fabian et al. (1973) when rats were fed degraded carrageenan. Wakabayashi et al. (1979) found that administration of a 10% degraded carrageenan diet induced metaplasia of the colorectum in nearly all rats examined after 12 months; colonic tumors were found in ~ 30% of these rats. Humans are no longer exposed to degraded carrageenan, though the native extract is used in many foods. The risk therefore seems to be minimal, yet it should be noted that progression to cancer did occur in animals fed the degraded form alone, in the absence of an overt chemical carcinogen.

Protein Pyrolysates

The "Maillard reaction" is the name given to the chemical reaction of sugars and amino acids when heated non-enzymatically to form brown-colored products responsible for the characteristic aroma of some cooked foods (Vuolo and Schuessler 1985). Early studies focused on the burnt and browned portions of meat and fish as sources of potential mutagenicity (Nagao et al. 1983). Protein pyrolysates, especially those of tryptophan and glutamine, are highly mutagenic and share structural similarity with several heterocyclic aromatic amines of known carcinogenicity, such as dimethyl-aminobiphenyl (Vuolo and Schuessler 1985). Recently identified pyrolysate mutagens are found in Table 2. 1,4-Dimethyl-5H-pyrido(4,3-6)indol-3-amine (Trp-P-1) was found by several Japanese investigators to be a strong hepatic and intestinal carcinogen (Matsukara et al. (1981), and 6-methyldipyrido(1,2-a:3,2-d)imidazole-2-amine (Glu-P-1) and dipyridol(1,2-a:3′,2′-d)imidazole-2-amine (Glu-P-2) induced tumors of the small and large bowel in F344 rats (Takayama et al. 1984). 2-Amino-3-methyl-imidazo[4,5-f]quinoline (IQ), found in broiled sardines and fried beef, is much more mutagenic than any of the other pyrolysates and was shown in the another study to be also carcinogenic for the colon, Zymbal's gland of the ear, and small bowel in male rats. Weisburger et al. (1985) found IQ to cause mammary carcinomas and neoplastic nodules in the liver of the Spraque-Dawley rat. Cohort studies by Ikeda et al. (1983) in Japan have linked the consumption of broiled fish and cancer at many sites though Kuratsume et al. (1986) considered that the link with gastric cancer was tenuous, at best, in a cohort study comparing cancer incidence at all sites in the Hiroshima area to that of Japanese Seventh Day Adventists. No reliable data are available concerning human risk of colorectal cancer with ingestion of burnt proteins.

Table 2. Mutagens and carcinogens from burnt foods

Compound	Chemical name	Food source
Trp-P-1	1,4-Dimethyl-5H-pyrido(4,3-6)indol-3-amine	Beef, dried sardine
Trp-P-2	1-Methyl-5H-pyrido(4,3-6)indol-3-amine	Beef, dried sardine
Glu-P-1	6-Methyldipyrido(1,2-a:3′,2′-d)imidazole-2-amine	Soybean
Glu-P-2	Dipyrido(1,2-a:3′,2′-d)imidazole-2-amine	Broiled fish
IQ	2-Amino-3-methylimidazo[4,5-f]quinoline	Fried beef and fish
MeJQ	2-Amino-3-dimethylimidazo[4,5-f]quinoline	Fried beef and fish

Endogenous Sources of Carcinogens

N-Nitroso Carcinogens

Nitrosation of amines derived from the ingestion of protein under certain conditions could evolve into the formation of N-nitrosamines that, as a single category, rank among of the most powerful alkylating carcinogens yet identified (Tannenbaum 1986). Nitrosamines could potentially form de novo by the combination of nitrite and amines under acidic conditions like that of the stomach (Bartsch and Montesano 1985). In fact, epidemiological evidence from studies of persons at risk for esophageal and stomach cancer suggests that high levels of nitrate or nitrite in the diet or drinking water may be associated with the prevalence of these cancers in Colombia and other South American countries as well as parts of China, Iran, and Japan. The carcinogenic activity of N-nitroso compounds has been well documented in animals (Preussman and Stewart 1984). Data linking nitrosamines with colorectal cancer in man are circumstantial. Indirect evidence comes only from the nitrosamine content of beer. The consumption of beer in some studies has correlated with colorectal cancer rates (Swann et al. 1984).

Fecal Mutagens

With the advent of microbial assays for mutagenicity, a possible explanation for large bowel cancer was sought by examining the feces of individuals for endogenous chemicals that were highly mutagenic. Bruce et al. (1977) first reported that fecal mutagens could be detected in the general population. Certain clues rapidly emerged that clearly implied difficulties in gaining structural information about the mutagens: the substances were present in very small amounts and the compounds degraded rapidly upon exposure to oxygen (Bruce et al. 1981). Structural identity co-emerged with novel chemical procedures for synthesis of the mutagens. In 1982 Bruce et al. renamed the mutagens "fecapentaenes" based on the structural elucidation. Prevalence studies of fecapentaenes in the general population compared to colorectal cancer patients tend to suggest only weakly that fecapentaene excreters are more common in a cancer-prone population, and persons with premalignant adenomatous polyps showed no correlation to fecal mutagenicity (Correa et al. 1981; Ferguson and Alley 1982). Other studies have identified at least two forms of fecal mutagens (Gupta et al. 1983). The general distribution of these, perhaps biologically differing mutagens, in cases vs. controls is presently unknown. What is known, is the observation that levels of fecal mutagenicity can be modulated by dietary interventions. Dion and Bruce (1982) reported that subjects supplemented daily with 400 mg each of vitamins C and E for 2 weeks significantly reduce fecal mutagen levels. In a study by Kuhnlein et al. (1983) fecal mutagenicity was higher when subjects consumed a meat diet compared to a cereal- and grain-rich diet. Though suggestive of a possible relationship to colon cancer, the demonstration of mutagens in the feces cannot as yet imply risk for the disease.

Oxidized Lipids

Dietary fats are thought to act as promoters of colon cancer, that is, they are not generally regarded as carcinogens per se. In some manner they accelerate the conversion of initiated cells to the malignant phenotype. Recently much attention has been drawn to the fact that lipids can undergo oxidation reactions that could generate superoxide, hydroxyl radicals, and hydrogen peroxide which could have carcinogenic potential (Ames 1986). Though preliminary in nature, Craven et al. (1986) have presented experimental data linking the release of reactive oxygen species from lipid peroxidation of unsaturated fatty acids to a similar release by bile salt-stimulated phospholipid breakdown in the colon. In their report, reactive oxygen species triggered colonic epithelial proliferation. Persistent colonic proliferation could signal a conversion of the mucosa to a preneoplastic state (Deschner 1987).

Infection with Schistosoma japonicum

Infestation with *S. japonicum* is endemic in many parts of Southeast Asia, particularly in China. Infection with the parasite often leads to chronic schistosomal colitis. Epidemiological and pathological studies suggest that this condition might be associated with an increased risk of large bowel cancer, although controversy exists. In China the mortality rate of colorectal cancer in the endemic area (the provinces adjoining of the Yangtze River into the South China Sea) is much higher than the national average (Li et al. 1981). A study of population-based correlation analyses in China revealed that the prevalence of the infestation with *S. japonicum* correlated highly with morbidity from colorectal cancer in Haining County of Zhejiang province in 1977–1979 (Zhong and Li 1984). A case-control study using regression analysis revealed that the relative risk of colorectal cancer significantly increased in association with schistosomiasis; a significant dose – response relationship with accumulated exposure to the schistosoma and colorectal cancer risk could be detected (Guo et al. 1987). Dysplastic changes in the colonic mucosa have been reported in documented cases of schistosomal colitis; these changes resemble those found in long-standing chronic ulcerative colitis, a condition often predisposing to the development of colon cancer (Chen et al. 1980, 1981).

Conclusions

Studies among populations infer that the risk for colon cancer is well varied. Epidemiological investigations point strongly to environmental factors as causal agents in the development of the disease and to other factors that are likely to protect individuals from acquiring colon cancer. It is difficult, even with the latest advances in analytical methods, to pinpoint a single environmental factor that would account for the prevalence of the disease in Western nations or explain the paucity of colorectal cancers in underdeveloped countries or the unusual anomaly of low risk in Japan. Even if certainties could be made, the questions of length of exposure, dose, and sequence in the carcinogenic process where putative dietary carcinogens exerted their influence would have to be identified. Almost as exciting as the search for the causative agents in the genesis of human colon cancer has been the identification of dietary factors present in the diet in small amounts that are *anticarcinogenic* (Wargovich 1988). Perhaps the identification of environmental factors conferring protection may in the long run prove to be more beneficial to the dream of attaining a cancer-free lifespan than the nearly impossible task of identifying possible cancer-causing chemicals in the human diet. In any event, the understanding of the molecular processes underlying the conversion of a normal cell to a cancer should provide the tools to tame this most common and difficult of the malignancies of the digestive tract.

References

Ames BN (1986) Food constituents as a source of mutagens, carcinogens, and anticarcinogens. In: Knudsen I (ed) Genetic toxicology of the diet. Less, New York, pp 3–32

Anderson LM, Deschner EE, Angel J, Hermann SL (1982) Murine colonic mucosal metabolism and cytotoxicity of benzo[a]pyrene. Oncology 39: 369–377

Anderson LM, Priest LJ, Deschner EE, Budinger JM (1983) Carcinogenic effects of intracolonic benzo[a]pyrene in B-naphthoflavone-induced mice. Cancer Lett 20: 117–123

Anderson W (1961) The antipeptic activity of sulfated polysaccharides. J Pharm Pharmacol 13: 139–147

Autrup H, Gafstrom RC, Brugh M, Lechner JF, Haugen A, Trump BF, Harris CC (1982) Comparison of benzo[a]pyrene metabolism in the bronchus, esophagus, colon, and duodenum from the same individual. Cancer Res 42: 934–938

Bartsch H, Montesano R (1985) Relevance of nitrosamines to human cancer. Carcinogenesis 5: 1381–1389

Bruce WR, Varghese AJ, Furrer R, Land PC (1977) A mutagen in the feces of normal humans. In: Hiatt HH, Watson JD, Winsten JA (eds) Origins of human cancer. Cold Spring Harbor, NY, pp 1641–1646

Bruce WR, Varghese AJ, Land PC, Krepinsky JF (1981) Properties of a mutagen isolated from feces. In: Bruce WR, Correa P, Lipkin M, Tannenbaum SR, Wilkins TD (eds) Gastrointestinal cancer: endogenous factors. Banbury report no 7. Cold Spring Harbor, NY, pp 227–238

Bruce WR, Baptista J, Che T, Furrer R, Gingerich JS, Grey AA, Gupta I, Krepinsky JJ, Yates P (1982) The mutagenic substance in human feces. General structure of "fecapentaenes". Naturwissenschaften 69: 557–558

Chen M (1980) Evolution of colorectal cancer in schistosomiasis: transitional mucosal changes adjacent to large intestinal carcinoma in colectomy specimens. Cancer 46: 1661–1675

Chen M (1981) Colorectal cancer and schistosomiasis. Lancet 1: 971–973

Cook JW, Hewett Cl, Heigher I (1933) II. Isolation of 1,2- and 4,5-benzopyrenes, perylene and 1,2-benzanthracene. J Am Chem Soc 55: 396–398

Correa P, Paschal J, Pizzolato P (1981) Fecal mutagens and colorectal polyps: preliminary report of an autopsy study. In: Bruce WR, Correa P, Lipkin M, Tannenbaum SR, Wilkins TD (eds) Gastrointestinal cancer: endogenous factors. Cold Spring Harbor, NY, pp 119–127 (Banbury report no 7)

Craven PA, Pfanstiel J, DeRubertis FR (1986) Role of reactive oxygen in bile salt stimulation of colonic epithelial proliferation. J Clin Invest 77: 850–859

Deschner EE (1987) Cell turnover and colon tumor development. Prev Med 16(4): 580–586

Dion PW, Bright-See EB, Smith CC, Bruce WR (1982) The effect of dietary ascorbic acid and alpha-tocopherol on fecal mutagenicity. Mutat Res 102(1): 27–37

Dipple A (1976) Polynuclear aromatic hydrocarbons. In: Searle CE (ed) Chemical carcinogens, ACS monograph 173. American Chemical Society, Washington, DC, pp 245–314

Fabian RJ, Abraham R, Coulston F, Golberg L (1973) Carrageenan-induced squamous meta-
    plasia of the rectal mucosa in the rat. Gastroenterology 65: 265–276
Ferguson LR, Alley PG (1982) Fecal mutagens from population groups within New Zealand at
    different risk of colorectal cancer. In: Sorsa M, Vainio H (eds) Mutagens in our environment.
    Liss, New York, pp 423–429
Gower JD, Wills ED (1986) The dependence of the rate of BP metabolism in the rat small
    intestinal mucosa on the composition of the dietary fat. Nutr Cancer 8: 151–161
Guo Z (1987) *Schistosoma japonicum* and colon cancer – an inquiry about the pathogenesis of
    colon cancer using the logistic regression model. Chung Hua Liu Hsing Ping Hsueh Tsa Chih
    8 (1): 21–24
Gupta I, Baptista J, Bruce WR, Che T, Furrer R, Gingerich JS, Grey AA, Marai L, Yates P,
    Krepinsky JJ (1983) Structure of fecapentaenes, the mutagens of bacterial origin isolated
    from human feces. Biochemistry 22: 241–245
Hirono I, Hachi H, Kato T (1970) A survey of acute toxicity of cycads and mortality rate from
    cancer in the Miyako Islands, Okinawa. Acta Pathol 20: 327–337
IARC (1973) IARC monograph on evaluation of carcinogenic risk of chemicals to man, vol 3:
    Certain polycyclic aromatic hydrocarbons and heterocyclic compounds. International Agen-
    cy for Research on Cancer, Lyon, France
Ikeda M, Yoshimoto K, Yoshimura T, Kono S, Kato H, Kuratsame M (1983) A cohort study
    on the possible association between broiled fish intake and cancer. Gann 74: 640–648
Kobiyashi A (1972) Cycasin in cycad materials used in Japan. Fed Proc 31: 1476–1477
Kuhnlein HV, Kuhnlein V, Bell PA (1983) The effect of short term dietary modification on
    human fecal mutagenicity activity. Mutat Res 113: 1–12
Kuratsune M, Ikeda M, Hayashi T (1986) Epidemiologic studies on possible health effects of
    intake of pyrolysates of foods with reference to mortality among Japanese Seventh-Day
    Adventists. Environ Health Perspect 67: 143–146
Laquer GL (1965) The induction of intestinal neoplasms in rats with the glycoside cycasin and
    its aglycone. Virchows Arch [A] 340: 151–153
Levin W, Wood A, Chang R, Ryan D, Thomas P (1982) Oxidative metabolism of polycyclic
    hydrocarbons to ultimate carcinogens. Drug Metab Rev 13: 555–580
Li JY (1981) Atlas of cancer mortality in the People's Republic of China – an aid for cancer
    control and research. Int J Epidemiol 10: 127–133
Lijinsky W, Ross AE (1967) Production of carcinogenic polynuclear hydrocarbons in the
    cooking of food. Food Cosmet Toxicol 5: 343–347
Lo MT, Sandi E (1978) Polycyclic aromatic hydrocarbons (polynuclears). Residue Rev
    69: 35–86
Matsubara N, Mori H, Hirono I (1978) Effect of colostomy on intestinal carcinogenesis bi-
    methylazoxymethanol acetate in rats. JNCI 61: 1161–1164
Matsukara N, Kawachi T, Morino K, Ohgaki H, Sugimura T, Takayama S (1981) Carcinogenic-
    ity in mice of mutagenic compounds from a tryptophan pyrolysate. Science 213: 346–347
Nagao M, Sato S, Sugimura T (1983) Mutagens produced by heating foods. In: Waller GR,
    Feather MS (eds) The Maillard reaction in foods and nutrition. American Chemical Society,
    Washington DC, pp 521–536 (ACS symposium series, no 215)
Preussman R, Stewart BW (1984) *N*-nitroso carcinogens. In: Searle CE (ed) Chemical carcino-
    gens, 2nd edn, vol 2. American Chemical Society, Washington DC, pp 643–828
Quaroni A, Isselbacher KJ (1981) Cytotoxic effects and metabolism of benzo[a]pyrene and
    7,12-dimethylbenz[a]anthracene in duodenal and ileal epithelial cell cultures. JNCI
    67: 1353–1362
Rubio CA, Nylander G, Santos M (1980) Experimental colon cancer in the absence of intestinal
    contents in Sprague-Dawley rats. JNCI 64: 569–572
Swann PF, Coe AM, Mace R (1984) Ethanol and dimethylnitrosamine and diethylnitrosamine
    metabolism and disposition in the rat. Possible relevance to the influence of ethanol on
    human cancer incidence. Carcinogenesis 5: 1337–1343
Takayama S, Masuda M, Mogami M, Ohgaki H, Sato S, Sugimura T (1984) Induction of
    cancers in the intestine, liver, and various other organs or rats by feeding mutagens from
    glutamic acid pyrolysate. Gann 75: 207–213
Tannenbaum SR (1986) Diet and exposure to *N*-nitroso compounds. In: Hayashi Y, Nagao M,

Sugimura T, Shozo T, Tomatis L, Wattenberg LW, Wogan GN (eds) Diet, nutrition, and cancer. Japan Scientific Societies Press, Tokyo, pp 67–75

Toth B (1979) Mushroom hydrazines: occurrence, metabolism, carcinogenesis and environmental implications. In: Miller EC, Miller JA, Hirono I, Sugimura T, Takayama S (eds) Naturally occurring carcinogens, mutagens and modulators of carcinogenesis. University Park Press, Baltimore, pp 111–125

Toth B (1980) Tumorigenesis by benzo[a]pyrene administered intracolonically. Oncology 37:77–82

Toth B, Erickson J (1986) Cancer induction in mice by feeding uncooked cultivated mushroom of commerce *Agaricus bisporus*. Cancer Res 46:4007–4011

Toth B, Nagel D (1978) Tumors induced in mice by N'-methyl-N-formylhydrazine in the false morel. *Gyromitra esculenta*. JNCI 60:201–204

Toth B, Patil K, Jae HS (1984) Carcinogenesis of 4-(hydroxymethyl)benzenediazonium ion (tetra fluoroborate) of *Agaricus bisporus*. Cancer Res 41:2444–2449

Vuolo LL, Schuessler JD (1985) Protein pyrolysate products. Environ Mutagen 7(4):577–598

Wakabayashi K, Fujimoto Y, Oohashi Y, Kuwabara N, Fukuda Y (1979) In: Miller EC et al. (eds) Naturally occurring carcinogens-mutagens and modulators of carcinogenesis. University Park Press, Baltimore, pp 127–138

Wargovich MJ (1988) New dietary anticarcinogens and prevention of gastrointestinal cancer. Dis Colon Rectum 31:72–75

Weisburger JH, Barnes WS, Tanaka T, Dime D (1985) Fried food mutagen 2-amino-3 -methyl-imidazo(4,5-)quinoline (IQ) is a powerful rodent carcinogen. Proc Am Assoc Cancer Res 26:73

Zhong X, Li SD (1984) *Schistosoma japonicum* and colorectal cancer: an epidemiological study in the People's Republic of China. Int J Cancer 34:315–318

Zedeck M, Sternberg SS (1974) A model system for studies of colon carcinogenesis by a single injection of methylazoxymethanol acetate. JNCI 53:1419–1421

Experimental Models of Colorectal Carcinogenesis

S. R. Hamilton

Department of Pathology and Oncology Center, The Johns Hopkins University School
of Medicine and Hospital, 600 North Wolfe Street, Baltimore, Maryland 21205, USA

Contents

Importance of Experimental Models of Colorectal Carcinogenesis

A large number of different experimental models of large bowel carcinogenesis have been used to study colorectal neoplasia (Autrup and Williams 1983; Rogers and Nauss 1985; Pozharisski et al. 1979; LaMont and O'Gorman 1978; Amberger 1986; Gilbert 1987). The importance of these models lies in their potential relevance to human colorectal neoplasia. Pathogenesis, diagnosis, and treatment have been addressed in experimental models.

Since the carcinogen(s) and modulating factors in human colorectal neoplasia are not yet known with certainty (Bruce 1986, 1987), appropriate use of models can be particularly helpful in obtaining clues to pathogenesis. Both risk factors and protective factors identified by epidemiologic and metabolic epidemiologic studies of human beings can be evaluated in the models. Enhancement of experimental colonic tumori-. genesis by presumed risk factors and suppression of tumorigenesis by presumed protective factors provide evidence which can help to form the basis for rational intervention in human beings. The models can also contribute to identification of the mechanisms by which modulating factors exert their effects.

Experimental Colonic Carcinogens

Numerous chemicals have been used as experimental colonic carcinogens (Weisburger and Fiala 1983; Shamsuddin 1983 a; Graftstrom 1983). Over the years, relatively few compounds have become "popular," while the rest are rarely used at present. The more commonly used experimental colonic carcinogens can be classified into two types: systemic, metabolically activated type and locally applied, direct-acting type.

Systemic, Metabolically Activated Colonic Carcinogens

The most commonly reported models of experimental colonic carcinogenesis (Table 1) use one of three related hydrazines: 1,2-dimethylhydrazine (DMH, which is administered as DMH dihydrochloride), azoxymethane (AOM), or methylazoxymethanol (MAM, which is administered as MAM acetate). AOM is the oxidation product of DMH and the parent compound of MAM. These compounds are usually given by subcutaneous injection. After absorption into the blood stream, they are distributed throughout the body, hence are "systemic." The explanation of organ specificity of tumorigenesis is uncertain, despite intensive investigation (Fiala et al. 1987; Weisburger and Fiala 1983). The compounds are known to be metabolized in the liver by pathways which include alcohol dehydrogenase and mixed function oxidases. MAM, representing the hepatic metabolite of DMH and AOM, appears to reach the colon via the blood stream rather than via bile, as evidenced by tumorigenesis in colonic segments from which the fecal stream was diverted before carcinogen administration. Metabolic activation and/or spontaneous decomposition of MAM eventually results in formation of the DNA adducts O^6- and 7-methylguanine in the colon and other organs (Rogers and Pegg 1977; Herron and Shank 1981). Formation of these adducts is the initiating event which leads ultimately to tumorigenesis in the colon, but also commonly in the small bowel and external auditory canal.

The occurrence of hepatic activation of these systemic carcinogens is an important consideration in the appropriate use of these models. Some modulating factors in the models affect hepatic metabolism, but these modulating effects are probably irrelevant to human colorectal neoplasia, as discussed in Modulation of Experimental Colonic Carcinogenesis below.

Table 1. Commonly used experimental colonic carcinogens

Systemic, metabolically activated compounds
    Hydrazines
        1,2-Dimethylhydrazine dihydrochloride (DMH)
        Azoxymethane (AOM)
        Methylazoxymethanol acetate (MAMA)
Locally applied, direct-acting compounds
    Alkylnitrosamides
        N-Methyl-N'-nitro-N-nitrosoguanidine (MNNG)
        N-Methyl-N-nitrosourea (MNU)

Locally Applied, Direct-Acting Colonic Carcinogens

N-Methyl-*N'*-nitro-*N*-nitrosoguanidine (MNNG) and *N*-methyl-*N*-nitrosourea (MNU) are the most commonly used compounds in this category. These alkyl-nitrosamides are given by intrarectal or intracolonic instillation, hence are "locally applied." In addition, these compounds result in DNA adduct formation without hepatic activation, hence are "direct acting." Carcinogens of this type have theoretical advantages over the systemic, metabolically activated colonic carcinogens. In particular, direct exposure of the colonic mucosa on the luminal aspect, absence of hepatic activation, and absence of extracolonic tumors may provide a model more analogous to the pathogenesis of human colorectal neoplasia.

Variables in Experimental Models of Colonic Carcinogenesis

Although experimental colonic carcinogenesis has the potential to contribute to understanding the human disease, the literature on the models is rife with conflicting results. Disparities are apparent between experimental and epidemiologic results, and even between results of investigators using apparently similar experimental models. Numerous variables, as shown in Table 2, affect the results of experimental studies.

Carcinogens

The differences in the carcinogen types and their implications are discussed in the previous section. Carcinogen dose affects the latent period and characteristics of tumorigenesis, i.e., higher doses generally lead to shorter latent periods, higher tumor incidence and prevalence, and greater multiplicity. Of particular note, inappropriately high or low doses of carcinogen may preclude detecting effects of modulating agents.

Table 2. Variables in experimental models of colonic carcinogenesis

Carcinogen	Endpoints
Type	Animal survival
Dose	Tumor characteristics
Route	Incidence
Schedule	Prevalence
Animal	Frequency
Species	Multiplicity
Strain	Size
Gender	Growth rate
Age	Mucosal markers for tumorigenesis
Diet	
Macronutrients	
Micronutrients	
Consumption	

For example, high-dose protocols may overwhelm modulators with weak suppressing effects, or produce so many tumors that enhancing effects of modulators cannot be detected. Route of carcinogen administration affects the organ specificity of some colonic carcinogens, e.g., oral DMH results in few colonic tumors but many liver tumors (Weisburger and Fiala 1983). Finally, most colonic carcinogens are given in multiple doses such that classic initiation and promotion phases do not exist in the models.

Experimental Animals

Animal characteristics also affect the models. Most studies use rodents, but different species respond differently to the same carcinogen protocol. Guinea pigs are relatively resistant to the systemic colonic carcinogens as compared with rats and mice. Even within a given species, different strains of rats or mice have different susceptibility to tumorigenesis with the same carcinogen protocol (Weisburger and Fiala 1983; Glickman et al. 1987a, b). Gender and age are also factors as males and younger animals are generally more susceptible.

Diets

Dietary constituents are a critical consideration in experimental models. Since diet plays a central role in human colorectal neoplasia, many studies in models are directed at manipulating dietary constituents (Visek 1986; Jacobs 1986; Kroes et al. 1986). Careful attention to macro- and micro-nutrients and to the level of dietary consumption is essential in interpretation of results. For example, reduced dietary intake alone has been shown to reduce tumorigenesis in some models (Reddy et al. 1987; Pollard and Luckert 1985). Thus, an unpalatable compound given in chow has the potential to reduce tumorigenesis by reducing dietary intake, rather than via direct effects of the compound itself. Pair-feeding of control animals is required in such circumstances. The importance of macro- and micronutrients as confounding variables in studies using the models is apparent from the large number of dietary factors which have been found to modulate experimental tumorigenesis (see Modulation of Experimental Colonic Carcinogenesis below).

Endpoints

Tumorigenesis is the end result of a complex series of events, particularly in the models using a systemic, metabolically activated carcinogen as illustrated for AOM in Fig. 1. Therefore, modulating agents can exert effects through a wide variety of mechanisms as will be discussed in Modulation of Experimental Colonic Carcinogenesis below. A modulator often has consistent effects on the various endpoints, but not always. Examples of effects on markers without altering tumorigenesis have been reported in the literature (Glickman et al. 1987a, b; Kingsnorth et al. 1986), as have effects on some tumor characteristics but not others in the same experiment (Nigro et al. 1987).

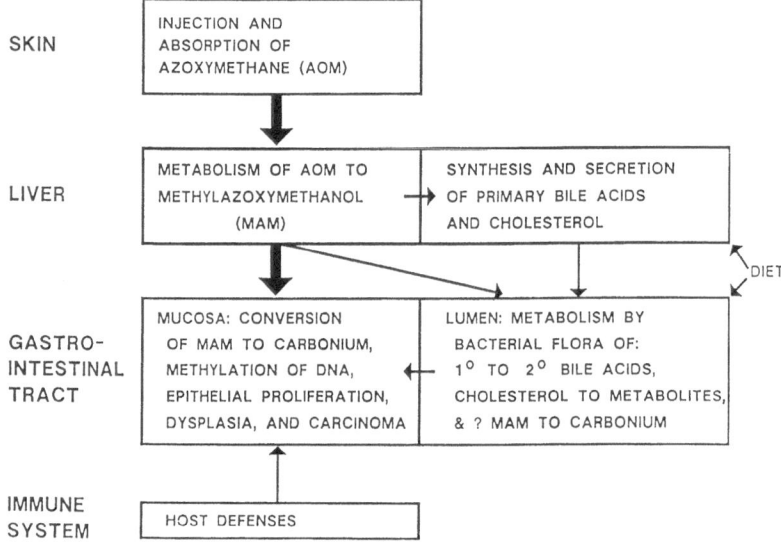

Fig. 1. Summary of events in AOM-treated rat model of colonic carcinogenesis. *Wide arrows* indicate transportation of compound from one site to another in blood stream; *narrow arrows* indicate influence of one aspect of the model on another aspect. The complexity of events leading to tumorigenesis is apparent. Such complexity provides multiple mechanisms by which a modulating agent can exert effects. Modulation of hepatic metabolism of the carcinogen is probably irrelevant to human colorectal neoplasia, whereas the mucosal events appear to be more analogous to the human disease

Optimization of Models

Consideration of these many variables leads to the conclusion that there is no one perfect model of colonic carcinogenesis. Rather, the variables should be defined to optimize the model for the study to be performed. In the case of modulating agents and factors, consistent findings in a variety of appropriate models provide the best evidence of the expected effects in human beings.

Morphogenesis of Experimental Colonic Carcinogenesis

Two aspects of morphogenesis can be considered in the models: the tumors themselves and the mucosa which is predisposed to tumorigenesis due to the effects of the carcinogen, i.e., premalignant mucosa.

Tumors

The morphologic characteristics of the carcinomas and their precursors in the models have been studied extensively (Teague 1983; Shamsuddin 1983 b; Nakamura and Kino

1985). Adenocarcinomas of the colon and small bowel (particularly the duodenum and proximal jejunum) and squamous carcinomas of the external auditory canal are seen with the hydrazine compounds (Figs. 2–4). The invasive carcinomas of the colon often show striking pathologic similarities to human colorectal carcinomas (Fig. 2): the experimental carcinomas are often moderately to well-differentiated gland-forming adenocarcinomas; they invade by direct extension into the subjacent colonic wall; and they produce lymph node and blood-borne metastases, particularly to the lungs, associated with involvement of angiolymphatic vessels.

There are two major dissimilarities between the experimental and human carcinomas of the large bowel. First, in the AOM-treated rat model, microglandular adenocarcinomas with prominent signet ring cells and extracellular mucin occur commonly in the lymphoid nodules of the ascending colon, cecum, and descending colon (Fig. 3). This histopathologic type of colorectal carcinoma is rare in human beings. Secondly, the liver is resistant to metastases in the model, whereas hepatic involvement is common in patients with metastatic colorectal carcinoma.

The morphogenesis of the tumors is controversial. Disagreements revolve around whether or not an adenoma-carcinoma sequence analogous to that in human beings occurs. In the AOM-treated rat model, the polyps which appear often show invasive carcinoma at the base, even when the polyps are small (Izbicki et al. 1985; Hamilton et al. 1986). The polyps are characterized histopathologically by dysplastic epithelium, but the appearances of the intramucosal glands are often similar to the epithelium of infiltrating carcinoma (Fig. 2) and different from adenomatous epithelium with its characteristic stratified, spindle-shaped nuclei (Izbicki et al. 1985). On the other hand, polyps in the DMH model have been reported to show adenocarcinomas arising in adenomas (Madara et al. 1983; Rubio et al. 1986). By contrast with the hydrazine models, the tumors in the MNU-treated rat model (Fig. 5) often show no invasive carcinoma.

Invasive gland-forming adenocarcinomas in all of the commonly used models typically arise in polyps with dysplastic epithelium, as do microglandular carcinomas developing in lymphoid nodules (Shinamoto and Vollmer 1987). Thus, a "dysplasia-carcinoma sequence" has been clearly demonstrated, and the carcinomas do not arise *de novo*. Whether the early, grossly evident dysplastic lesion is a benign neoplasm (adenoma) or a malignant neoplasm without identifiable invasion (carcinoma *in situ*) or with only mucosal invasion (intramucosal carcinoma) seems often to be in the eye of the beholder. Some investigators use the presence or absence of invasion in polyps as the only criterion to distinguish carcinomas and adenomas, respectively. The distinctions may be moot as regards the utility of experimental colonic carcinogenesis as a model for human colorectal neoplasia.

Premalignant Colonic Mucosa

The characteristics of the premalignant colonic mucosa induced by the chemical carcinogens in the models have also been studied intensively. Serial sacrifice protocols have been particularly useful in such studies (Mayer et al. 1987). The immediate precursor to grossly visible tumors appears to be microscopic foci of epithelial dysplasia in crypts of grossly normal colonic mucosa (Hamilton et al. 1982). Abnormal crypt

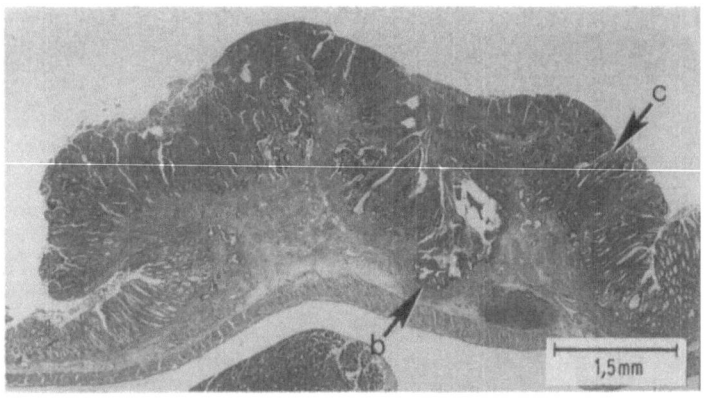

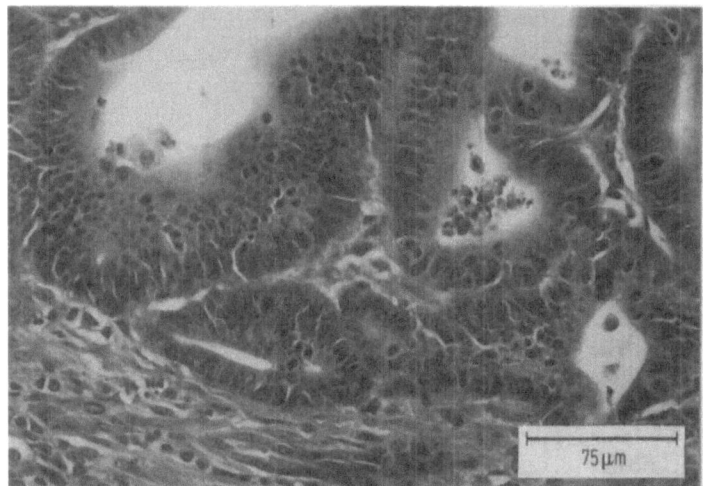

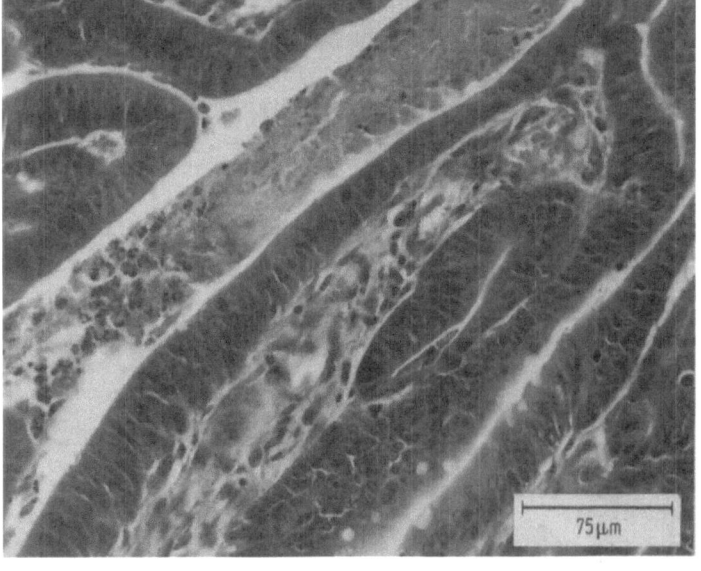

epithelial proliferation is found throughout the colon (Lipkin 1983; Tutton and Barkla 1983), along with changes in biochemical characteristics such as elevated ornithine decarboxylase activity (Luk et al. 1986) and prostaglandin production (Pugh et al. 1986), changes in mucin histochemistry with appearance of altered carbohydrate moieties (Shioda et al. 1987), and changes in ultrastructural characteristics (Pan et al. 1985; Traynor et al. 1986). Some of the abnormalities, such as altered mucin histochemistry, appear to be secondary to altered epithelial proliferation (Chabot and Colacchio 1985). On the other hand, some of these abnormalities are probably pathogenetic precursors to tumorigenesis. For example, inhibition of increased colonic mucosal ornithine decarboxylase activity by the specific inhibitor difluoromethylornithine suppresses tumorigenesis (Kingsnorth et al. 1983; Rozhin et al. 1984; Tempero et al. 1986; Nigro et al. 1986; Benrezzak et al. 1987; Luk et al. 1987; Nigro et al. 1987). A number of the alterations found in the models are under investigation as markers of increased colorectal cancer risk in human beings.

Modulation of Experimental Colonic Carcinogenesis

An incredible number of agents and factors have been shown to modulate experimental colonic carcinogenesis, as summarized in Table 3. It seems highly unlikely that all of these modulators would affect human colorectal neoplasia. Of note, conflicting results have been obtained for some modulators, e.g., dietary ethanol (Seitz et al. 1984; Nelson and Samelson 1985; McGarrity et al. 1986a, b; Garzon et al. 1986; Hamilton et al. 1987a, b) in that both enhancement and suppression of tumorigenesis have been found in experimental models. Thus, knowledge of the mechanisms of action of modulators is needed before the results can be generalized to human beings.

Modulators can be considered from the standpoint of the phase of the models which they affect (Table 4). The effects of some modulators are limited to one phase, whereas others have more global effects. Knowledge of the phase(s) affected can help to direct investigations of mechanism and to assess likelihood that the modulator will affect tumorigenesis in human beings. For example, modulators such as pyrazole which block metabolic activation of systemic colonic carcinogens and thereby inhibit tumorgenesis are unlikely to inhibit human colorectal neoplasia, since the modulated induction phase events are probably irrelevant to pathogenesis of the human disease.

Fig. 2a–c. Tumor of mid-descending colon in AOM-treated rat. a Adenocarcinoma invades deeply into the submucosa, approaching the muscularis propria in the central portion of the tumor in area indicated by b. *Scale in lower right corner* represents 1.5 mm. b and c Designated areas (*b, c*) at higher magnification. b Area of deep invasion indicated in a shows well-differentiated gland-forming adenocarcinoma with subjacent desmoplasia. The histopathologic characteristics are similar to many human colorectal carcinomas. *Scale in lower right corner* represents 75 µm. c Intramucosal component of tumor indicated in a is histopathologically similar to deeply invasive adenocarcinoma shown in b, without evidence of adenomatous epithelium characterized by stratified, spindle-shaped nuclei. *Scale in lower right corner* represents 75 µm

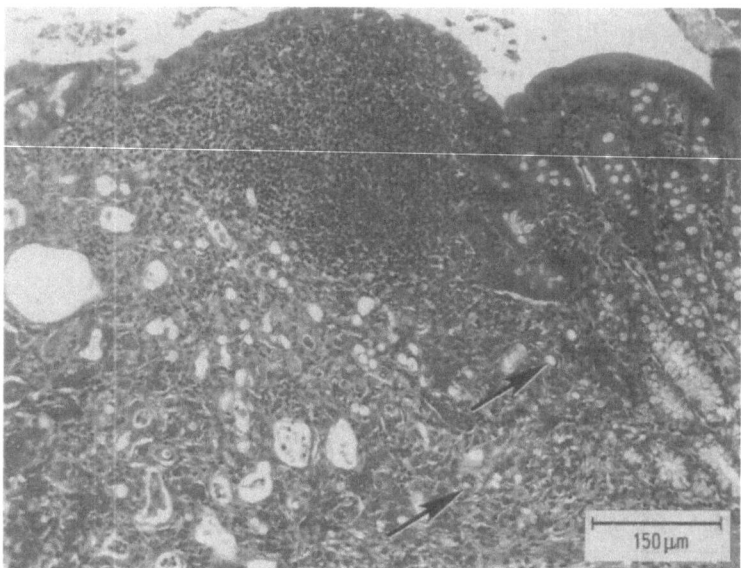

Fig. 3. Tumor of lymphoid nodule in ascending colon of AOM-treated rat. The microglandular adenocarcinoma shows prominent signet ring cells (*arrows*), and abundant extracellular mucin is often present, although not in this example. This histopathologic type of tumor is uncommon in human beings. The colonic mucosa adjoining the tumor shows the characteristic prominence of mucinous epithelial cells in the crypt bases, a histologic finding which is dissimilar from the ascending colon of human beings. *Scale in lower right corner* represents 150 μm

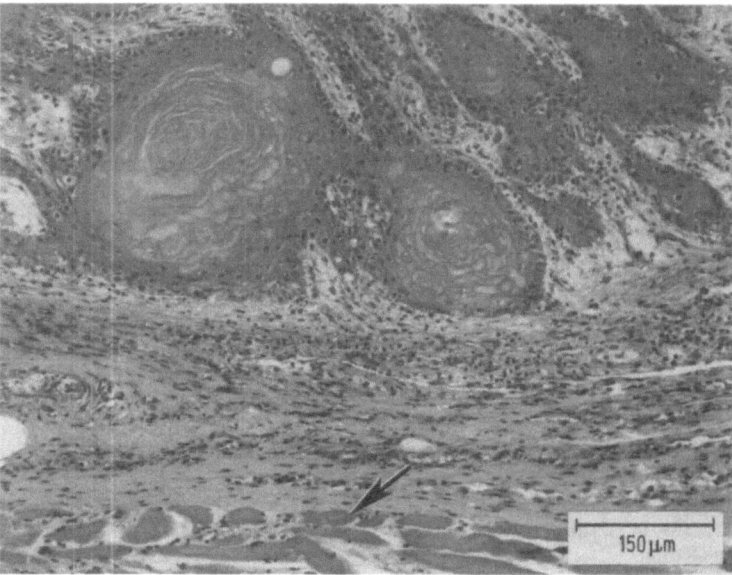

Fig. 4. Tumor of external auditory canal in AOM-treated rat. The strikingly well-differentiated squamous carcinoma compresses skeletal muscle fibers (*arrow*) of neck muscle. *Scale in lower right corner* represents 150 μm

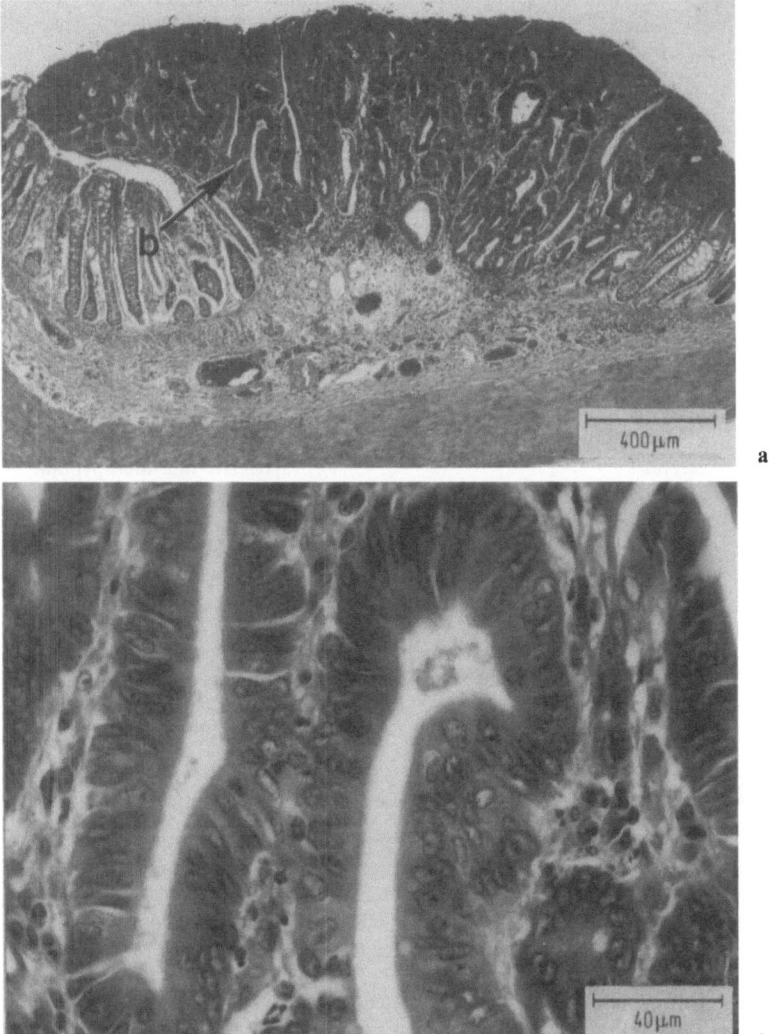

Fig. 5a, b. Tumor of distal descending colon in MNU-treated rat. **a** Invasion through the muscularis mucosae into superficial submucosa is evident in the central portion of the tumor. Area indicated by *b* is shown at higher magnification in **b**. *Scale in lower right corner* represents 400 μm. **b** Intramucosal component of tumor indicated in **a** shows moderately differentiated adenocarcinoma histopathologically similar to many human colorectal carcinomas. *Scale in lower right corner* represents 40 μm

Table 3. Examples of reported modulators of experimental colonic carcinogenesis

Modulators	Reported effects of modulators	
	Suppression of tumorigenesis	Enhancement of tumorigenesis
Dietary factors	Low fat	"Western" diet
	High fiber (wheat bran and cellulose)	High fat
	Beta-carotene and retinoic acid analogue	Low fiber
	Vitamin A deficiency	High fiber (pectin, corn bran,
	Supplementation with selenium,	carageenan, agar, Meta-
	calcium, vitamin C, vitamin E	mucil, alfalfa)
	Fish oil	Vitamin C deficiency
	Ethanol and beer	Copper deficiency
	Food restriction	Ethanol
	Diallyl sulfide (garlic)	Selenium deficiency
	Lactobacillus acidophilus	
	Beta-sitosterol	
Exogenous	Secretin	Vasoactive intestinal peptide
hormones		Gastrin
Drugs and	Difluoromethylornithine	Deoxycholate
chemicals	Chemotherapeutic agents	Carbon black
	Interleukin 2	Protamine
	Disulfiram and similar compounds	Butyrate
	Pyrazole	Butylated hydroxytoluene
	Warfarin	Cyproterone (anti-androgen)
	Butylated hydroxytoluene	Neomycin
	Butylated hydroxyanisole	
	Indomethacin	
	Ethoxyquin	
	Antibiotics	
	Lactulose	
Surgial	Diversion of fecal stream	Cholecystectomy
manipulation	Castration	Enterectomy
		Suture line
Miscellaneous		Experimental colitis

Table 4. Phases in experimental models of colonic carcinogenesis

Phase	Characteristics and events	Examples of modulator
Pre-induction phase	Baseline state of animal; carcinogen susceptibility	Nonspecific injury stimulating colonic epithelial proliferation ultimately enhancing tumorigenesis, e.g., suture line
Induction phase	Multiple doses of carcinogen; activation and catabolism, initiating events of DNA adduct formation and repair	Competitive inhibitors of carcinogen metabolism suppressing tumorigenesis, e.g., ethanol
Post-induction latent phase	After carcinogen administration; grossly normal colonic mucosa with epithelial proliferative abnormalities and dysplasia	Inhibitor of epithelial proliferation suppressing tumorigenesis, e.g., difluoromethylornithine
Tumor growth phase	Presence and growth of visible tumors	Cytotoxic agents suppressing tumor growth, e.g., 5-fluorouracil

Table 5. Comparison of experimental models and human colorectal neoplasia

	Experimental colonic carcinogenesis		Human colorectal neoplasia
	Systemic metabolically activated carcinogen	Locally applied direct acting carcinogen	
Mechanisms of carcinogenesis			
Systemic route of carcinogen exposure, hepatic activation	+	−	− (?)
Luminal route of carcinogen exposure	−	+	+ (?)
Genetic susceptibility to tumorigenesis	+	+	+
Modulation of tumorigenesis			
Modulation by luminal mechanisms	+	+	+
Modulation by hepatic metabolic mechanisms	+	−	− (?)
Morphogenesis of tumors			
Dysplasia-carcinoma sequence	+	+	+
Adenoma-carcinoma sequence	+/−	+/−	+
Mucosal markers for tumorigenesis	+	+	+
Morphology of colonic tumors			
Gland-forming adenocarcinomas	+	+	+
Microglandular adenocarcinoma in lymphoid nodules	+	−	−
Character of metastases			
High prevalence	+	−	+
Hepatic metastases common	−	−	+
Extracolonic tumors			
Small bowel tumors	+	−.	−
Extraintestinal tumors	+	−	+ (?)

Relevance to Human Colorectal Neoplasia

The ultimate criterion by which the experimental models of colonic carcinogenesis should be judged is relevance to the human disease. The models using systemic, metabolically activated carcinogens or locally applied, direct-acting carcinogens are compared with human large bowel neoplasia in Table 5. Epidemiologic studies suggest that different etiologic and pathogenetic factors are involved in carcinoma of the rectum as compared with the colon (Weisburger and Wynder 1987). The precise relationship of the various experimental models to human tumors of various anatomic sites in the large bowel is uncertain at present. In part, this uncertainty relates to the anatomic and histopathologic differences between the ascending and descending colon in rodents (Fig. 3) and human beings (Hamilton 1984). Nonetheless, the comparison shows that with appropriate usage the models can continue to make important contributions to research on colorectal neoplasia.

Acknowledgements. Secretarial assistance was provided by Mrs. N. Folker. The photomicrographs were taken by Mr. R. E. Lund, R.B.P. Technical assistance was provided by Mrs. C. L. Hamilton, Mr. J. Floyd, Ms. S. Golightly, Mrs. L. Hartka, Dr. Y. Chaudhry, and Ms. E. Natuzzi.

References

Amberger H (1986) Different autochthonous models of colorectal cancer in the rat. J Cancer Res Clin Oncol 111:157–159

Autrup H, Williams GM (eds) (1983) Experimental colon carcinogenesis. CRC, Boca Raton

Benrezzak O, Nigam VN, Madarnas P (1987) Increased survival of CD1 mice bearing dimethylhydrazine-induced primary colon and anal cancers by diffluoromethylornithine with concomitant increase in angiosarcoma incidence. Anticancer Res 7:251–258

Bruce WR (1986) What chemicals are responsible for colon cancer? J Cell Physiol [Suppl] 4:47–49

Bruce WR (1987) Recent hypotheses for the origin of colon cancer. Cancer Res 47:4237–4242

Chabot JA, Colacchio TA (1985) Early colonic dysplasia: comparison of differential mucin staining and tritiated thymidine labelling. Am J Surg 149:133–139

Fiala ES, Sohn OS, Puz C, Czerniak R (1987) Differential effects of 4-iodopyrazole and 3-methylpyrazole on the metabolic activation of methylazoxymethanol to a DNA-methylating species by rat liver and rat colon mucosa in vivo. J Cancer Res Clin Oncol 133:145–150

Garzon FT, Seitz HK, Simanowski UA, Berger MR, Schmahl D (1986) Enhancement of acetoxymethylmethylnitrosamine (AMMN)-induced colorectal tumors following chronic ethanol consumption in rats (Abstract). Gastroenterology 90:1424

Gilbert JM (1987) Experimental colorectal cancer as a model of human disease. Ann R Coll Surg Engl 69:48–53

Glickman LT, Senterman MK, Fleiszer DM (1987a) 1,2-Dimethylhydrazine-induced nuclear aberrations in A/J and C57BL/6J mouse colonic crypts. JNCI 79:499–507

Glickman LT, Suissa S, Fleiszer DM (1987b) Proliferative characteristics of colonic crypt cells in C57BL/6J and A/J mice as predictors of subsequent tumor formation. Cancer Res 47:4766–4770

Grafstrom RC (1983) Metabolism of chemical carcinogens by intestinal tissue. In: Autrup H, Williams GM (eds) Experimental colon carcinogenesis. CRC, Boca Raton, pp 63–82

Hamilton SR (1984) Structure of the colon. Scand J Gastroenterol 18 (Suppl 93):13–23

Hamilton SR, Stephens RB, Natuzzi E, Boitnott JK, Yardley JH (1982) Morphologic analogy of intestinal tract carcinogenesis in adenomatous polyposis and the azoxymethane-treated rat model (Abstract). Lab Invest 46:33A–34A

Hamilton SR, Zhang S, O'Ceallaigh D, McAvinchey D (1986) Growth characteristic of autochthonous experimental colonic tumors as assessed by serial colonoscopic measurement in rats. Gastroenterology 91:1511–1520

Hamilton SR, Hyland J, McAvinchey D, Chaudhry Y, Hartka L, Kim HT, Cichon P, Floyd J, Turjman N, Kessie G, Nair PP, Dick J (1987a) Effects of chronic dietary beer and ethanol consumption on experimental colonic carcinogenesis by azoxymethane in rats. Cancer Res 47:1551–1559

Hamilton SR, Sohn OS, Fiala ES (1987b) Effects of timing and quantity of chronic dietary ethanol consumption on azoxymethane-induced colonic carcinogenesis and azoxymethane metabolism in Fischer 344 rats. Cancer Res 47:4305–4311

Herron DC, Shank RC (1981) In vitro kinetics of O^6-methylguanine and 7-methylguanine formation and persistence in DNA of rats treated with symmetrical dimethylhydrazine. Cancer Res 41:3967–3972

Izbicki JR, Hamilton SR, Izbicki W, Blochl H, Dornschneider G, Adamek L, Kusche J (1985) Lack of evidence for adenoma-carcinoma sequence in chemically induced colonic carcinogenesis in rats. Dig Surg 2:143–151

Jacobs LR (1966) Modification of experimental colon carcinogenesis by dietary fibers. Adv Exp Med Biol 206:105–118

Kingsnorth AN, King WW, Diekema KA, McCann PP, Ross JS, Malt RA (1983) Inhibition of ornithine decarboxylase with 2-difluoromethylornithine: reduced incidence of dimethyl-hydrazine-induced colon tumors in mice. Cancer Res 43: 2545–2549

Kingsnorth AN, LaMuraglia GM, Ross JS, Malt RA (1986) Vanadate supplements and 1,2-dimethylhydrazine-induced colon cancer in mice: increased thymidine incorporation without enhanced carcinogenesis. Br J Cancer 53: 683–686

Kroes R, Beems RB, Bosland MC, Bunnik GS, Sinkeldam EJ (1986) Nutritional factors in lung, colon, and prostate carcinogenesis in animal models. Fed Proc 45: 136–141

LaMont JT, O'Gorman TA (1978) Experimental colon cancer. Gastroenterology 75: 1157–1169

Lipkin M (1983) Cell proliferation in colon carcinogenesis. In: Autrup A, Williams GM (eds) Experimental colon carcinogenesis. CRC, Boca Raton, pp 139–154

Luk GD, Hamilton SR, Yang P, Smith JA, O'Ceallaigh D, McAvinchey D, Hyland J (1986) Kinetic changes in mucosal ornithine decarboxylase activity during azoxymethane-induced colonic carcinogenesis in the rat. Cancer Res 46: 4449–4452

Luk GD, Zhang S-Z, Smith JA, Hamilton SR (1987) Effects of timing and dose of difluorome-thylornithine on azoxymethane-induced colonic carcinogenesis in the rat (Abstract). Gastroenterology 92: 1511

Madara JL, Harte P, Deasy J, Ross D, Lahey S, Steele G (1983) Evidence for an adenoma-carcinoma sequence in dimethylhydrazine-induced neoplasms of rat intestinal epithelium. Am J Pathol 110: 230–235

Mayer D, Trocheris V, Hacker HJ, Viallard V, Murat JC, Bannasch P (1987) Sequential histochemical and morphometric studies in preneoplastic and neoplastic lesions induced in rat colon by 1,2-dimethylhydrazine. Carcinogenesis 8: 155–161

McGarrity TJ, Via EA, Colony PC (1986a) Changes in tissue sialic acid content and staining in dimethylhydrazine (DMH)-induced colorectal cancer: effects of ethanol (Abstract). Gastroenterology 90: 1543

McGarrity TJ, Erwin B, Pegg AE, Colony PC (1986b) Polyamine levels in dimethylhydrazine (DMH)-induced colorectal cancer: effects of chronic alcohol (Abstract). Gastroenterology 90: 1543

Nakamura S, Kino I (1985) Morphogenesis of experimental colonic neoplasms induced by dimethylhydrazine. In: Pfeiffer CJ (ed) Animal models for intestinal disease. CRC, Boca Raton, pp 99–122

Nelson RL, Samelson SL (1985) Neither dietary ethanol nor beer augments experimental colon carcinogenesis in rats. Dis Colon Rectum 28: 460–462

Nigro ND, Bull AW, Boyd ME (1986) Inhibition of intestinal carcinogenesis in rats: effect of difluoromethylornithine with piroxicam or fish oil. JNCI 77: 1309–1313

Nigro ND, Bull AW, Boyd ME (1987) Importance of the duration of inhibition of intestinal carcinogenesis by difluoromethylornithine in rats. Cancer Lett 35: 153–158

Pan Q, Hamilton SR, Hyland J, Boitnott JK (1985) Effects of carcinogen dosage on experimental colonic carcinogenesis by azoxymethane: an ultrastructural study of grossly normal colonic mucosa. JNCI 74: 689–698

Pollard M, Luckert PH (1985) Tumorigenic effects of direct- and indirect-acting chemical carcinogens in rats on a restricted diet. JNCI 74: 1347–1349

Pozharisski KM, Likhachev AJ, Climashevski BF, Shaposhnikov JD (1979) Experimental intestinal cancer research with special reference to human pathology. Adv Cancer Res 30: 165–237

Pugh S, Gellister JS, Williams SC, Lewin MR, Barton TP, Clark CG, Boulos PB (1986) Prostaglandin E2 (PGE2) changes precede tumor formation in the dimethylhydrazine (DMH) colon cancer model in rats (Abstract). Dig Dis Sci 10 (Suppl): 363S

Reddy BS, Wang CX, Maruyama H (1987) Effect of restricted caloric intake on azoxymethane-induced colon tumor incidence in male F344 rats. Cancer Res 47: 1226–1228

Rogers AE, Nauss KM (1985) Rodent models for carcinoma of the colon. Dig Dis Sci 30 (Suppl): 87S–102S

Rogers KJ, Pegg AE (1977) Formation of O^6-methylguanine by alkylation of rat liver, colon, and kidney DNA following administration of 1,2-dimethylhydrazine. Cancer Res 37: 4082–4087

Rozhin J, Wilson PS, Bull AW, Nigro ND (1984) Ornithine decarboxylase activity in the rat and human colon. Cancer Res 44: 3226–3230

Rubio CA, Nylander G, Wahlin B, Sveander M, Duvander A, Alun ML (1986) Monitoring the histogenesis of colonic tumors in the Sprague-Dawley rat. J Surg Oncol 31:225–228

Seitz HK, Cyzgan P, Waldher R, Veith S, Raedsch R, Kassmodel H, Kommerell B (1984) Enhancement of 1,2-dimethylhydrazine-induced rectal carcinogenesis following chronic ethanol consumption in the rat. Gastroenterology 86:886–891

Shamsuddin AKM (1983a) In vivo induction of colon cancer dose and animal species. In: Autrup H, Williams GM (eds) Experimental colon carcinogenesis. CRC, Boca Raton, pp 51–62

Shamsuddin AKM (1983b) Comparative pathology – human large intestinal cancer and animal models. In: Autrup H, Williams GM (eds) Experimental colon carcinogenesis. CRC, Boca Raton, pp 125–138

Shinamoto F, Vollmer E (1987) Changes in intestinal mucosa above lymph follicles during carcinogenesis in rats. A light and electron microscopic study. J Cancer Res Clin Oncol 113:41–50

Shioda Y, Brown WR, Ahnen DJ (1987) Serial observations of colonic carcinogenesis in the rat. Premalignant mucosa binds *Ulex europeus* agglutinin. Gastroenterology 92:112–117

Teague CA (1983) Morphological changes during chemical induction of colon cancer. In: Autrup H, Williams GM (eds) Experimental colon carcinogenesis. CRC, Boca Raton, pp 107–124

Tempero M, Nishioka K, Wolfrey W, Zetterman R (1986) Chemoprevention with difluorome-thylornithine (DFMO) during and after carcinogen exposure in colon cancer (Abstract). Proc Am Assoc Cancer Res 27:126

Traynor OJ, Costa NL, Wood CB (1986) A scanning electron microscopy study of changes in rat colonic mucosa during carcinogenesis. J Surg Res 41:529–537

Tutton RPJM, Barkla DH (1983) Regulation of cell kinetics and colon cancer. In: Autrup H, Williams GM (eds) Experimental colon carcinogenesis. CRC, Boca Raton, pp 199–214

Visek WJ (1986) Dietary protein and experimental carcinogenesis. Adv Exp Med Biol 206:163–186

Weisburger JH, Fiala ES (1983) Experimental colon carcinogens and their mode of action. In: Autrup H, Williams GM (eds) Experimental colon carcinogenesis. CRC, Boca Raton, pp 27–50

Weisburger JH, Wynder EL (1987) Etiology of colorectal cancer with emphasis on mechanism of action and prevention. In: DeVita VT, Hellman S, Rosenberg SA (eds) Important advances in oncology. Lippincott, Philadelphia, pp 197–220

Colonic Microsomal Enzymes and Their Role in Colorectal Carcinogenesis

H. W. Strobel, D. K. Hammond, and T. B. White

Department of Biochemistry and Molecular Biology, P.O. Box 20708, Houston, Texas 77225, USA

Contents

Introduction

The metabolism of drugs and carcinogens by microsomal enzymes in mammalian tissues has been elucidated and characterized by many investigators over the last 30 years. The hepatic microsomal system has been studied most extensively because it is the most active system of all the various tissues and it appears to metabolize the broadest range of substrates (Brodie et al. 1958; Gillette 1966; Lu and West 1978; Nebert and Gonzales 1987; Nelson and Strobel 1987). In general, drug and carcinogen metabolism occurs in two phases: an oxidative phase (phase I), catalyzed by the cytochromes P-450; and a conjugative phase (phase II), catalyzed by a variety of enzymes such as the glutathione S-transferases and others.

The cytochromes P-450-dependent mixed function oxidase is the nicotinamide-adenine-dinucleotide phosphate, reduced form (NADPH) requiring electron transfer system of the endoplasmic reticulum which catalyzes drug and carcinogen metabolism. The other major oxidative system of endoplasmic reticulum, the cytochrome b_5 system, requires NADH as its source of electrons and supports fatty acid desaturation. The drug metabolism system consists of the cytochrome P-450 isozymes and NADPH cytochrome P-450 reductase which transfers electrons from NADPH to the cytochromes P-450 (Lu et al. 1969; Dignam and Strobel 1975). Reducing equivalents for the cytochrome P-450 system can also be obtained from NADH or NADPH through cytochrome b_5 (reviewed by Peterson and Prough 1986). Following the cytochrome P-450-catalyzed oxidative phase, the conjugative phase begins; epoxide hydratase facilitates the linkage between the oxidative and conjugative phases for some substrates.

Although drug metabolism studies have focused on the hepatic microsomal system, the primary site of activation of some orally ingested compounds may well be the colon or other areas of the digestive tract. The study of activating systems of the colon has often made use of the colon-specific model carcinogens 1,2-dimethylhydrazine and azoxymethane. Fiala (1977) and Fiala et al. (1987) have suggested a scheme for the activation of these compounds to the active carcinogen involving catalysis by cytochrome P-450. These studies stemmed in part from earlier work showing that colon cancer could be induced in rodents by the natural plant product cycasin (methylazoxymethanol β-glucoside; Weisburger 1971, 1973). The active component of cycasin was identified by Druckrey (1970) as methylazoxymethanol (MAM) which can be produced by the cytochrome P-450 system from azoxymethane or 1,2-dimethylhydrazine (Fiala 1977), as well as through release from the β-glucoside linkage by glycosidases of the bacteria present in the lumen of the colon. These studies with model carcinogens have pointed to a role for colonic activation enzymes in the process of colon carcinogenesis. The putative role of these enzymes is examined in this chapter.

Results and Discussion

A general scheme suggesting the involvement of various microsomal enzymes in colonic carcinogenesis is shown in Fig. 1. Dietary and/or blood-borne precarcinogens may be activated by the cytochromes P-450, especially those in the 3-methylcholanthrene and phenobarbital-inducible families present in colonic tissue. One or more cytochrome P-450-dependent steps may be involved in metabolism of a compound to an active form or forms of a carcinogen. Cytochrome P-450-catalyzed reactions require reducing equivalents which are usually provided to the reaction by cytochrome P-450 reductase from NADPH. A growing body of evidence from various

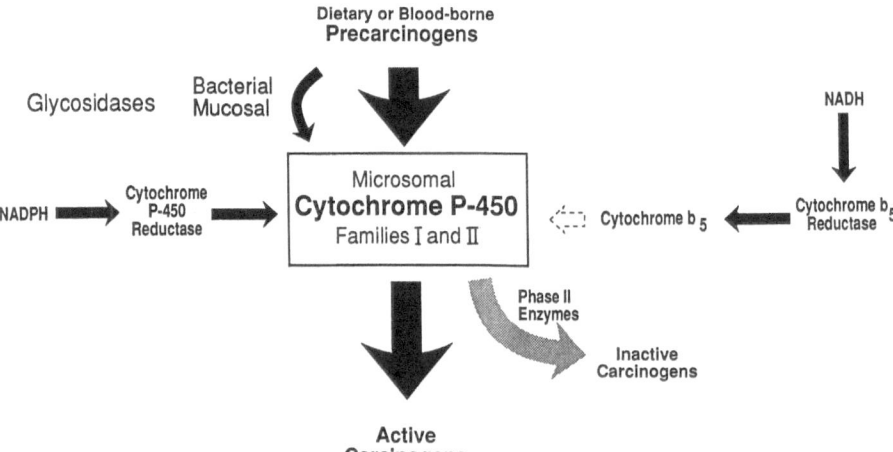

Fig. 1. Scheme showing component enzymes which may be involved in the conversion of precarcinogens to active carcinogens in colon tissue

tissues, however, suggests that the cytochrome b_5: cytochrome b_5 reductase system may in some cases provide electrons to cytochrome P-450 as suggested in the scheme (Lu and West 1978). Metabolism of precarcinogens by cytochromes P-450 may directly activate these substrates to carcinogenic products. The cytochrome P-450-dependent activation of substrates to carcinogenic products may be aided by epoxide hydratase.

Some of the multiple forms of colonic cytochrome P-450 may produce products from a substrate which are inactive as carcinogens. The scheme indicates that phase II drug metabolism enzymes such as the glutathione S-transferases, etc., also play a role in rendering potential carcinogens harmless to the colon cell. Epoxide hydratase action may facilitate detoxification of metabolic intermediates. These phase II reactions contribute significantly to detoxification of chemicals in other tissues, e.g., liver. On the other hand, the scheme suggests a possible interaction whereby glycosides might be hydrolyzed releasing a carbohydrate moiety and a precarcinogen or carcinogen for metabolism by the cytochrome P-450 system.

Cytochrome P-450 Activation of Carcinogens

Autrup et al. (1977) provided good evidence that colon cells were able to activate carcinogens by showing that radiolabeled benzo[a]pyrene and 1,2-dimethylhydrazine or metabolites were bound covalently to colon macromolecules after incubation of human colon explant segments in organ culture with the carcinogens. Fang and Strobel (1978a) used the Ames mutagenesis system with *Salmonella typhimurium* strain TA100 (Ames et al. 1973) to show that rat colonic microsomes were able to activate 2-aminoanthracene and benzo[a]pyrene to mutagenic products. This demonstration that carcinogens and mutagens can be activated by colonic mucosa not just by hepatocytes was recently confirmed by Oravec et al. (1986) who demonstrated that rat colon epithelial cells metabolized 1,2-[^{14}C]dimethylhydrazine into products mutagenic for human P3 teratoma cells as well as into ^{14}C-labeled alkali-soluble volatile products (presumably CO_2).

Newaz et al. (1983) demonstrated that human colon microsomes from segments of human large bowel metabolized 1,2-dimethylhydrazine through an enzymatic process inhibitable with carbon monoxide or SKF-525A. These results suggest that the enzymatic catalyst in human colon segment microsomes is cytochrome P-450, but these authors were unable to demonstrate cytochrome P-450 directly by carbon monoxide difference spectroscopy. By using a cell line derived from a human colon tumor Fang and Strobel (1982) directly demonstrated not only the presence of cytochrome P-450 in microsomes prepared from a human colon tumor cell line but also the induction of hydroxylation activity of the carcinogen benzo[a]pyrene by pretreatment of the cells in culture with phenobarbital or benzanthracene. Newaz et al. (1983) later demonstrated that pretreatment of human colon tumor cells with phenobarbital plus hydrocortisone markedly increased (282% of control) the rate of activation of the colon-specific carcinogen 1,2-dimethylhydrazine. Thus the case for cytochrome P-450 activation of carcinogens in colon tissue is based on the work of a number of laboratories using adduct formation studies in explant culture, activation and mutagenesis studies in vitro, plus inhibition and induction studies in tissue culture. These data all support the posit that activation of model colon carcinogens and polycyclic aromatic hydrocarbons to their mutagenic or carcinogenic adduct-forming metabolites can be catalyzed through the agency of colonic cytochromes P-450.

Evidence in Support of Scheme 1

Cytochrome P-450 Distribution. Early work from this laboratory (Fang and Strobel 1978 b) demonstrated the presence and activity of a cytochrome P-450 mixed function oxidase system in rat colon microsomes. The data presented by those workers also suggested the presence of multiple forms of cytochrome P-450 based on the differential induction of activities following treatment of rats with phenobarbital or β-naphthoflavone and the differential sensitivities of hydroxylation activities to the inhibitors SKF525A and 7,8-benzoflavone. Using antibodies to purified rat hepatic isozymes, four different forms of cytochrome P-450 were subsequently shown by radial immunodiffusion to be present in colonic microsomes from rats treated with β-naphthoflavone or phenobarbital (Strobel et al. 1983). Kaku et al. (1985) partially purified three forms of cytochrome P-450 from rabbit colonic microsomes and demonstrated their hydroxylation activities in reconstituted systems toward a variety of substrates including prostaglandins, fatty acids of varying chain lengths, N-alkyl drugs, and the carcinogen benzo[a]pyrene.

Evidence for the presence of cytochromes P-450 in human colon tissue comes from several lines of experimentation. Human colon microsomal preparations were examined for the presence of particular forms of cytochrome P-450 using antibodies to rat liver cytochromes P-450 by the Western blot technique. Evidence for the presence of form 4 (form d, P-450lA2) was reported by Strobel et al. (1983) using rabbit antibodies to form 4 purified from rat liver. In the same set of experiments form 5 (form c, P-450lA1) could not be detected by the Western blot technique. In both of these experiments microsomes from human colon obtained at autopsy were used as enzyme source. Since evidence of drug use or alcohol consumption were used as exclusion criteria for selection of colons, the resultant microsomal preparations approximate the control (untreated) state and therefore probably reflect the expression of this isoform under basal or "normal" conditions. On the other hand, little is known about the effects of individual variation on the expression of cytochrome P-450 in human colon. Additionally, the immunological cross reactivity between human colonic forms and rabbit antibodies prepared to rat liver forms may limit detectability of forms present in colon. Indeed, it is likely that other forms are present in human colon microsomes that are not detectable in the systems used for these studies.

More recently our laboratory has turned to the use of cDNA probes for the expression of forms of cytochrome P-450 in colonic tissue in order to take advantage of the sensitivity of this technique. We have also utilized the human colon tumor cell line LS174T to study the induction properties of human colonic cytochromes P-450 in a readily manipulable system free of complications caused by the presence of mucus. This strategy has led to the demonstration of the responsivity of cytochrome P-450 form c (P-450lA1) to induction with benzanthracene pretreatment of LS174T

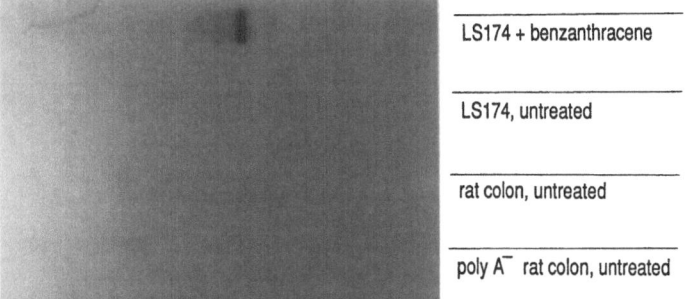

LS174 + benzanthracene

LS174, untreated

rat colon, untreated

poly A⁻ rat colon, untreated

Fig. 2. Northern analysis of rat colon tissue and human colon tumor cell line LS174T. RNA isolated from LS174T cells either untreated or benzanthracene treated was enriched for Poly A-containing molecules. Poly A-enriched RNA (20 μg) was loaded into lanes 1 (LS174T + benzanthracene) and 2 (LS174T, untreated) of a 1% agarose formaldehyde gel. Poly A-enriched RNA (50 μg) from normal rat colon was loaded into lane 3, and RNA which did not bind to oligo (dT) cellulose was loaded into lane 4 (10 μg). Following electrophoresis, the RNA was transferred to a gene screen plus filter and probed with a ^{32}P-random primed plasmid (pA8) containing a portion of the DNA coding for rat cytochrome P-450 form c (P-4501A1). Hybridization was performed at 42 °C for 18 h at a probe concentration of 2×10^6 cpm/ml. The filter was exposed to Kodak AR film for 18 h at room temperature

cells as shown in Fig. 2. Using a radiolabeled DNA probe, a single band was detected in poly A-enriched RNA from cells after induction with benzanthracene but not from untreated colon tumor cells. No hybridization was detectable in poly A-enriched RNA prepared from untreated rat colon tissue consistent with the absence of any immunologically detectable form c in human colon cells (Strobel et al. 1983). The absence of any hybridization band in the lane loaded with poly A⁻ RNA from untreated rat colon confirms the specificity of the probe. This study provides the first demonstration of inducer-triggered expression of poly A⁺ RNA in human colon LS174T cells. This approach will doubtless identify other cytochromes present in human colon tumor cells and responsive to inducer-modulated expression. Further, this methodology may provide the sensitivity needed to specify the isoforms of cytochrome P-450 which are involved in the discrete aspects of carcinogen activation and chemotherapeutic agent metabolism.

Reducing Equivalents for the Cytochrome P-450 System

As shown in Fig. 1, cytochrome P-450 accepts electrons from NADPH through NADPH cytochrome P-450 reductase. The cytochrome P-450 reductase is the primary source of reducing equivalents for the cytochromes P-450 as has been shown by reconstituting drug-metabolizing activities from solubilized and purified components (Lu et al. 1969; Dignam and Strobel 1975; Yasukochi and Masters 1976). In other experiments the role of cytochrome P-450 reductase was demonstrated by selective removal of reductase activity from microsomes with steapsin protease and restoration of near total microsomal activity by adding back purified detergent-solubilized cytochrome P-450 reductase (Gum and Strobel 1979).

Table 1. Induction of cytochrome P-450/cytochrome b_5 ratio in various tissues

Tissue	Treatment	$[b_5]/[P\text{-}450]$
Liver (rat)	Control	0.35
	Phenobarbital	0.17
	β-Naphthoflavone	0.2
LS174T cells	Control	2.5
	Phenobarbital	3.0

Cytochrome P-450 reductase activity has been clearly demonstrated in human colon microsomes, and its inducibility in human colon tumor cells has been shown (Fang and Strobel 1982; Strobel et al. 1986). When added to human colon microsomes, rabbit antibody to rat cytochrome P-450 reductase substantially inhibits dimethylhydrazine metabolism in the presence of NADPH (Strobel et al. 1986). These data point to the central role of cytochrome P-450 reductase in presenting reducing equivalents to the cytochrome P-450 system.

The scheme presented in Fig. 1 also suggests that reducing equivalents from NADH may also be utilized in cytochrome P-450-mediated reactions in the colon. While it is not clear whether both, only one, or none of the required electrons are provided from NADH, several lines of evidence suggest that components of the NADH system may supply some of the electrons in the colonic system. One line of evidence supportive of a role for cytochrome b_5 in colonic cytochrome P-450 activities is shown in Table 1. The data presented in this table show that, unlike hepatic microsomes, the LS174T cells show a much higher ratio of cytochrome b_5 to cytochrome P-450 in control cells. Further, cytochrome b_5 responds more to phenobarbital induction of the cells than does cytochrome P-450. Another piece of evidence derives from the inhibition of dimethylhydrazine metabolism by human colon microsomes using NADPH by the addition of rabbit antibody to rat liver cytochrome b_5 (Strobel et al. 1986). The substantial inhibition by anticytochrome b_5 (35%) illustrates the possible role of cytochrome b_5 in electron transfer in colonic metabolism. These lines of evidence taken together with the demonstration of cytochrome b_5 reductase activity in human colon and human colon tumor cells point to the possible involvement of colonic cytochrome b_5 in cytochrome P-450-mediated catalysis.

Phase II Activities and Other Enzymes

Phase II drug metabolism activities include a variety of enzymes leading to the conjugation of hydroxylated substrate intermediate with acceptor molecules such as glutathione, uridine diphosphate (UDP)-glucuronic acid or others. Epoxide hydratase, often included within this broadly defined group, has been demonstrated to be present in rat colonic mucosal microsomes (data not shown). This enzyme, which hydrates epoxides to catechol derivatives, may play a role in fostering conjugation reactions and thereby reducing the carcinogenic potential of some of the initial substrates hydroxylated by colonic cytochromes P-450. Although little evidence now exists to support this possibility, the weight of evidence from the liver and other tissues requires the inclusion of these alternatives in the colonic metabolic scheme.

The role of glycosidases and the possibility of metabolite exchange between the colonic mucosal cells and the bacterial content of the colon must also be considered. The presence of glycosidases in bacteria in the colon is known. The role proposed for bacterial glycosidases in the release of the partially activated carcinogen methyl-azoxymethanol from cycasin illustrates the importance of bacterial enzymes in the metabolism of potential carcinogens (Weisburger 1973). It is possible that compounds activated and conjugated by colonic cells might be deconjugated or further converted by bacterial glycosidase or similar enzymes following elimination from colonic mucosal cells. Thus a combination of mucosal cell and bacterial processes might together eventuate in the formation of active ultimate carcinogens. On the other hand, the bacterial glycosidases or mucosal phase II enzymes might foster inactivation and elimination of potentially toxic or carcinogenic metabolites.

Since the exact causes of cancer of the colon are not known, it is likely that multiple chemical and enzymatic steps are involved in the process of colon carcinogenesis. The cytochrome P-450 system is a likely enzymatic first step in the activation for some, though not all, candidate carcinogens. The multiple isozymes which comprise this family of enzymes enable this mixed function oxidase system to catalyze with some facility the metabolism of a variety of structurally dissimilar compounds. Thus the initial steps in activation of many compounds can be fostered. Similarly, the wide range of phase II enzymes provides alternative pathways for the products of initial cytochrome P-450-catalyzed phase I oxidative reactions. These multiple enzyme steps thus offer many possible metabolic routes, some of which ultimately produce active metabolites which are ultimate carcinogens through adduct formation with cellular macromolecules. Inclusion of bacterial enzymes in this consideration further increases the possibilities for metabolic activation and metabolism of initial substrates.

At this point in time an examination and description of the expression and control of expression of the various cytochromes P-450 and other enzymes in colon is needed to assess the differences in these parameters in young and old individuals, in normal individuals and in those with conditions which predispose to colon cancer (e.g., hereditary polyposis). We already know that expression of certain cytochromes P-450 such as P-450 form c (P-450lA1) increase markedly with aging in rats (Sun and Strobel 1986). It may be that changes associated with aging or disease states bring about alterations in the expression of some of the enzymic components of this system which eventuate in carcinogenesis or in at least an increased potential to activate precar-cinogens presented to the colon by diet or environment.

Acknowledgement. This work was supported by grant CA42995 from the National Cancer Institute DHHW and a grant from the W. S. Farish Foundation.

References

Ames BN, Lee FD, Durston WE (1973) An improved bacteria test system for the detection and classification of mutagenesis and carcinogens. Proc Natl Acad Sci USA 70: 782–786

Autrup H, Harris CC, Stoner GD, Jesudason ML, Trump B (1977) Binding of chemical carcinogens to cultured human colon. J Natl Cancer Inst 59: 351–354

Brodie BB, Gillette JR, LaDu BN (1958) Enzymatic metabolism of drugs and other foreign compounds. Rev Biochem 27: 427–454

Dignam JD, Strobel HW (1975) Preparation of homogeneous NADPH-cytochrome P-450 reductase from rat liver. Biochem Biophys Res Commun 63: 845–852

Druckrey H (1970) Production of colonic carcinomas by 1,2-dialkylhydrazines and azoxy-alkanes. In: Burdette WJ (ed) Carcinoma of the colon and antecedent epithelium. Thomas, Springfield IL, pp 267–279

Fang WF, Strobel HW (1978a) Activation of carcinogens and mutagens by rat colonic mucosa. Cancer Res 38: 2939–2944

Fang WF, Strobel HW (1978b) The drug and carcinogen metabolism system of rat colon microsomes. Arch Biochem Biophys 186: 128–138

Fang WF, Strobel HW (1982) Effects of cyclophosphamide and polycyclic aromatic hydrocarbons on cell growth and mixed function oxidase activity in a human colon tumor cell line. Cancer Res 42: 3676–3681

Fiala ES (1977) Investigations into the metabolism and mode of action of the colon carcinogens 1,2-dimethylhydrazine and azoxymethane. Cancer 40: 2436–2445

Fiala ES, Sohn OS, Hamilton SR (1987) Effects of chronic dietary ethanol on in vivo and in vitro metabolism of methylazoxymethanol and on methylazoxymethanol-induced DNA methylation in rat colon and liver. Cancer Res 47: 5939–5943

Gillette JR (1966) Biochemistry of drug oxidation and reduction by enzymes in hepatic endoplasmic reticulum. Adv Pharmacol 4: 219–261

Guengerich FP (1979) Isolation and purification of cytochrome P-450, and the existence of multiple forms. Pharmacol Ther 6: 99–121

Gum JR, Strobel HW (1979) Purified NADPH-cytochrome P-450 reductase: interaction with hepatic microsomes and phospholipid vesicles. J Biol Chem 254: 4177–4185

Kaku M, Kusunose E, Yamamoto S, Ichihara K, Kusunose M (1985) Multiple form of cytochrome P-450 in rabbit colon microsomes. J Biochem (Tokyo) 97: 663–670

Lu AYH, West SB (1978) Reconstituted mammalian mixed function oxidases: requirements, specificities and other properties. Pharmacol Ther 2: 337–358

Lu AYH, Junk KW, Coon MJ (1969) Resolution of the cytochrome P-450 containing ω-hydroxylation system of liver microsomes into three components. J Biol Chem 244: 3714–3721

Nebert DW, Gonzales FJ (1987) P-450 genes: structure, evolution and regulation. Annu Rev Biochem 56: 945–993

Nelson DR, Strobel HW (1987) Evolution of cytochrome P-450 proteins. Mol Biol Evol 4: 572–593

Newaz SN, Fang WF, Strobel HW (1983) Metabolism of the carcinogen 1,2-dimethylhydrazine by isolated human colon microsomes and human colon tumor cells in culture. Cancer 52: 794–798

Oravec CT, Jones CA, Huberman E (1986) Activation of the colon carcinogen, 1,2-dimethylhydrazine in a rat colon cell-mediated mutagenesis assay. Cancer Res 46: 5068–5071

Peterson JA, Prough RA (1986) Cytochrome P-450 reductase and cytochrome b_5 in cytochrome P-450 catalysis. In: Ortiz de Montellano, PR (ed) Cytochrome P-450: structure, mechanism and biochemistry. Plenum, New York, pp 89–117

Strobel HW, Newaz SN, Fang WF, Lau PP, Oshinsky RJ, Stralka DJ, Salley FF (1983) Evidence for the presence and multiple forms of cytochrome P-450 in colonic microsomes from rats and humans. In: Rydström J, Montelius J, Bengtsson M (eds) Extrahepatic drug metabolism and chemical carcinogenesis. Elsevier Science, Amsterdam, pp 57–66

Strobel HW, Fang WF, Takazawa RS, Stralka DJ, Newaz SN, Kurzban GP, Nelson DR, Beyer RS (1986) Cytochromes P-450 and the activation and inactivation of mutagens and carcinogens. In: Shankel DM, Hartman PE, Kada T, Hollaender A (eds) Antimutagenesis and anticarcinogenesis mechanisms. Plenum, New York, pp 61–71

Sun J, Strobel HW (1986) Aging affects the drug metabolism systems of rat liver, kidney, colon and lung in a differential fashion. Exp Gerontol 21: 523–534

Weisburger JH (1971) Colon carcinogens: their metabolism and mode of action. Cancer 28: 60–70

Weisburger JH (1973) Chemical carcinogens and their mode of action in colonic neoplasia. Dis Colon Rectum 16: 431–437

Yasukochi Y, Masters BSS (1976) Some properties of a detergent-solubilized NADPH-cytochrome c reductase purified by biospecific affinity chromatography. J Biol Chem 251: 5337–5344

Mucosal Cellular Regeneration and Colorectal Carcinogenesis

U. A. Simanowski [1], N. A. Wright [2] and H. K. Seitz [1]

[1] Department of Medicine, University of Heidelberg, Bergheimerstr. 58, D-6900 Heidelberg, FRG
[2] Department of Histopathology, Hammersmith Hospital, Royal Postgraduate Medical School, Du Cane Road, London W12 0HS, UK

Contents

Introduction

Altered cellular regeneration is the prominent feature that distinguishes cancer from normal tissue. Therefore it is of paramount importance to understand cell regeneration and its regulation in normal colonic mucosa during carcinogenesis and in carcinomas if we want to design and evaluate new therapeutic measures. Cell proliferation and its measurement has been the domaine of histology. However, recent years have seen increasing attempts to link molecular biology to cell cycle events and regulation of cell proliferation, which will be dealt with elsewhere.

Cell proliferation in the normal colon is located at the bases of colonic crypts, the putative stem cell compartment comprising the lowermost crypt cell positions (Fig. 1). From here the crypt cells migrate upwards towards the lumen of the colon, whereby proliferative indices decrease and cells differentiate into resorptive and goblet cells (Fig. 1). Much of our knowledge of colonic mucosal cell proliferation during carcinogenesis comes from the use of murine experimental models, the most applied of which is the 1,2-dimethylhydrazine (DMH) model.

Target Cells of Carcinogenesis

Gut epithelia are rapidly renewing cell populations with short transit times of the colonic crypt cells. In the mouse colon the reported transit times range from 32 to 233 h (Wright and Alison 1984) before cells are lost to the intestinal lumen. This relatively short time during which intestinal cells can be exposed to carcinogens contrasts sharply with the long induction periods of approximately 6 months in experimental carcinogenesis. It is largely because of this that a stem cell compartment

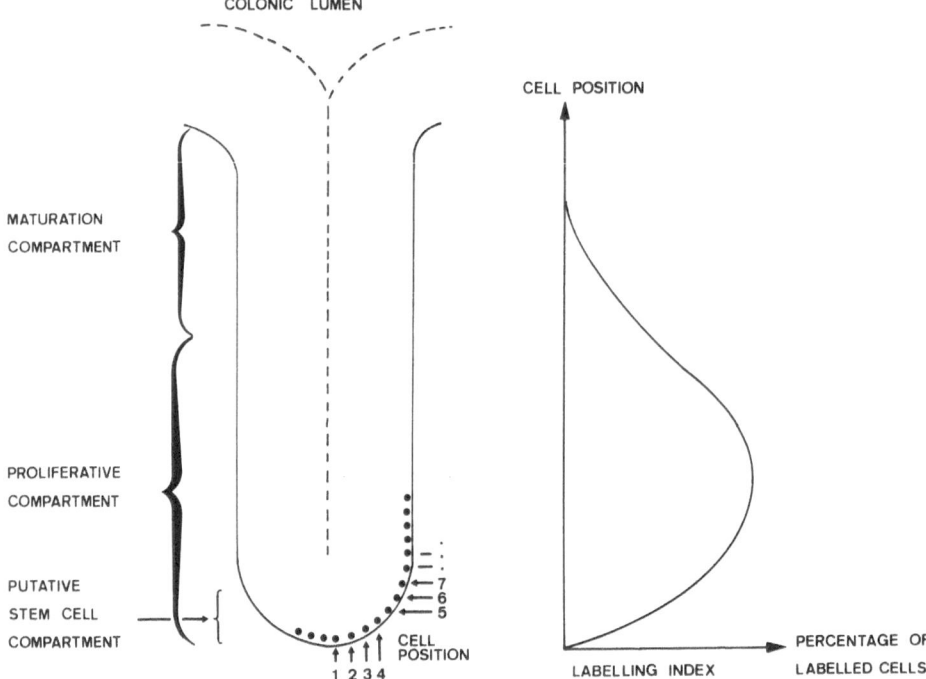

Fig. 1. Schematic presentation of a colonic mucosal crypt, defining crypt cell positions. The graph on the *right* shows the crypt cell position-related labelling index

in intestinal crypts is hypothesized. There are many different connotations of these putative stem cells, and no consistent definition of intestinal stem cells or experimental isolation or labelling has yet been achieved. However, there are some basic assumptions to make the stem cell hypothesis work, and there is a large body of indirect experimental evidence indicating their properties:

– They may be clonogenic (Withers 1967a, b; Withers and Elkind 1969).
– There are two subpopulations, i.e., functional and potential stem cells (Cairnie 1976; Steel 1977).
– They are slowly cycling (Wright 1978).
– They are pluripotent (Cheng and Leblond 1974).
– They are radiosensitive (Potten 1977).
– They possess mechanisms for protecting their genome (Potten et al. 1978).

For a detailed discussion of stem cell characteristics and their role in carcinogenesis see Wright and Alison (1984), Zajicek (1984), Bykorez and Ivashcheno (1984), and Potten and Hendry (1983).

Acute Effects of Carcinogens

The initial reaction of the gut mucosa to carcinogen treatment is an inhibition of DNA synthesis. Most observations apply equally to the small intestinal and the colonic mucosa. Methylazoxymethanol (MAM) produces a marked reduction in both DNA and RNA synthesis which is evident within 1 h, but maximal over the initial 24 h after treatment (Zedeck et al. 1970; Lohrs et al. 1969), and in some cases, lasting as long as 48 h in the mouse (Deschner 1978). Histological examination shows that there is prominent necrosis of crypt cells in both large and small intestinal mucosa, extensive within 6 h of treatment, and recovering over the next 24 h (Zedeck et al. 1970). Sunter (1980, 1981) has described an essentially similar sequence of microscopic and cell-proliferative changes in the intestinal crypts of rats treated with DMH. The damage appears localized to that region of the crypt where actively proliferating cells are found. Zedeck et al. (1977) have suggested that the severity and distribution of acute mucosal changes parallels the distribution pattern of the neoplasms which arise if treatment with the carcinogen is continued, and Sunter (1981) has also concurred that the cytotoxic effects are most marked in the distal colon where most tumors appeared to arise. Within 24 h of DMH injection, mouse colonic crypt cells show widespread necrosis (Deschner 1978); crypts become reduced in size, and some cells appear atypical, with multinucleate forms and abnormal mitoses. Chromosomal and nuclear aberrations like gaps, breaks, exchanges, additional micronuclei, disintegration of nuclei, and mitochondrial injury can be observed (Muratani et al. 1985; Wargovich et al. 1983; Pan et al. 1985). There is thus little doubt that carcinogens produce a prominent necrogenic effect on proliferative gastrointestinal cells in the early period.

In human colonic mucosa, maintained in organ culture, several carcinogens inhibit or stimulate DNA synthesis, but in the doses used do not induce toxic changes either in tissue taken from cancerous or noncancerous colons (Mak et al. 1979; Mikol and Lipkin 1984).

Not unreasonably, there follows a prominent and presumably compensatory proliferative response, both in mice (Deschner 1978) and in rats (Sunter 1981), with elevation of both labelling and mitotic indices at 36–48 h, resulting in crypt hyperplasia at about 4 days after treatment. During this hyperplastic period there is an evident increase in the crypt growth fraction in both species, indicated by changes in the distribution of labelled cells in the crypt, with DNA-synthesizing cells high in the crypt (Deschner 1978; Sunter 1981). This early response is, however, relatively rapidly curtailed, and by about 7 days after treatment, both morphology and kinetic state appear normal again.

Later Response to Carcinogen Treatment; the Phase of Promotion?

Chronic treatment with suitable carcinogens leads to a variety of hyperplastic changes in colonic as well as other gastrointestinal epithelia (Altmann and Snow 1984), i.e., a generalized mucosal change occurs, and it is widely considered that the dysplastic changes which eventually lead to invasive carcinoma result, in some way, from the hyperplastic mucosa. There may be, however, a tendency for dysplastic foci as well as early mucosal damage to develop preferably in mucosa overlaying lymphoid plaques (Shimamoto and Vollmer 1987; Wargovich et al. 1983). In most studies there is a latent phase before hyperplasia occurs (Chang 1978), but in mice, Richards (1977) and Thurnherr et al. (1973) have described hyperplastic changes as early as 14 and 38 days of treatment, respectively; this becomes severe and widespread at about 100 days of continued carcinogen treatment, and dysplastic changes ensue soon after. Although most workers in the mouse DMH colonic cancer model are in agreement about the sequence of events during this stage, in the rat disparate reports are evident; Pozharisski (1975) and Pozharisski et al. (1982) noted a generalised expansion of the proliferative compartment without changes in the crypt length, although the advisability of three-dimensional studies is emphasised by the finding that the crypt circumference ("the column count") is increased, thus ensuring an increase of the crypt population (Tutton and Barkla 1976; Sunter et al. 1981). Weibecke et al. (1973) considered that the hyperplasia was localised towards the tips of the mucosal folds, and it was in these areas of hyperplasia that the earliest atypical changes occurred. Other studies (Maskens 1976; Sunter 1981), however, indicate that, as in the mouse, there is a progressive hyperplasia, increasing with the duration of carcinogen treatment. Most studies concur that the chronic DMH model, in both rats and mice, is associated with a diffuse crypt hyperplasia in both small and large intestines.

The changes of intracrypt cell kinetics during this phase are interesting. Although the pattern of differentiation (i.e., into vacuolated columnar, mucous, and endocrine cells) does not seem to be perturbed, these expanded hyperplastic crypts are hyperproliferative with increased labelling indices (Chang 1978, 1980; Deschner 1974, 1978; Barthold and Jonas 1977). There are, however, conflicting results: Haase et al. (1973) could not demonstrate a generalised increase in proliferative rate, and in Richards' (1977) study labelling indices remained elevated for the first 16 weeks of treatment only, falling to control values at 26 weeks. The increased labelling index is generally associated with an expansion in the proliferative compartment, produced by an upward movement of the cut-off position towards the intestinal lumen, although the shape of the distribution did follow the normal pattern in these hyperplastic crypts (Sunter 1980, 1981; Pozharisski 1975; Pozharisski et al. 1982; Weibecke et al. 1973). The labelling indices at lower crypt cell positions, however, remain the same or are even reduced (Thurnherr et al. 1973). Because of the increased crypt size, the upward expansion of the proliferative compartment is not necessarily associated with an increase in the growth fraction of these hyperplastic crypts. It may actually be reduced, and the absolute numbers of proliferating cells per crypt is either unchanged or little increased (Maskens 1976). Nevertheless, the net effect of the several kinetic changes is an increase in the cell production rate (Sunter 1981).

Analysis of the cell cycle in hyperplastic crypts during colonic carcinogenesis has given incongruous results: in the mouse there is no apparent decrease in cell cycle duration or of its component phases (for a detailed review of these data see Wright and Alison 1984, pp 812ff). In the rat colon, during chronic DMH administration, crypt cells showed a general decrease in cell cycle times, although the kinetic behaviour of small intestinal crypt cells was unchanged (Sunter 1981). The decrease of cell cycle times was most marked in the descending colon, with no change at all in the caecum. The reduction of mitotic indices in these crypts coupled with an increased cumulated birth rate indicates that chronic DMH treatment results in a profound reduction of the duration of mitosis (Sunter et al. 1981). The claim of Tutton and Barkla (1976) that the normally small basal zone of slowly cycling cells was expanded in DMH-treated rat colon, based on metaphase-arrest experiments, would not appear to be substantiated in either rat small intestine or colon, by detailed cell positional FLM (fraction of labelled mitoses) studies (Sunter 1980, 1981).

Other changes, possibly related to the quantitative and/or qualitative carcinogen-induced alterations of mucosal cell proliferation include changes in mucin and sialo-mucin production and distribution and lymphocyte infiltration (James et al. 1983; Wargovich et al. 1983). Ultrastructurally enlarged nucleoli, reduced numbers of goblet cells and apical cytoplasmic vacuoles in the upper third of the crypts can be found (Pan et al. 1985).

We thus have evidence that chronic carcinogen treatment causes a large increase in population size, and that this increase is widespread in the target organ. It occurs at some time removed from the initial (compensatory?) proliferative response to acute cell death initiated by the first carcinogen injections and is continuous right up to and indeed past the appearance of the first neoplasms. Hyperplasia and kinetic changes are persistent even 4 months after cessation of carcinogen treatment, indicating a fixed (mutation-based?) alteration of the mucosa (Barthold 1981). Although we have no evidence that the changes seen are any different from those in non-carcinogen-associated hyperplasia, there are features which have been said to indicate carcinogen-specific hyperplasia: while it is conceivable that the change in the distribution of labelled cells might result from a specific failure to repress DNA synthesis and is caused by the carcinogen (Deschner 1974), it may be reasonable to propose that the distribution change is the end result of an adaptive process, with an early increase in growth fraction without crypt length changes, followed by a fall in the growth fraction but an increase in the number of proliferative cells, evoked by an increase in crypt population size, a kinetic situation resembling coeliac disease (Wright et al. 1973). Sunter (1980) considered that, since the birth rate (measured by metaphase arrest) in proliferative cell positions was decreased, whereas the cell cycle time tended to remain unchanged, the decrease in the crypt growth fraction was associated with a reduction in the growth fraction *within the proliferative compartment itself*, resulting in the situation that normally proliferative cell positions contain nonproliferating cells. This situation resembles the hypoproliferative mucosa in starvation (Al-Dewachi et al. 1975). This observation, coupled with the prolonged cell cycle time data of Chang et al. (1979) and the possible expansion of the slowly cycling basal cell compartment in rat colonic crypts (Tutton and Barkla 1976), possibly indicates the evolution of a more slowly cycling subpopulation of (transformed?) cells. On the other hand, there is distinct evidence, in the rat colon, that the progressive hyperplasia associated with prolonged DMH treatment produces an increase in the crypt cell production rate (Sunter 1980, 1981). We might try to explain both findings by proposing that out of a generalised hyperplasia evolves a slowly cycling transformed cell which gives rise to the resultant tumours, were it not for the fact that in the rat model, at least, the cells in the established tumours show prominent reductions in their cell cycle time (Sunter 1981; Maskens 1976; Schauer et al. 1971). We must conclude that the best data to date do indicate a sustained hyperplasia during carcinogenesis, with a progressive reduction in the cell cycle time until, with the evolution of frankly neoplastic cells, the cell cycle time is decreased enough to confer a definite carcinogenic advantage, at least in colon cells. There are suggestions that the transformed subpopulation might be more slowly cycling which, however, cannot yet be substantiated. The hyperplasia which occurs with carcinogen treatment probably cannot be distinguished from routine gut hyperplasias, apart from reports that labelled cells are found on the surface of the colon (Pozharisski et al. 1982) and that label-retaining cells appear (Nakamura et al. 1979), which would not be expected in non-neoplastic hyperplasia.

Effects of Mucosal Proliferative Status on Carcinogenesis

Following from this, if hyperplasia is considered important, what are the effects of hyperplasia itself upon tumorigenesis? Stimulation of cell regeneration generally enhances carcinogenesis. This was found to be true after ligature insertion in the rat caecum (Pozharisski 1975), after large bowel transection and reanastomosis (Roe et al. 1987), in *Citrobacter freundii*-infected mice (Barthold and Jonas 1977) and after cholic acid feeding (Cohen et al. 1980). The work of Williamson (1979) and Williamson and Malt (1980) has approached the concept of hyperplasia and carcinogenesis in the DMH/azoxymethane rat model on a systematic basis. It appeared that the compensatory responses to manoeuvres such as small bowel resection were accompanied by hyperplastic changes in the colon. Resected animals showed an increase in the prevalence of colonic tumors on DMH treatment. It thus appears that the initial proliferative status of the colonic mucosa is an important parameter in carcinogenesis in the colon. This seems to be a general principle of intestinal carcinogenesis in experimental models as well as in the human intestine. Hyperproliferation linked with an increased cancer risk are found in the human small bowel in coeliac disease (Wright et al. 1973; Swinson et al. 1983), and in the human colon in a variety of conditions: ulcerative colitis (Bleiberg et al. 1970; Collins et al.1987), familial polyposis syndromes, Peutz-Jeghers syndrome, juvenile polyposis and familial colon cancer without polyposis (Lipkin 1981, 1984). Lipkin (1984) reported an extended proliferative compartment in those conditions, with labelled cells displaced towards the colonic lumen, and utilised this feature to identify high-risk populations. Subsequently it was demonstrated that this proliferative pattern was present in animals particularly susceptible to chemical carcinogenesis (Deschner et al. 1983, 1984), and in the rectal mucosa of chronically ethanol-fed rats (Simanowski et al. 1986) where ethanol is cocarcinogenic (Seitz et al. 1984).

The cause of the association of hyperproliferation with tumorigenesis is naturally interesting; from first principles, if the carcinogenic event is a somatic mutation which is arguably proliferation dependent, then increasing the proliferative rate will increase the chances of a mutation. Pozharisski (1975) speculated that induced hyperplasia could act by "an increased entry of stem cells into the cell cycle". Although Pozharisski evidently assumed that all proliferating enterocytes were stem cells and did not demonstrate that there was an increased proliferative rate in the presumptive stem cell zone (i.e, the crypt base), this hypothesis would of course be consistent with the concept that functional stem cells need periods of G_0 to effect genetic housekeeping, without which irreparable damage to stem cell DNA (which may possess an immortal DNA strand) may occur (Cairns 1975; Potten et al. 1978).

There are other instances where this association between stimulated mucosal proliferation and enhanced carcinogenesis holds as well: after colostomy closure in the distal colon (Terpstra et al. 1981), following jejunoileal bypass surgery (Bristol et al.

1982), in the vicinity of colonic suture lines (Williamson et al. 1982; Barkla and Tutton 1983), after bile acid application (Cohen et al. 1980; Deschner et al. 1981; Rainey et al. 1986), in increased faecal bulk due to dietary fibre (Jacobs 1983, 1984; Jacobs and Lupton 1986; Goodlad et al. 1987) and after abdominal irradiation (Sharp et al. 1985; Sandler and Sandler 1985). These instances represent mucosal states where proliferation is increased because of functional demand and/or compensatory due to injury-related cell death. This must be distinguished from increased mucosal proliferation due to changes in cell cycle regulation either in normal tissue or as part of malignant transformation. At this point it becomes crucial, although extremely difficult, to decide what the causes of the stimulation of cell proliferation are and what is merely expression of the subsequent, regulatory mechanisms. Epidermal growth factor may be involved on either side (Schattenkerk et al. 1981; Malt et al. 1987; Kingsnorth et al. 1985; Maley et al. 1986; Finney et al. 1987), as well as oncogenes (Weinberg 1985), growth hormone and/or somatomedins (Clemmons and van Wyk 1981; Ituarte et al. 1984), and other so-called growth factors (Baserga 1981).

Perhaps supporting the hypothesis that induced hyperproliferation leads to increased carcinogenesis are the observations that reductions in the proliferative rate lead to decreased incidences of tumours in most sites; there have been several studies in which animals with defunctioned bowel segments have been treated with colonic carcinogens (Cleveland et al. 1967; Wittig et al. 1971; Gennaro et al. 1973; Rubio 1980). Most of these studies have concluded that the reduced incidence was due to the lack of the carcinogen or promoter in the faecal stream, but since defunctioning does lead to hypoplasia and atrophy, an alternative explanation could be the reduced proliferative rate, a view, which is substantiated by observations following total parenteral nutrition and DMH treatment (Heitman et al. 1983).

Inhibition of proliferation may therefore be one important principle of tumour protection. Candidates for this approach are retinoids (Jetten 1984; Sporn and Roberts 1983), calcium (Bird et al. 1986; Appleton et al. 1987; Lipkin and Newmark 1985), guar gum (Jacobs 1987), selenium (Rampal et al. 1986), ornithine decarboxylase inhibitors (Kingsnorth et al. 1982; Luk and Yang 1987; Hosomi et al. 1987), plant sterols (Deschner et al. 1982a, b) and antioxidants (Deschner and Wattenberg 1982); the effect of the latter, however, may well be transmitted via its potential to inhibit colonic alcohol dehydrogenase, thus leading to reduced acetaldehyde-dependent mucosal damage (Seitz et al. 1987). Some of these factors may be involved in the tumour protection or rather diminished tumour promotion attributable to a "healthy" fibre-rich diet, since faecal bulk itself can stimulate mucosal proliferation and tumour development (see above).

On the other hand, reduced cellular proliferation may, however, reflect different underlying mechanisms: bile acids, generally implicated in tumour promotion, have not invariably been demonstrated to increase proliferation; there have been reports of unchanged or decreased proliferative activity following administration of cocarcinogenic bile acids (Weidema et al. 1985; Simanowski et al. 1987). Because of possible interaction of the tumour promoter with nucleic acids and consequent hinderance of the normal cell cycle, reduced proliferation may in these instances indicate tumour promotion instead of protection (Suzuki and Bruce 1986; Galloway et al. 1987). We cannot just measure changes in cell proliferation, we must search for the underlying mechanism.

References

Al-Dewachi HS, Wright NA, Appleton DR, Watson AJ (1975) The effect of starvation and refeeding on cell population kinetics in the rat small bowel mucosa. J Anat 119:105–116

Altmann GG, Snow AD (1984) Effects of 1,2-dimethylhydrazine on the number of epithelial cells present in the villi, crypts, and mitotic pool along the rat small intestine. Cancer Res 44:5522–5531

Appleton GV, Davies PW, Bristol JB, Williamson RCN (1987) Intraluminal calcium decreases colonic tumor yield and crypt cell production rates in the adapting colonic epithelium. Proc Annu Meet Am Assoc Cancer Res 28:135

Barkla DH, Tutton PM (1983) The influence of surgical transection and anastomosis on the rate of cell proliferation in the colonic epithelium of normal and DMH-treated rats. Carcinogenesis 4:1323–1325

Barthold SW (1981) Relationship of colonic mucosal background to neoplastic proliferative activity in dimethylhydrazine-treated mice. Cancer Res 41:2616–2620

Barthold SW, Jonas AM (1977) Morphogenesis of early 1,2-dimethylhydrazine-induced lesions and latent period of colon carcinogenesis in mice by a variant of *Citrobacter freundii*. Cancer Res 37:4352–4360

Baserga R (ed) (1981) Tissue growth factors. Springer, Berlin Heidelberg New York

Bird RP, Schneider R, Stamp D, Bruce WR (1986) Effect of dietary calcium and cholic acid on the proliferative indices of murine colonic epithelium. Carcinogenesis 7:1657–1661

Bleiberg H, Mainguet P, Galant P, Chretien J, Dupont-Marisse N (1970) Cell renewal in the human rectum; in vitro autoradiographic study on active ulcerative colitis. Gastroenterology 58:851–855

Bristol J, Wells M, Williamson RCN (1982) Jejunoileal bypass stimulates cell proliferation and enhances experimental carcinogenesis in rat large bowel. Proc Am Assoc Cancer Res 23:233

Bykorez AI, Ivashchenko YD (1984) Gastrointestinal stem cells and their role in carcinogenesis. Int Rev Cytol 90:309–373

Cairnie AB (1976) Homeostasis in the small intestine. In: Cairnie AB, Lala PK, Osmond DG (eds) Stem cells of renewing cell populations. Academic, New York, pp 67–78

Cairns J (1975) Mutation selection and the natural history of cancer. Nature 225:197–200

Chang WWL (1978) Histogenesis of symmetrical 1,2-dimethylhydrazine-induced neoplasms of the colon in the mouse. JNCI 60:1415–1418

Chang WWL (1980) Pathogenesis and biological behaviour of 1,2-dimethylhydrazine-induced colonic neoplasms in the mouse. In: Appleton DR, Sunter JP, Watson AJ (eds) Cell proliferation in the gastrointestinal tract. Pitman Medical, London, pp 273–297

Chang WWL, Mack KM, MacDonald PDM (1979) Cell population kinetics of 1,2-dimethylhydrazine-induced colonic neoplasms and their adjacent colonic mucosa in the mouse. Virchows Arch [B] 30:149–161

Cheng H, Leblond CP (1974) Origin, differentiation and renewal of the four main epithelial cell types in the mouse small intestine. V. Unitarian theory of the origin of the four epithelial cell types. Am J Anat 141:537–562

Clemmons DR, van Wyk JJ (1981) Somatomedin: physiological control and effects on cell proliferation. In: Baserga R (ed) Tissue growth factors. Springer, Berlin Heidelberg New York, pp 161–208

Cleveland JC, Litvak SF, Cole JW (1967) Identification of the route of action of the carcinogen 3,2-dimethyl-aminobiphenyl in the induction of intestinal metaplasia. Cancer Res 27:708–712

Cohen BI, Raicht RF, Deschner EE, Takahashi M, Sarwal AN, Fazzini E (1980) Effect of cholic acid feeding on N-methyl-N-nitrosourea-induced colon tumors and cell kinetics in rats. JNCI 64:573–578

Collins RH, Feldman M, Fordtran JS (1987) Colon cancer, dysplasia, and surveillance in patients with ulcerative colitis; a critical review. N Engl J Med 316:1654–1658

Deschner EE (1974) Experimentally induced cancer of the colon. Cancer 34:824–828

Deschner EE (1978) Early proliferative effects induced by six weekly injections of 1,2-dimethylhydrazine in epithelial cells of mouse distal colon. Z Krebsforsch 91:205–216

Deschner EE, Wattenberg LW (1982) The proliferative effect of dietary butylated hydroxy-anisole on methylazoxymethanol treated colonic mucosa. Cancer Lett 16:197–202

Deschner EE, Cohen BI, Raicht RF (1981) Acute and chronic effect of dietary cholic acid on colonic epithelial cell proliferation. Digestion 21:290–296

Deschner EE, Cohen BI, Raicht RF (1982a) The kinetics of the protective effect of beta-sitosterol against MNU-induced colonic neoplasia. J Cancer Res Clin Oncol 103:49–54

Deschner EE, Cohen BI, Raicht RF (1982b) The acute effect of beta-sitosterol on colonic epithelial cell proliferation: implications for MNU-induced neoplasia. Cell Tissue Kinet 15:102

Deschner EE, Long FC, Hakissian M, Herrmann SL (1983) Differential susceptibility of AKR, C57BL/6J, and CF1 mice to 1,2-dimethylhydrazine-induced colonic tumor formation predicted by proliferative characteristics of colonic epithelial cells. JNCI 70:279–282

Deschner EE, Long FC, Hakissian M, Cupo SH (1984) Differential susceptibility of inbred mouse strains forecast by acute colonic proliferative response to methylazoxymethanol. JNCI 72:195–198

Finney KJ, Ince P, Appleton DR, Sunter JP, Watson AJ (1987) A trophic effect of epidermal growth factor (EGF) on rat colonic mucosa in organ culture. Cell Tissue Kinet 20:43–56

Galloway DJ, Jarrett F, Boyle P, Indran M, Carr K, Owen RW, George WD (1987) Morphological and cell kinetic effect of dietary manipulation during colorectal carcinogenesis. Gut 28:754–763

Gennaro AR, Villaneauva R, Sukon-Haman Y, Vathanphas V, Rosemond GP (1973) Chemical carcinogenesis in transposed intestinal segments. Cancer Res 33:536–541

Goodlad RA, Lenton W, Ghatei MA, Adrian TE, Bloom SR, Wright NA (1987) Proliferative effect of "fibre" on the intestinal epithelium: relationship to gastrin, enteroglucagon and PYY. Gut 28:221–226

Haase P, Cowen DM, Knowles E, Cooper EH (1973) Evaluation of dimethylhydrazine-induced tumours in mice as a model system for colorectal cancer. Br J Cancer 28:530–543

Heitmann DW, Grubbs BG, Heitmann TO, Cameron IL (1983) Effects of 1,2-dimethyl-hydrazine treatment and feeding regimen on rat colonic epithelial cell proliferation. Cancer Res 43:1153–1162

Hosomi M, Lirussi F, Stace NH, Vaja S, Murphy GM, Dowling RH (1987) Mucosal polyamine profile in normal and adapting (hypo- and hyperplastic) intestine: effects of DFMO treatment. Gut 28:103–107

Ituarte EA, Petrini J, Hershman JM (1984) Acromegaly and colon cancer. Ann Intern Med 101:627–628

Jacobs LR (1983) Enhancement of rat colon carcinogenesis by wheat bran consumption during the stage of 1,2-dimethylhydrazine administration. Cancer Res 43:4057–4061

Jacobs LR (1984) Stimulation of rat colonic crypt cell proliferative activity by wheat bran consumption during the stage of 1,2-dimethylhydrazine administration. Cancer Res 44:2458–2463

Jacobs LR (1987) Inhibition of duodenal carcinogenesis and crypt cell proliferation in rats fed guar gum. Fed Proc 46:585

Jacobs LR, Lupton JR (1986) Relationship between colonic luminal pH, cell proliferation, and colon carcinogenesis in 1,2-dimethylhydrazine treated rats fed high fiber diets. Cancer Res 46:1727–1734

James JT, Shamsuddin AM, Trump BF (1983) Comparative study of the morphologic, histochemical, and proliferative changes induced in the large intestine of ICR/Ha and C57BL/Ha mice by 1,2-dimethylhydrazine. JNCI 71:955–964

Jetten AM (1984) Modulation of cell growth by retinoids and their possible mechanisms of action. Fed Proc 43:134–139

Kingsnorth AN, King WW, MacCann PP, Diekema K, Ross JS, Malt RA (1982) Difluorome-thylornithine (DFMO) diminishes 1,2-dimethylhydrazine-induced colonic carcinogenesis in mice. Gastroenterology 82:1100

Kingsnorth AN, Abu-Khalaf M, Ross JS, Malt RA (1985) Potentiation of 1,2-dimethyl-hydrazine-induced anal carcinoma by epidermal growth factor in mice. Surgery 97:696–700

Lipkin M (1981) Early identification of population groups at high risk for gastrointestinal cancer. In: Malt RA, Williamson RCN (eds) Colonic carcinogenesis. MTP Press, Lancaster, pp 31–46

Lipkin M (1984) Method for binary classification and risk assessment of individuals with familial polyposis based on ³H-TdR labelling of epithelial cells in colonic crypts. Cell Tissue Kinet 17:209–222

Lipkin M, Newmark H (1985) Effect of added dietary calcium on colonic epithelial cell proliferation in subjects at high risk for familial colonic cancer. N Engl J Med 313:1381–1384

Lohrs U, Weibecke B, Eder M (1969) Morphologische und autoradiographische Untersuchung der Darmschleimhautveränderungen nach einmaliger Injektion von 1,2-Dimethylhydrazin. Z Gesamte Exp Med 151:297–307

Luk GD, Yang P (1987) Polyamines in intestinal and pancreatic adaptation. Gut 28:95–101

Mak KM, Slater GI, Hoff MB (1979) Inhibition of DNA synthesis by carcinogens in human colon mucosa in organ culture. JNCI 63:1305–1312

Maley MAL, Agrez MV, House AK (1986) Growth factor-induced proliferative responses of human and DMH-induced rat colorectal tumour cell lines. Aust J Exp Biol Med Sci 64:445–451

Malt RA, Chester JF, Gaissert HA, Ross JS (1987) Augmentation of chemically induced pancreatic and bronchial cancers by epidermal growth factor. Gut 28:249–251

Maskens AP (1976) Histogenesis and growth pattern of 1,2-dimethylhydrazine induced rat colon adenocarcinoma. Cancer Res 36:1585–1592

Muratani A, Shiraishi N, Maeda S, Ueda N, Saito Y, Sugiyama T (1985) Chromosome aberrations in epithelial cells of the digestive tract of rats induced by 1-methyl-3-nitro-1-nitroso-guanidine. Cancer Genet Cytogenet 14:37–44

Mikol YB, Lipkin M (1984) Effects of carcinogens on indices of cell proliferation in human colonic epithelial cells. Proc Annu Meet Am Assoc Cancer Res 25:78

Nakamura S, Kino I, Naito Y (1979) Cell renewal of the colonic mucosa of ICR mice with N,N-dimethylhydrazine dihydrochloride (DMH) treatment. Meeting abstract. Proceedings of the 38th annual meeting of the Japanese Cancer Association, Tokyo, September, p 321

Pan Q, Hamilton SR, Hyland J, Boitnott JK (1985) Effects of carcinogen dosage on experimental colonic carcinogenesis by azoxymethane: an ultrastructural study of grossly normal colonic mucosa. JNCI 74:689–698

Potten CS (1977) Extreme sensitivity of some intestinal crypt cells to X and gamma irradiation. Nature 269:518–521

Potten CS, Hendry JH (1983) Stem cells in murine small intestine. In: Potten CS (ed) Stem cells, their identification and characterisation. Churchill Livingstone, Edinburgh, pp 155–199

Potten CS, Hume WJ, Reid P, Cairns J (1978) The segregation of DNA in epithelial stem cells. Cell 15:899–906

Pozharisski KM (1975) Morphology and morphogenesis of experimental epithelial tumours of the intestine. JNCI 54:1115–1135

Pozharisski KM, Klimashevski VF, Gushchin VA (1982) Study of kinetics of epithelial cell populations in normal tissues of the rat's intestines and in carcinogenesis. II. Changes in kinetics of enterocyte populations in the course of experimental intestinal tumour induction in rats. Exp Pathol 21:165–179

Rainey JB, Maeda M, Williamson RCN (1986) The tropic effect of intrarectal deoxycholate on rate colorectum is unaffected by oral metronidazole. Cell Tissue Kinet 19:485–490

Rampal P, Nano JL, Veyres B, Rampal A, François E (1986) Prevention of chemically induced colon cancer by dietary selenium in rats. Dig Dis Sci (New Series) 31 (Suppl 10):247S

Richards TC (1977) Early changes in the dynamics of crypt cell populations in mouse colon following administration of 1,2-dimethylhydrazine. Cancer Res 37:1680–1685

Roe R, Fermor B, Williamson RCN (1987) Proliferative instability and experimental carcinogenesis at colonic anastomoses. Gut 28:808–815

Rubio CA (1980) Experimental colon cancer in the absence of intestinal contents in Sprague Dawley rats. JNCI 64:569–572

Sandler RS, Sandler DP (1983) Radiation-induced cancers of the colon and rectum: assessing the risk. Gastroenterology 84:51–57

Schattenkerk ME, DeVries JE, Li AK, Ford WD, Ross JS, Jeppsson BW, Jamieson CG, Malt RA (1981) Decreased dimethylhydrazine-induced colonic neoplasia after submandibular sialodenectomy in male mice. Proc Am Assoc Cancer Res 222:106

Schauer A, Kunze E, Boscler K (1971) Generationszeitzyklus von 1,2-Dimethylhydrazin-induzierten Adenokarzinomen des Rattenkolon. Naturwissenschaften 58:221–229

Seitz HK, Czygan P, Waldherr P, Veith S, Raedsch R, Käsmodel H, Kommerell B (1984) Enhancement of 1,2-dimethylhydrazine induced rectal carcinogenesis following chronic ethanol consumption in the rat. Gastroenterology 86:886–891

Seitz HK, Simanowski UA, Garzon FT, Peters TJ (1987) Letter to the editor. Hepatology 7:616

Sharp JG, Crouse DA, Jackson JD, Mann SL, Murphy BO (1985) Abdominal irradiation is a potent promoter of dimethylhydrazine induced colon tumors in rats. Proc Am Assoc Cancer Res 26:144

Shimamoto F, Vollmer E (1987) Changes in intestinal mucosa above lymph follicles during carcinogenesis in rats. A light and electron microscopic study. J Cancer Res Clin Oncol 113:41–50

Simanowski UA, Seitz HK, Baier B, Kommerell B, Schmidt-Gayk H, Wright NA (1986) Chronic ethanol consumption selectively stimulates rectal cell proliferation in the rat. Gut 27:278–282

Simanowski UA, Seitz HK, Czygan P, Hörner M, Waldherr R, Weber E, Kommerell B (1987) Chronic ursodeoxycholic acid- and chenodeoxycholic acid-feeding-induced changes of colon mucosal cell proliferation in rats. INCI 79:163–166

Sporn MB, Roberts AB (1983) Role of retinoids in differentiation and carcinogenesis. Cancer Res 43:3034–3040

Steel GG (1977) Growth kinetics in tumors. Oxford University Press, Oxford

Sunter JP (1980) Experimental carcinogenesis and cancer in the rodent gut. In: Appleton DR, Sunter JP, Watson AJ (eds) Cell proliferation in the gastrointestinal tract. Pitman Medical, London, pp 255–277

Sunter JP (1981) Cell proliferation studies on normal, carcinogenic-damaged and neoplastic intestinal epithelia. MD thesis, University of Newcastle upon Tyne, United Kingdom

Sunter JP, Watson AJ, Appleton DR (1981) Kinetics of the non-neoplastic mucosa of the large bowel of dimethylhydrazine-treated rats. Br J Cancer 44:35–44

Suzuki K, Bruce WB (1986) Increase by deoxycholic acid of the colonic nuclear damage induced by known carcinogens in C57BL/6J mice. JNCI 76:1129–1132

Swinson CM, Slavin G, Coles EC, Booth CC (1983) Coeliac disease and malignancy. Lancet I:111–115

Terpstra OT, Peterson Dahl P, Williamson RCN, Ross JS, Malt RA (1981) Colostomy closure promotes cell proliferation and dimethylhydrazine-induced carcinogenesis in rat distal colon. Gastroenterology 81:475–480

Thurnherr N, Deschner EE, Stonehill EH, Lipkin M (1973) Induction of adenocarcinomas of the colon in mice by weekly injections of 1,2-dimethylhydrazine. Cancer Res 33:940–945

Tutton PJM, Barkla DH (1976) Cell proliferation in the descending colon of dimethylhydrazine-treated rats and in dimethylhydrazine-induced adenocarcinomata. Virchows Arch [B] 21:147–160

Wargovich MJ, Medline A, Bruce WB (1983) Early histopathologic events to evolution of colon cancer in C57BL/6 and CF1 mice treated with 1,2-dimethylhydrazine. JNCI 71:125–131

Weibecke B, Krey U, Eder M (1973) Morphological and experimental investigations on experimental carcinogenesis and polyp development in the intestinal tract of rats and mice. Virchows Arch [A] 360:179–193

Weidema WF, Deschner EE, Cohen BI, DeCosse JJ (1985) Acute effects of dietary cholic acid and methylazoxymethanol acetate on colonic epithelial cell proliferation; metabolism of bile salts and neutral sterols in conventional and germfree SD rats. JNCI 74:665–670

Weinberg RA (1985) The action of oncogenes in the cytoplasm and nucleus. Science 230:770–776

Williamson RCN (1979) Hyperplasia and neoplasia of the intestinal tract. Ann R Coll Surg Engl 61:341–348

Williamson RCN, Malt RA (1980) Promotion of intestinal carcinogenesis by adaptive mucosal hyperplasia. In: Appleton DR, Sunter JP, Watson AJ (eds) Cell proliferation in the gastrointestinal tract. Pitman, London, pp 303–315

Williamson RCN, Davies PW, Bristol JB, Wells M (1982) Intestinal adaption and experimental carcinogenesis after partial colectomy; increased tumour yields are confined to the anastomosis. Gut 23:316–325

Withers HR (1967a) Recovery and repopulation in vivo by mouse skin epithelial cells during fractionated irradiation. Radiat Res 32:227–234

Withers HR (1967b) The effect of oxygen and anesthesia on radiosensitivity in vivo of epithelial cells of mouse skin. Br J Radiol 40:335–344

Withers HR, Elkind MM (1969) Radiosensitivity and fractionation response of crypt cells in mouse jejunum. Radiat Res 38:598–613

Withers HR, Elkind MM (1970) Microcolony survival assay for cells of mouse intestinal mucosa exposed to irradiation. Int J Radiat Biol 17:261–267

Wittig G, Wildner GP, Zeibarth D (1971) Der Einfluß der Ingesta auf die Kanzerisierung des Rattendarmes durch Dimethylhydrazin. Arch Geschwulstforsch 37:105–115

Wright NA (1978) The cell population kinetics of repopulating cells in the intestine. In: Lord BI, Potten CS, Cole RJ (eds) Stem cells and tissue homeostasis. Cambridge University Press, Cambridge, pp 335–358

Wright NA, Alison M (1984) The biology of epithelial cell populations. Clarendon, Oxford

Wright NA, Watson A, Morley A, Appleton D, Marks J (1973) Cell kinetics in flat avillous mucosa of the human small intestine. Gut 14:701–710

Zajicek G (1984) Neoplasia – a stem cell pathology. Med Hypotheses 13:125–136

Zedeck MS, Grab DJ, Sternberg SS (1977) Differences in the acute response of the various segments of the rat intestine to treatment with the intestinal carcinogen methyl-azoxymethanol. Cancer Res 37:32–36

Zedeck MS, Sternberg SS, Poynter RW, McGowan J (1970) Biochemical and pathological effects of methylazoxymethanol acetate, a potent carcinogen. Cancer Res 30:801–812

The Control of Cell Proliferation in Colonic Epithelium

N. A. Wright

Department of Histopathology, Royal Postgraduate Medical School, Hammersmith Hospital, London W12 0NN, UK

Contents

The colonic epithelium forms one of the great renewal systems of the mammalian body, together with the small intestine and stomach. There is considerable evidence that cell proliferation is ultimately concerned with the process of carcinogenesis (see Simanowski/Wright, this volume), and here we consider how cell production is organised and controlled in the colon.

Morphological Considerations

The basic organisation of crypt systems in the intestine is similar, and largely independent of site (Wright and Alison 1984). Cell production occurs in tubular crypts, themselves housed in a supporting matrix of connective tissue, the lamina propria. There is much current interest in epithelio-mesenchymal interactions in gut development and maintenance, and an intimate relationship exists between epithelial cells and the myofibroblasts which clothe, the crypt.

Within the crypts, there are several cell lineages to be considered: those of the mucus or goblet cell lineage are of considerable importance, secreting mucus in sufficient amounts to facilitate elimination of dehydrated faeces by lubrication of the mucosal surface. They appear in the lower portion of the crypt, and increase in number as the surface is approached. The mature goblet cell contains a large superficial theca, filled with mucus. The absorptive and secretory columnar cells, or colonocytes, are highly polarised cells, with packed apical microvilli and numerous mitochondria. Colonic endocrine cells, recognised by their numerous neurosecretory granules, are found predominantly towards the crypt base, are responsible for the production of a large number of peptide hormones and are thus important in the integrated function of the intestine. In animals such as mice, a vacuolated cell is seen which contains membrane-bound vacuoles and is found in the lower half of the crypt. These cells lose their vacuoles as they mature and give rise to typical columnar cells on the surface. Caveolated cells, with long microvilli and basal cytoplasmic processes, are also seen. Their function is as yet unknown.

The Organisation of Cell Production in the Colon

In common with gastrointestinal tissues, the colonic crypt is readily divided into proliferative and functional compartments, cells being born in the proliferative compartment and migrating into the functional compartment (Fig. 1). Between these two is a half-way house where cells are losing their proliferative capabilities and acquiring the characteristics of mature functional cells; this area of the crypt is usually termed the maturation compartment.

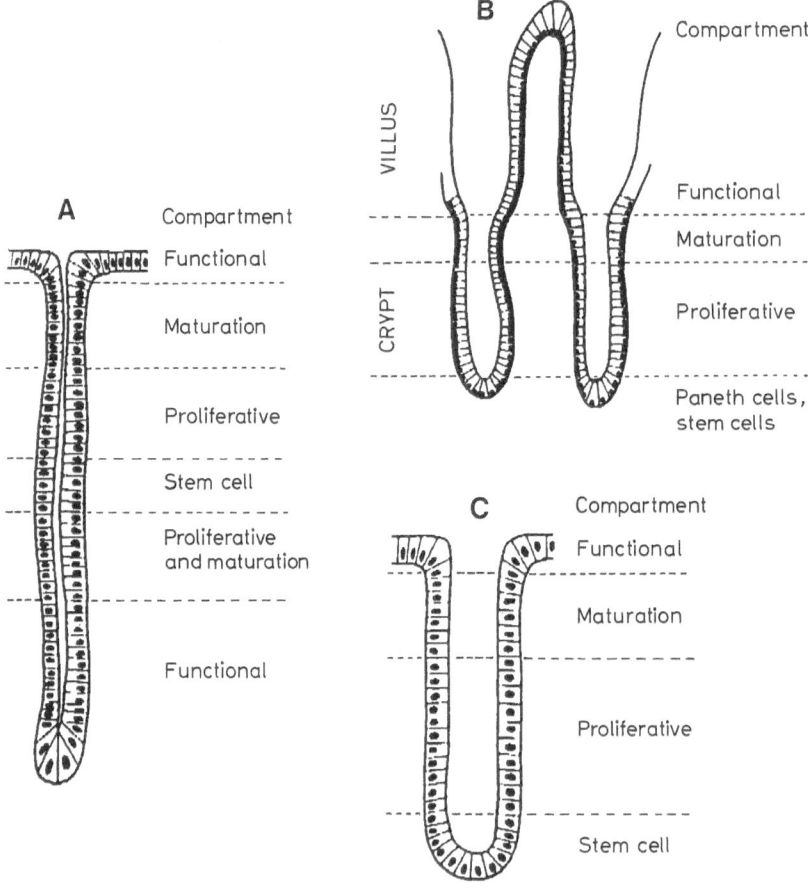

Fig. 1 A−C. The compartmental organisation of colonic crypts (C) resembles that of gastric glands (A) and small intestinal crypts (B). (From Wright and Alison 1984)

Colonic crypts are closed systems; there is no epithelial cell ingress from outside. Hence the origin of the cell flux is the base of the crypt. Current thought, based largely on morphological observations, places the important stem cells here, housed in a defined stem cell zone (Bjerknes and Cheng 1981) or stem cell compartment. All cell lineages are considered to originate in this zone, coming from a multipotential stem cell – the unitarian hypothesis of Chang and Leblond (1971a). Until recently, conclusive evidence for this was lacking, but Ponder et al. (1985) have shown that, ultimately at any rate, crypts are clonal in origin, i.e. derived from a single cell in development. Williams and Williams (1988) have also produced evidence that repopulation of crypts in adults is also the property of a single cell. Although these studies have not been definitive about the origin of endocrine cells from the putative single, multipotential stem cell, recent work by Kirkland (1988) has shown that single cells, cloned from a human colorectal carcinoma, give rise to all main colonic cell lineages, demonstrating the clonal origin of these cells. The factors which commit stem cell progeny to a particular line of differentiation are not presently known: however, the colonocytic cell lineage maintains proliferative capacity, giving rise to most of the proliferative activity seen in the colonic crypt. Mucous cells, once committed to differentiation, do retain some proliferative capability, but endocrine cells do not appear to proliferate after achieving recognisable endocrine habitus, and are fed exclusively from an undifferential basal crypt stem cell (Chang and Leblond 1971b).

Thus a picture emerges of a tubular crypt system which contains several cell lineages, each performing important functions, that are the clonal progeny of an undifferentiated basal crypt stem cell. The important conclusion for colonic carcinogenesis that emerges from this concept is that even if early neoplastic lesions are shown to be monotypic, as has proved to be the case using such markers as glucose-6-phosphate dehydrogenase haplotypes, or restriction fragment length polymorphisms (Fearon et al. 1987), it cannot be concluded that such neoplasms are monoclonal. Because of the clonal and therefore monotypic nature of individual crypts, all that can be said is that such tumours are monocryptal, thereby incriminating at least 600 cells in the process.

While there is a considerable amount of information about the rate of cell production in the colon of experimental animals, there are few data in the literature about such rates in humans. In the rat, colonocytic cells appear to divide about every 50 h, depending on site, and DNA synthesis takes about 9 h. The proliferative compartment occupies some 30% of the crypt, and about 7% of the crypt population is labelled by a single injection of tritiated thymidine. In man, indirect calculations indicate that colonocytes divide once every 70–90 h and DNA synthesis lasts between 10–15 h: about 15% of the crypt population is labelled with a flash exposure to tritiated thymidine.

Proliferative Responses in Colonic Epithelia

As we have seen, the initial response to carcinogens in the colon is the establishment of a new, hyperproliferative state, which appears mandatory for the carcinogenic process. The manner in which the colon mounts such a response is important: there is evidence that proliferative responses in the colonic crypts are mediated by changes in several of the mechanisms available for modulating changes in cell production. Thus the duration of the cell cycle is reduced after carcinogen treatment (Sunter et al. 1978) and in the recovery of the colonic mucosa after damage induced by ischaemia (Rijke et al. 1979 a). Reciprocally, a prolonged cell cycle has been shown to partially cause the hypoplasia which accompanies prolonged colonic bypass (Rijke et al. 1979 b). In the hyperplasia accompanying carcinogen treatment there is an increase in the size of the proliferative compartment (Wright and Alison 1984); interestingly enough, in mucosae at high risk of producing colorectal neoplasms there is an expansion of the proliferative compartment, demonstrated by the occurrence of flash-thymidine-labelled cells or mitoses further up the crypt than is usual (Weibecke et al. 1974; Lipkin 1974), an indication of the failure of these cells to repress DNA synthesis. An increase in the overall crypt population size is also a powerful mediator of an increased crypt cell production rate (Rijke 1980), while a reduction in crypt size promotes the hypoplasia of prolonged bypass (Rijke et al. 1979 b).

Control of Cell Proliferation in the Colon

We know of many experimental manipulations which will modulate the cell production rate in the colon, and administration of many exogenous agents which will similarly change colonic cell proliferation. However, it is also true to say that we do not know what controls colonic cell proliferation in physiological conditions, although there are several hypotheses, in which there are several discrete themes: attention was formerly focussed on negative feedback control of cell proliferation, by which loss of functional surface epithelium induces an increase in cell production rate in the crypts, which continues until the defective number of cells is made good. This implies that some transfer of information must occur between surface epithelial cells and the proliferative compartment, and suggestions of a tissue-specific chalone which selectively represses cell production have met with something less than enthusiasm. In any case, while the evidence for a negative feedback loop in the small intestine is strong (Wright and Al-Nafussi 1982), definitive evidence for its presence in the colon, correlating functional cell number with the number of proliferative cells and their rates of cell production (Wright and Alison 1984), is lacking.

There is general agreement that the presence of luminal contents is essential for maintenance of mucosal mass; starvation or bypass of the colon produces a reduction in colonic cell proliferation and mucosal epithelial cells which is reversed by refeeding or reversal of the bypass operation. There are perhaps two possible mechanisms which could account for such an observation:

1. The presence of luminal contents itself could stimulate cell production via the putative mechanisms of luminal nutrition and/or mucosal workload. Luminal nutrition is a concept usually reserved for the small intestine, and refers to the possibility that when luminal nutrients are absorbed, the mucosal epithelial cells are able to derive energy for cell division from these absorbed substances. The concept of tissue workload defining mass was strongly advocated by Goss (1964) and, in the microcosm of the intestine, has been interpreted as meaning that work expended in absorption or

secretion is somehow translated into a need for epithelial cell replacement. Where the small intestine is concerned, there is certainly a linear relationship between water absorption and crypt cell production rate in various growth situations (Goodlad et al. 1987a); but in the colon no such correlation has yet been mooted. Moreover, where the small bowel is concerned, Clarke (1975) could find no consistent evidence for either luminal nutrition or mucosal workload as a force motif for cell renewal.

However, it has been known for some time that the products of fermentation can be utilised by gut epithelial cells as nutrients (Sakata et al. 1980), and it is well known that hindgut fermentation occurs in both animals and man. A major component of the fermentation process are the short-chain fatty acids, such as butyrate. Recent experiments by Goodlad and colleagues (Goodlad et al. 1987b) have produced evidence that hindgut fermentation and cell production are closely correlated: a selection of fibres were shown to stimulate colonic cell proliferation in rats in a manner directly related to their content of fermentable fibre. Thus stimulation of colonic cell proliferation was found to be abolished by maintaining the rats in gnotobiotic or germ-free conditions, in which case no hindgut fermentation occurs. There is thus evidence that short-chain fatty acids, produced by hindgut fermentation, do stimulate colonic cell proliferation.

2. The second way in which food in the lumen could stimulate cell proliferation is by the production of a local or systemic hormone which stimulates cell proliferation. For example, feeding stimulates production of enteroglucagon, a hormone produced mainly in the terminal ileum, and which has been proposed as an intestinal growth hormone, mainly with the small intestine in mind. Indeed, there is a close correlation between crypt cell production rates in the small intestine and blood levels of enteroglucagon in a variety of adaptive situations (Al-Mukhtar et al. 1982a). However, more recent work has indicated that colonic regeneration is not associated with increases in blood enteroglucagon levels (Bristol et al. 1987).

There are very few instances where peptide hormones which are associated with gut epithelia have been infused into experimental animals or humans and shown to have a stimulatory effect on cell proliferation in the colon. One notable exception is epidermal growth factor (EGF). The human homologue of mouse epidermal growth factor is urogastrone (EGF/URO) produced in the salivary and Brunners glands; it is a 53-amino-acid peptide, highly homologous with EGF. Recent studies have shown that recombinant EGF/URO, infused into rats maintained on total parenteral nutrition, is a highly potent mitogen for colonic epithelium. Doses of 15 µg/rat/day by maintained intravenous infusion were able to stimulate crypt cell production rates in the colon at levels well above those seen in animals maintained by oral feeding, arguably the most prominent proliferative response described to date in colonic epithelium (Goodlad et al. 1987c). Increased doses produced a substantial hyperplastic response in the colonic epithelium. As yet there is no evidence that EGF/URO is involved in the physiological control of cell proliferation in the colon, but it is clear that growth factors can mediate powerful proliferative responses in the colon, and this field is likely to expand considerably over the next few years.

There has been considerable discussion about the role of so-called second messengers in gastrointestinal, including colonic, cell proliferation. Cyclic nucleotides and polyamines are undoubtedly involved in the mediation of adaptive responses in the colon: EGF/URO stimulates ornithine decarboxylase (ODC) and polyamine production in the intestine, an effect abolished by difluoromethylornithine (DFMO), a competitive inhibitor of ODC (Goodlad et al. 1988). DFMO has also been claimed to abolish the proliferative response to small intestinal resection, and ODC and polyamine production is also increased during carcinogenesis and also in colonic neoplasms themselves. It does therefore appear that ODC and polyamine synthesis are intimately involved in the production of proliferative responses. Studies on inositol lipids and diacylglycerol in intestinal responses have not been conclusive, but early evidence indicates that calcium, closely concerned with the transfer of intracellular information, can modify cell proliferation rates in the colon (Lipkin and Newmark 1985). Many other influences are often incriminated as mediators of cell proliferation in the colon, including various types of prostaglandins, induced changes in blood flow, neurotransmitters and changes in bacterial flora. At this point, a word of warning about experimental technique might be worthwhile: few studies are accompanied by stringent analysis of the effects of changes in food intake or feeding patterns evoked by the various treatments, and in many cases the end point for measuring the cell proliferation rate is less than optimal (Al-Mukhtar et al. 1982b; Wright and Alison 1984). For these reasons, much care must be taken before accepting many of the claims in this difficult and controversial field.

Conclusions

The several factors which influence the rate of cell proliferation in the colon are known, the organisation of colonic crypt systems is beginning to be understood and we are starting to dissect the nature of colonic stem cells. Several factors which modulate cell proliferation in the colon are known, and we stand at the threshold of the molecular biological era of gastrointestinal cell proliferation. The next years could see signal advances in this field.

References

Al-Mukhtar MYT, Sagor GR, Ghatei MA, Polak JM, Koopmans HS, Bloom SR, Wright NA (1982a) The relationship between gastrointestinal hormones and cell proliferation in models of intestinal adaptation. In: Robinson JWL, Dowling HR, Reicken EO (eds) Mechanisms of intestinal adaptation. MTP Press, Lancaster, pp 243–253

Al-Mukhtar MYT, Polak J, Bloom SR, Wright NA (1982b) The search for appropriate measurements of proliferative and morphological status in studies of intestinal adaptation. In: Robinson JWL, Dowling HR, Reicken EO (eds) Mechanisms of intestinal adaptation. MTP Press, Lancaster, pp 3–28

Bjerknes M, Cheng H (1981) The stem cell zone in the small intestinal epithelium. III. Evidence from columnar, enteroendocrine and mucous cells in the adult mouse. Am J Anat 166:76–92

Bristol JB, Ghatei MA, Smith JA, Bloom SR, Williamson RCN (1987) Elevated plasma enteroglucagon alone fails to alter distal colonic carcinogenesis in rats. Gastroenterology 92:617–627

Chang WWL, Leblond CP (1971a) A unitarian theory of the origin of the three populations of epithelial cells in the mouse large intestine. Anat Rec 169:293

Chang WWL, Leblond CP (1971b) Renewal of the epithelium in the descending colon of the mouse. I. Presence of three epithelial cell populations: vacuolated columnar, mucous and argentaffin. Am J Anat 131:73–100

Clarke RM (1975) Intestinal function and epithelial replacement. MD thesis, University of Cambridge

Fearon ER, Hamilton SR, Vogelstein B (1987) Clonal analysis of human colorectal tumours. Science 238:193–196

Goodlad R, Plumb J, Wright NA (1987a) Epithelial cell proliferation and intestinal absorptive function during starvation and refeeding in the rat. Clinical Science 74:301–306

Goodlad RA, Lenton W, Ghatei MA, Adrian TE, Bloom SR, Wright NA (1987b) Proliferative effects of fibre on the intestinal epithelium; relationship to plasma gastrin, enteroglucagon and PYY levels. Gut 28:221–226

Goodlad RA, Wilson TG, Lenton W, Wright NA, Gregory H, McCullagh KC (1987c) The proliferative effects of urogastrone (epidermal growth factor) on the intestinal epithelium. Gut 28:37–44

Goodlad RA, Smith W, Lenton W, Gregory H, Wright NA (1989) Epidermal growth factor/urogastrone stimulates gut growth via an ornithine decarboxylase-dependent mechanism. Clin Sci (in press)

Goss RJ (1964) Adaptive growth. Logos, London

Kirkland S (1988) Clonal origin of columnar, mucous and endocrine cell lineages in human colorectal epithelium. Cancer 61:1359–1363

Lipkin M (1974) Phase 1 and phase 2 proliferative lesions of colonic epithelial cells in premalignant diseases leading to colonic cancer. Cancer 34:878–888

Lipkin M, Newmark H (1985) Effect of added dietary calcium on colonic epithelial cell proliferation in subjects at high risk for familial colonic cancer. N Engl J Med 313:1381–1384

Ponder BAJ, Schmidt GH, Wilkinson MA, Wood MJ, Monk M, Reid A (1985) Derivation of mouse intestinal crypts from single progenitor cells. Nature 313:689–691

Rijke RPC (1980) Some speculations on control mechanisms of cell proliferation in intestinal epithelium. In: Appleton DR, Sunter JP, Watson AJ (eds) Cell proliferation in the gastrointestinal tract. Pitman Medical, London, pp 57–65

Rijke KPC, Garte R, Lagendoen NJ (1979a) Epithelial cell kinetics in the descending colon of the rat. 1. The effect of ischaemia-induced cell loss. Virchows Arch [B] 31:15–22

Rijke RPC, Garte R, Lagendoen NJ (1979b) Epithelial cell kinetics in the descending colon. 2. The effect of experimental bypass. Virchows Arch [B] 31:23–30

Sakata T, Hitosaka K, Shiomara Y, Tawate H (1980) The stimulatory effect of butyrate on epithelial cell proliferation in the lumen of the sheep, and its mediation by insulin; differences between in vivo and in vitro studies. In: Appleton DR, Sunter JP, Watson AJ (eds) Cell proliferation in the gastrointestinal tract. Pitman Medical, London, pp 123–137

Sunter JP, Wright NA, Watson AJ (1978) Kinetics of changes in the crypts of the jejunal mucosa of dimethylhydrazine-treated rats. Br J Cancer 37:662–672

Weibecke B, Brandts A, Eder M (1974) Epithelial proliferation and morphogenesis of hyperplastic, adenomatous and villous polyps of the human colon. Virchows Arch [A] 364:35–49

Williams GT, Williams ED (1988) Evidence that colonic crypts are maintained by a single stem cell. Nature 334:87–88

Wright NA, Alison MR (1984) The biology of epithelial cell populations, vol 2. Clarendon, Oxford, pp 540–869

Wright NA, Al-Nafussi A (1982) Kinetics of villous cell populations in the mouse small intestine. II. Negative feedback after death of proliferative cells. Cell Tissue Kinet 15:618–622

Arachidonic Acid Metabolism and Colorectal Cancer

F. R. DeRubertis and P. A. Craven

Department of Medicine, VA Medical Center, and University of Pittsburgh, University Drive C, Pittsburgh PA 15240, USA

Contents

Introduction

Normal colonic epithelium is characterized by a relatively rapid and constant rate of renewal. As replicating cells at the base of the crypt migrate toward the surface, division ceases, and differentiation occurs with eventual sloughing of senescent cells into the lumen (Lipkin 1974). Under normal conditions, cell division is confined to the lower two-thirds of the colonic crypt (Lipkin 1974). However, studies of patients with ulcerative colitis, familial polyposis, or high dietary fat intake, and of rodents exposed to chemical carcinogens (Deschner et al. 1983; Lipkin 1973; Lipkin et al. 1985) have correlated an increased risk of colon cancer with both enhanced epithelial replication and expansion of the proliferative zone of colonic crypts. The factors which control the normal growth and differentiation of colonic epithelial cells and which lead to proliferative abnormalities in populations at a high risk for colonic cancer are not well understood. Among the local factors implicated in control of colonic epithelial growth are arachidonic acid and its metabolites (Bull et al. 1984; Craven and DeRubertis, 1988; DeRubertis et al. 1985; Lipkin and Newmark 1985; Tutton and Barkla 1980; Wargovich et al. 1984). Arachidonic acid per se, reactive oxygen species, formed as intermediate products during arachidonate oxygenation, and end products of the cyclo-oxygenase (prostaglandins and thromboxane) and lipoxygenase [leukotrienes and hydroxyeicosatetraenoic acids (HETEs)] pathways of arachidonate oxygenation may alter colonic epithelial growth by (a) activating cellular second messenger systems involved in the control of cell replication (Anderson

et al. 1986; Craven and DeRubertis, in press), (b) injuring colonocytes with consequent enhanced rates of cell loss and a compensatory increase in proliferation (Wargovich et al. 1984; Szelenzi et al. 1986; Romano et al. 1987; Balaa and Goldgar 1986)
(c) altering the genome via a free radical mechanism (Cerutti 1985; Weitzman et al.
1985), or through a combination of these processes.

In colon, as in other tissues, the influence of arachidonate and its metabolites on
cell growth and neoplastic transformation is complex. When present at high concentrations within the colonic lumen, many fatty acids, including arachidonate, cause
epithelial cell injury with a compensatory increase in proliferative activity (Wargovich
et al. 1984). Increased Ca^{2+} intake leads to formation of insoluble Ca^{2+} salts of fatty
acids and suppresses the actions of fatty acids to induce colonocyte injury and reactive
proliferation (Lipkin and Newmark 1985; Wargovich et al. 1984). In addition to this
pathway, however, recent evidence suggests that low concentrations of arachidonate
and other unsaturated fatty acids (Craven and DeRubertis, 1988) or fatty acid
hydroperoxides (Bull et al. 1984) may increase colonic epithelial proliferative activity
without causing cellular injury. As discussed in detail below, this most likely occurs
through activation of cellular second messenger systems which modulate growth.

Indeed, many of the cellular actions of arachidonate and its metabolic products
noted above (prostaglandins, leukotrienes, HETEs, and reactive oxygen species) are
most likely mediated by activation of second messenger systems. Specifically, the
phosphoinositide (protein kinase C, calcium) and the adenylate cyclase-cyclic adenosine monophosphate (cAMP)-signalling pathways are both responsive to arachidonate and/or one or more of its oxygenation products. These pathways are illustrated schematically in Fig. 1. As shown, activation of the colonic epithelial phospholipase C system by an intraluminal stimulus of growth such as bile salts (Bull et al. 1983;
DeRubertis et al. 1984; Deschner et al. 1981) results in hydrolysis of phosphati-

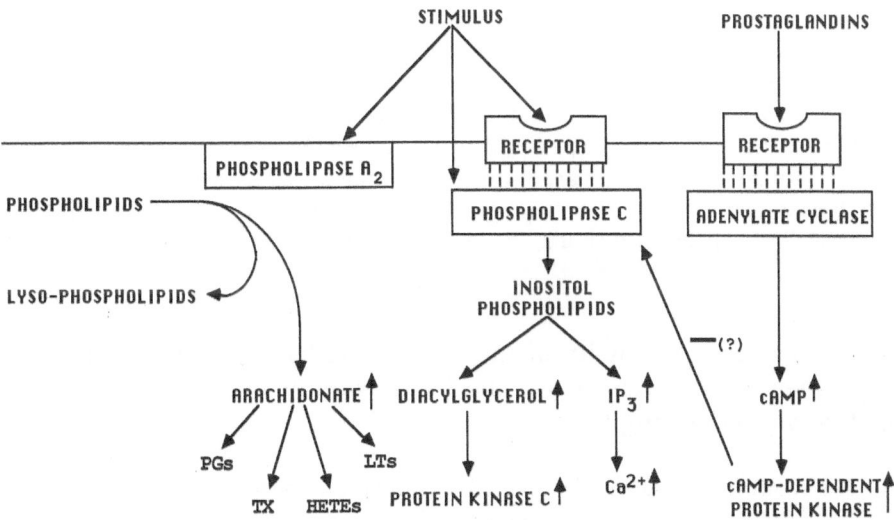

Fig. 1. Potential and observed consequences of stimulation of colonic mucosal phospholipid
breakdown

dylinositol-4,5-bisphosphate (PIP_2) and production of diacylglycerol and inositol-1,4,5-bisphosphate (IP_3) (Craven et al. 1987a). IP_3 is a key mobilizer of intracellular Ca^{2+} (Nishizuka et al. 1984). Diacylglycerol activates protein kinase C by reducing its requirement for Ca^{2+} and phospholipid (Nishizuka et al. 1984). The increase in cell Ca^{2+} and activation of protein kinase C are thought to act synergistically to initiate proliferative activity, possibly by alteration of NA^+/H^+ exchange and cellular pH (Berridge et al. 1985) or phosphorylation of nuclear proteins (Halsey et al. 1987). In this regard, numerous studies in cultured cell systems have linked enhanced inositol lipid hydrolysis and activation of protein kinase C to rapid growth (Anderson et al. 1985; Berridge et al. 1985; Halsey et al. 1987). Phospholipid hydrolysis through the phospholipase C or A2 pathway also leads to release of arachidonate, enhanced synthesis of prostaglandin and lipoxygenase products, and generation of reactive oxygen species (Fig. 1), all of which may alter the proliferative activity of colonocytes. Of interest, some of the products of phospholipid hydrolysis per se, including leukotrienes, HETEs, and arachidonate, have been reported to augment inositol phospholipid hydrolysis in colonic epithelium (Craven and DeRubertis, 1988) and in other tissues (Anderson et al. 1986; Kragballe et al. 1985; Setty et al. 1986). This may serve to amplify the response to the initial stimulus.

As is also illustrated in Fig. 1, an increase in prostaglandin synthesis activates colonic mucosal adenylate cyclase, and increases cellular cAMP. Increases in cAMP and activation of the cAMP-dependent protein kinase induced by prostaglandins or other agonists suppress proliferative activity of colonic epithelium (Craven et al. 1983). In several cell systems (Bianca et al. 1986; Takenawa et al. 1986; Watson et al. 1984), cAMP has also been shown to suppress inositol phospholipid hydrolysis. Thus the cAMP and inositol phospholipid signalling pathway may have reciprocal and integrated actions in the regulation of colonic epithelial proliferation, and both pathways may be activated by arachidonate or its metabolites. This review will focus on the roles of several putative primary signals to colonic epithelial cell growth which are derived from or linked to enhanced membrane phospholipid turnover. The consequences of enhanced membrane phospholipid turnover include release of arachidonate with the subsequent generation of prostanoids, lipoxygenase products, and reactive oxygen, and the concurrent activation of the protein kinase C and cAMP second messenger systems. As discussed below, reactive oxygen species, which in colonocytes are generated in part during oxygenation of released arachidonate, have also been implicated as mediators of colonocyte injury and proliferation and in DNA damage. These effects in turn may be involved in neoplastic transformation.

Differences in the Activity of the cAMP and Protein Kinase C Signalling System and Eicosanoid Production in Proliferating and Non-proliferating Colonocytes

Studies conducted in superficial (nonproliferating) and deep (proliferating) colonic epithelial cells isolated from normal rat colon have identified clear differences in eicosanoid production and in two of the major cellular second messenger systems which have been implicated in the regulation of the growth of these and other cells

Table 1. Comparison of proliferating and nonproliferating colonic epithelial cells[a]

	Proliferative : surface cells
DNA synthesis	5.0
cAMP content	0.4
Activated cAMP-dependent protein kinase	0.5
Synthesis of prostaglandins	0.3
Synthesis of HETEs, leukotrienes	3.0
Activated protein kinase C	2.0

[a] Studies were conducted in isolated superficial and proliferative cells. The results shown represent the ratio of values obtained in proliferative to those in surface cells.

(Craven and DeRubertis 1981; Craven and DeRubertis 1983; Craven and DeRubertis 1986; Craven and DeRubertis 1987; DeRubertis and Craven 1987). Table 1 summarizes the findings with regard to eicosanoid production and to cellular levels of cAMP, the state of activation of the cAMP-dependent protein kinase and protein kinase C systems. As illustrated in Table 1, DNA synthesis was five-fold higher in isolated colonic proliferative versus surface epithelial cells. Prostaglandin synthesis, cAMP content, and the state of activation of the cAMP-dependent protein kinase system were all reduced in the proliferating colonocytes compared to the surface cells. By contrast, the content of leukotrienes and HETEs and the state of activation of protein kinase C were all higher in proliferating compared to the surface epithelial cells.

Recent studies conducted in our laboratory have demonstrated the presence of protein kinase C activity in colonic epithelium and suggested a role for this enzyme in the control of colonic epithelial growth (Craven et al. 1987a; Craven and DeRubertis 1987). Exposure of colonic epithelium to bile salts, to arachidonate or other unsaturated fatty acids, or to the known activators of protein kinase C [12-O-tetradecanoyl phorbol-13-acetate (TPA) or 1-oleoyl-2-acetyl-glycerol (OAG)] either in vitro or by intracolonic instillation in vivo, induced a rapid (10 min) translocation of soluble protein kinase C activity to the particulate cell fraction, an index of enzyme activation. Activation of protein kinase C by bile salts, arachidonate, TPA, or OAG in vivo preceded and was correlated as a function of concentration with increases in proliferative activity of colonic mucosa. Although controversial (Jacobs 1983), recent evidence suggests that a high fat intake stimulates the proliferative activity of colonic epithelium (Lipkin et al. 1985). This change may increase the susceptibility of the epithelium to malignant transformation (Lipkin et al. 1983). The enhanced rate of epithelial proliferation, associated with a high fat intake, may be linked to the effects of increased colonic excretion of bile salts and fatty acids. Both bile salts and fatty acids have now been shown to activate the inositol phospholipid/protein kinase C pathway, and the latter may represent the intracellular signal which initiates proliferation of colonocytes (Craven and DeRubertis, 1988; Craven et al. 1987a).

A role for protein kinase C in the control of the basal rate of proliferative activity of colonic epithelial cells as well as in increases in proliferation induces by TPA, bile salts, and arachidonate is supported by studies with 1-(5-isoquinolinyl)-2-methyl-piperazine (H-7), an inhibitor of protein kinase C activity (Craven and DeRubertis

1987). Thus, treatment of rats with H-7 inhibited the basal rate of DNA synthesis in proliferating colonic epithelial cells and suppressed the enhancement of proliferative activity observed in colonocytes that were exposed to TPA, bile salts or arachidonate.

The above findings, taken together, suggest that as colonocytes migrate from the lower regions of the crypt toward the surface, activation of cAMP-dependent protein kinase and inactivation of protein kinase C may signal the termination of cell replication. Increases in the cAMP content of nonproliferating superficial colonocytes with the corresponding activation of cAMP-dependent protein kinase may be due in part to a higher rate of local production of prostanoids by these cells, many of which increase cAMP (Craven and DeRubertis 1981). The role, if any, of lipoxygenase products, which are preferentially generated by proliferating colonocytes, as determinants of proliferative activity is at present uncertain. However, stimulation of cell growth by lipoxygenase products has been reported (Anderson et al. 1986; Setty et al. 1986). Of interest, in some cells, a reciprocal relationship has been observed between cAMP-dependent protein kinase and protein kinase C during cellular replication. In these instances, activation of protein kinase C and inactivation of cAMP-dependent protein kinase occurs during active proliferation (Anderson et al. 1985). The results in Table 1 suggest that such a reciprocal relationship exists between cAMP-dependent protein kinase and protein kinase C activities in colonocytes with different proliferative activities. Figure 1 illustrates one reported interaction between the cAMP and protein kinase C system which may modulate cell growth or other cell functions, namely the action of cAMP to inhibit inositol phospholipid turnover. Other interactions between these two signalling systems probably exist.

Influence of Prostaglandin Analogues and Inhibitors of Prostaglandin Synthesis on Colonic Epithelial Proliferation

Studies in small intestinal and fundic mucosa (Eastwood and Quimby 1982; Kuwayama and Eastwood 1985) have consistently demonstrated that treatment of rats with aspirin or indomethacin stimulates tritiated thymidine ([^{3}H]dThd) incorporation into DNA. Similarly, studies from our laboratory have demonstrated that treatment of rats with indomethacin or aspirin for 1 – 5 days stimulates proliferation of colonic epithelium (DeRubertis et al. 1985). Concurrent treatment with the stable PGE_2 analogue 16,16-dimethyl PGE_2 did not alter basal DNA synthesis, suppressed indomethacin-induced increases in colonic mucosal DNA synthesis, and prevented the extension of the proliferative zone otherwise induced by 5 days of treatment with indomethacin (DeRubertis et al. 1985). These studies support a role for endogenous prostaglandin synthesis in the tonic suppression of basal proliferative activity of gastrointestinal epithelium. The failure of the PGE_2 analogue to alter basal rates of DNA synthesis may reflect maximal prostaglandin suppression by local endogenous colonic prostanoids.

Nevertheless, some studies employing analogues of PGE_2 have suggested that prostaglandins are trophic to the gastrointestinal epithelium. Thus, treatment of rats with analogues of PGE_2 causes thickening of gastrointestinal mucosa (Gilbertson et al. 1984; Halter et al. 1984; Tutgat et al. 1986). The mechanism by which thickening occurs is controversial with some studies demonstrating stimulation (Dembinski and Konturek 1985; Gilbertson et al. 1984; Halter et al. 1984), no effect (Baumgartner et al. 1985; DeRubertis et al. 1985; Tutgat et al. 1986); or inhibition (Fich et al. 1985) by PGE_2 analogues of [^{3}H]dThd incorporation into gastrointestinal mucosal DNA. In the case of colonic mucosa, PGE_2 analogues have been found to have no effect on the basal rate of [^{3}H]dThd incorporation into mucosal DNA when examined in vivo (DeRubertis et al. 1985; Gilbertson et al. 1984; Tutton and Barkla 1980) and to suppress [^{3}H]dThd incorporation into DNA in vitro (DeRubertis et al. 1985; Alpers and Philpott 1975). Some of these conflicting results may be explained by an action of PGE_2 analogues to reduce cell loss rather than an action to stimulate cell division. Thus, in a recent study conducted in jejunal, corpus, and antral mucosa (Uribe et al. 1986), administration of a PGE_2 analogue was found to have no effect on [^{3}H]dThd incorporation into DNA when examined at 45 min after [^{3}H]dThd injection, but to have a marked enhancing effect on labeling index by 3 days after [^{3}H]dThd injection due to retention of cells in the mucosa of prostaglandin analogue-treated rats. In contrast to the [^{3}H]dThd labeling index, the mitotic index was suppressed or unchanged in the mucosa of rats treated with the PGE_2 analogue for 3–5 days. This study clearly suggests that the apparent trophic actions of PGE_2 analogues on gastrointestinal mucosa are related to enhanced retention of gastrointestinal epithelial cells rather than to increased proliferative activity.

Enhanced proliferation of colonic epithelium is associated with an increased risk of colon cancer in both man and experimental animals (Lipkin et al. 1983). Nevertheless, treatment of rats with indomethacin (up to 20 weeks) had previously been reported to suppress colon tumor formation (Metzger et al. 1984; Narisawa et al. 1984; Pollard and Luckert 1983). This effect has often been presumed to be due to suppression of colonic prostaglandin synthesis. However, in none of these earlier reports had a reduction in colonic prostaglandin synthesis in response to the dose of indomethacin employed actually been documented. Indeed, in one instance, concurrent treatment with exogenous PGE_2 failed to prevent the putative anticarcinogenic effect of indomethacin (Narisawa et al. 1984). In view of these considerations, studies were conducted to assess: (a) whether sustained increases in the proliferation of normal colonic epithelium occur in response to chronic (6–20 weeks) administration of aspirin or indomethacin; (b) the relationship between changes in mucosal proliferative activity and alterations in colonic prostanoid production; and (c) whether the doses of indomethacin previously reported to suppress tumor initiation (1 mg kg^{-1} day^{-1} in drinking water for 1 week) or tumor promotion (3 mg kg^{-1} day^{-1} in drinking water for 20 weeks) in response to chemical carcinogens alter either colonic prostaglandin synthesis or mucosal proliferative activity (Craven et al., in press). The results demonstrated that treatment of rats for 1–20 weeks with 1 or 3 mg kg^{-1} day^{-1} indomethacin in the drinking water had no effect on colonic prostanoid production or colonic mucosal proliferative activity. Subcutaneous indomethacin (3 mg kg^{-1} day^{-1}) for 2 weeks suppressed colonic prostanoid production by 50% and increased colonic mucosal proliferative activity but induced an inflammatory response in colon (Craven et al., in press). Higher doses of indomethacin were toxic and associated with high mortality.

In contrast to indomethacin, administration of aspirin (50 mg kg^{-1} day^{-1} subcutaneously) for 2–20 weeks markedly suppressed colonic prostanoid production

(90%–100%) without evident colonic injury or inflammation as reflected by light microscopy, and with no obvious systemic toxicity. This dose of aspirin in the rat is equivalent to a dose of 10–12 aspirin tablets per day in adult man, a dose employed frequently on a chronic basis in the treatment of rheumatoid arthritis and related disorders. Chronic suppression of colonic prostanoid synthesis with aspirin (2–20 weeks) was associated with a sustained stimulation of [^{3}H]dThd incorporation into colonic mucosal DNA, which was demonstrable both in vivo and ex vivo in short-term cultured explants of colon. Autoradiographic studies conducted at 20 weeks demonstrated an increase in labeling index throughout the entire crypt column and an increase in the position of the highest labeled cell. Addition of either exogenous PGE$_2$ (the major prostanoid product of colon) which increases the endogenous cAMP content of colonocytes, or the addition of 8-bromo-cAMP (8-Br-cAMP) suppressed the enhanced rates of mucosal DNA synthesis of incubated colon segments from aspirin-treated rats. These findings thus support a physiologic role for local prostaglandins as negative modulators of the proliferative activity of colonic mucosa. They also suggest that the action of prostaglandins on proliferation may be mediated at least in part through changes in cellular cAMP. Chronic treatment of rats with aspirin provides a model for future evaluation of the influence of sustained suppression of colonic prostaglandin production and the associated sustained increase in mucosal proliferative activity on colonic carcinogenesis.

Roles of Lipoxygenase Products and Prostaglandins in the Acute Stimulation of Colonocyte Proliferation by Bile Salts

Acute exposure of colonic epithelium to bile salts in vivo increases the proliferative activity of colonic epithelium, as assessed by increases in mucosal ornithine decarboxylase (ODC) and [^{3}H]dThd incorporation into mucosal DNA (Bull et al. 1983; DeRubertis et al. 1984). Chronic exposure of colonic epithelium to high concentrations of bile salts increases proliferative activity, induces an extension of the proliferative zone (Deschner et al. 1981) and promotes tumor formation in response to administration of chemical carcinogens in experimental animals (Reddy et al. 1977). One of the earliest and most striking effects of exposure of colonic epithelium to bile salts is an increase in phospholipid hydrolysis which leads to a release of arachidonate, enhanced synthesis of prostaglandins, thromboxane and lipoxygenase products, generation of reactive oxygen moieties (DeRubertis et al. 1984; Craven et al. 1986a, 1987b), and release of diacylglycerol, the putative endogenous activator of protein kinase C (Craven et al. 1987a). These events are illustrated schematically in Fig. 1. Accordingly, the role of increases in each of these moieties in the acute stimulation of proliferative activity by bile salts was examined.

Prior treatment of rats with indomethacin suppressed to undetectable levels basal and deoxycholate (DOC)-induced increases in colonic prostanoid and thromboxane production, but enhanced accumulation of lipoxygenase products in colon. Indomethacin also enhanced basal and DOC-induced increases in colonic mucosal [^{3}H]dThd incorporation into DNA, thus indicating that DOC-induced increases in prostanoids and thromboxane were not responsible for the stimulation of colonic mucosal proliferation by DOC. In contrast to indomethacin, treatment of rats with phenidone or esculetin, which inhibited the production of both lipoxygenase and cyclo-oxygenase products, as reflected by marked declines in colonic 12-HETE, PGE_2, and TXB_2 production, suppressed bile salt-induced increases in mucosal ODC and [^{3}H]dThd incorporation into mucosal DNA. The results of the above studies, taken together, suggested a role for release of arachidonate and its subsequent oxygenation via the lipoxygenase pathway in the mediation of bile salt-induced increases in colonic epithelial proliferative activity. However, these studies did not delineate the potential role of reactive intermediates of arachidonate oxidation generated via either the cyclo-oxygenase or lipoxygenase pathways versus end products of the lipoxygenase pathway in the stimulation of colonic epithelial proliferation by bile salts.

Role of Reactive Oxygen Species in the Mediation of Colonic Epithelial Cell Injury and Proliferative Activity

Numerous previous studies have demonstrated that reactive oxygen species are mutagenic and cause DNA damage (Brawn and Fridovich 1985; Jackson et al. 1987; Moody and Hassan 1982). Recent evidence implicates reactive oxygen species as mediators of the growth-enhancing and tumor-promoting effects of phorbol esters in skin and hepatocytes (Kensler et al. 1983; Armato et al. 1984) and in cell transformation by activated neutrophils (Weitzman et al. 1985). Bile salts stimulate reactive oxygen generation (Craven et al. 1986a), possibly by stimulating arachidonate release and increasing oxidation through the lipoxygenase pathway (Kukreja et al. 1986; Mornett et al. 1974; Lilius and Laakso 1982). Bile salts also cause colonic epithelial injury and superficial cell lysis (Chadwick et al. 1979; Craven et al. 1986b), and it is likely that cell injury is linked to the observed increase in colonic epithelial proliferation which follows. Recent studies with the membrane-permeable superoxide dismutase mimetic Cu II (3,5-diisopropylsalicylic acid)$_2$ (CuDIPS) support a role for reactive oxygen production, possibly generated through the lipoxygenase pathway, in the mediation of bile salt-induced increases in colonocyte proliferation (Craven et al. 1986a). CuDIPS had previously been shown to inhibit phorbol ester-induced increases in ODC and tumor promotion in skin (Kensler et al. 1983). In studies in colon, CuDIPS suppressed bile salt-induced increases in both reactive oxygen production and colonic epithelial proliferation. CuDIPS was without influence on the production of PGE_2 or the lipoxygenase products 5,12- and 15-HETE or LTB_4 by colonic epithelium (Craven et al. 1986a). Further evidence for an action of reactive oxygen to increase proliferative activity of colonic mucosa was obtained from the stimulatory effect of direct intracolonic instillation of the xanthine-xanthine oxidase superoxide generating system on mucosal proliferative activity. These studies support a role for reactive oxygen, possibly generated through the lipoxygenase pathway, in the mediation of bile salt-induced increases in colonocyte proliferation.

The colonic mucosa of patients with ulcerative colitis is characterized by cell injury, inflammation, and enhanced proliferative activity (Lipkin 1974). Similar to the bile salt model described above, generation of reactive oxygen species is most likely also increased in colonic mucosa of patients with ulcerative colitis due to inflammatory cell infiltration (Bleiberg et al. 1970). Mucosal injury and accelerated cell loss may be responsible for a compensatory increase in proliferative activity seen in patients with ulcerative colitis, as in the rodent bile salt model above. Recent studies employing sulfasalazine and its therapeutically active metabolite 5-aminosalicylic acid (5-ASA) have provided further support for a link between increased generation of reactive oxygen species and bile salt-induced colonocyte injury and the subsequent increases in proliferative activity (Craven et al. 1987b). The results of these studies have demonstrated that intracolonic instillation of sulfasalazine or 5-ASA prevents bile salt-induced mucosal injury and the subsequent increases in proliferative activity. Sulfasalazine and 5-ASA also prevented mucosal injury and blocked the increase in proliferative activity induced by intracolonic instillation of the superoxide generating system xanthine-xanthine oxidase. Moreover, the actions of bile salts to increase reactive oxygen formation by colonic mucosal scrapings or isolated crypt epithelium were blocked by sulfasalazine and 5-ASA. Studies with the xanthine-xanthine oxidase superoxide generating system further demonstrated that sulfasalazine and 5-ASA were scavenging reactive oxygen, rather than inhibiting its generation. An excellent correlation was found between the ability of sulfasalazine and 5-ASA to suppress reactive oxygen production and to prevent bile salt-induced mucosal injury and increases in proliferative activity (Craven et al. 1987b). The ability of sulfasalazine and 5-ASA to scavenge reactive oxygen may thus play an important role in their therapeutic effects on inflammatory bowel disease. As noted above, reactive oxygen species have been implicated as mutagens and potential co-carcinogenic agents through their ability to cause DNA damage. It is thus tempting to speculate that the increased generation of reactive oxygen species which occurs with exposure of colonic mucosa to bile salts and with inflammatory cell infiltration in ulcerative colitis may be involved in the increased risk of colon cancer induced by both bile salts and inflammatory bowel disease. At least in the instance of bile salts, increased generation of reactive oxygen species is in part derived during the oxygenation of released arachidonate.

In summary, arachidonic acid and its metabolic products may modulate the growth and neoplastic transformation of colonic epithelium through multiple pathways and actions. A better understanding of these processes should provide considerable insight into the mechanism by which dietary factors such as fat intake and concurrent disorders such as inflammatory bowel disease increase the risk of colon cancer.

Acknowledgement. This work was supported by Grant CA 31 680 from the National Cancer Institute through the Large Bowel Cancer Project.

References

Alpers DH, Philpott GW (1975) Control of deoxyribonucleic acid synthesis in normal rabbit colonic mucosa. Gastroenterology 69:951–959

Anderson WB, Estival A, Tapiovaara H, Gopalkrishma R (1985) Altered subcellular distribution of protein kinase C: possible role in tumour promotion and the regulation of cell growth, relationship to changes in adenylate cyclase activity. Adv Cyclic Nucleotide Protein Phosphorylation Res 19:287–306

Anderson T, Schlegel W, Monod A, Krause KH, Stendahl O, Lew DP (1986) Leukotriene B4 stimulation of phagocytes results in the formation of inositol 1,4,5 trisphosphate. Biochem J 240:333–340

Armato U, Andreis PG, Romano F (1984) Exogenous Cu, Zn superoxide dismutase suppresses the stimulation of neonatal rat hepatocyte growth by tumor promoters. Carcinogenesis 12:1547–1555

Balaa MA, Goldgar DE (1986) Lipoxygenase enzyme inhibitors diminish ethanol damage to the rat stomach. Clin Res 34:436A

Baumgartner A, Koelz HR, Halter F (1986) Indomethacin and turnover of gastric mucosal cells in the rat. Am J Physiol 250:6830–6835

Berridge MJ, Brown DD, Irvine RF, Heslop JP (1985) Phosphoinositides and cell proliferation. J Cell Sci [Suppl] 3:187–198

Bianca VD, DeTogni P, Grzeskowiak M, Vicentini LM, DiVirgilio F (1986) Cyclic AMP inhibition of phosphoinositide turnover in human neutrophils. Biochim Biophys Acta 886:441 –447

Bleiberg H, Mainguet P, Galand P, Claretien J, Dupont-Mariesse N (1970) Cell renewal in the human rectum: in vitro autoradiographic study on active ulcerative colitis. Gastroenterology 58:851–855

Brawn MK, Fridovich I (1985) Increased superoxide radical production evokes inducible DNA repair in *E. coli*. J Biol Chem 260:922–925

Bull AW, Marnett LJ, Dawe EJ, Nigro ND (1983) Stimulation of deoxythymidine incorporation in the colon of rats treated intrarectally with bile acids and fats. Carcinogenesis 4:207–210

Bull AW, Nigro ND, Golembieski WA, Crissman JD, Marnett LJ (1984) In vivo stimulation of DNA synthesis and induction of ornithine decarboxylase in rat colon by fatty acid hydroperoxides, autooxidation products of unsaturated fatty acids. Cancer Res 44:4924–4928

Cerutti PA (1985) Active oxygen and promotion. In: Fischer SM, Slaga TJ (eds) Arachidonic acid metabolism and tumor promotion. Martinus Nijhoff Publishing, Boston, pp 132–168

Chadwick VS, Gaginella TS, Carlson GL, DeBongnie JC, Phillips SF, Hofmann AF (1979) Effects of molecular structure on bile acid-induced alterations in absorptive function, permeability and morphology in the perfused rabbit colon. J Lab Clin Med 94:661–674

Craven PA, DeRubertis FR (1981) Cyclic nucleotide metabolism in rat colonic epithelial cells with different proliferative activities. Biochim Biophys Acta 676:155–169

Craven PA, DeRubertis FR (1983) Patterns of prostaglandin synthesis and degradation in isolated superficial and proliferative colonic epithelial cells compared to residual colon. Prostaglandins 26:583

Craven PA, DeRubertis FR (1986) Profiles of eicosanoid production by superficial and proliferative colonic epithelial cells and subepithelial colonic tissue. Prostaglandins 32:387–399

Craven PA, DeRubertis FR (1987) Subcellular distribution of protein kinase C in colonic epithelial cells with different proliferative activities. Cancer Res 47:3434–3438

Craven PA, DeRubertis FR (1988) Role of activation of protein kinase C in the stimulation of colonic epithelial proliferation by unsaturated fatty acids. Gastroenterology 95:676–685

Craven PA, Saito R, DeRubertis FR (1983) Role of local prostaglandin synthesis in the modulation of proliferative activity of rat colonic epithelium. J Clin Invest 72:1365–1375

Craven PA, Pfanstiel J, DeRubertis FR (1986a) Role of reactive oxygen in bile salt stimulation of colonic epithelial proliferation. J Clin Invest 77:850–859

Craven PA, Pfanstiel J, Saito R, DeRubertis FR (1986b) Relationship between loss of colonic surface epithelium induced by deoxycholate and initiation of the subsequent proliferative response. Cancer Res 46:5754–5759

Craven PA, Pfanstiel J, DeRubertis FR (1987a) Role of activation of protein kinase C in the stimulation of colonic epithelial proliferation and reactive oxygen formation by bile salts. J Clin Invest 79:532–541

Craven PA, Pfanstiel J, Saito R, DeRubertis FR (1987b) Actions of sulfasalazine and 5-aminosalicylic acid on deoxycholate induced increases in colonic epithelial cell loss and proliferative activity. Gastrenterology 92:1998–2008

Craven PA, Thornburg K, DeRubertis FR (1988) Sustained increase in the proliferation of rat colonic mucosa during chronic treatment with aspirin. Gastroenterology 94:567–575

Dembinski A, Konturek SJ (1985) Effects of E, F and I series prostaglandins and analogues on growth of gastroduodenal mucosa. Am J Physiol 248:G170–G175

DeRubertis FR, Craven PA (1987) Physiologic cessation of colonic epithelial proliferation is associated with inactivation of protein kinase C and activation of cAMP dependent protein kinase. Clin Res 35:589A

DeRubertis FR, Craven PA, Saito R (1984) Bile salt stimulation of colonic epithelial proliferation: evidence for involvement of lipoxygenase products. J Clin Invest 74:1614–1624

DeRubertis FR, Craven PA, Saito R (1985) 16,16 Dimethyl prostaglandin E_2 suppresses the increases in the proliferative activity of rat colonic epithelium induced by indomethacin and aspirin. Gastroenterology 89:1054–1063

Deschner EE, Cohen BI, Raicht RF (1981) Acute and chronic effect of dietary cholic acid on colonic epithelial cell proliferation. Digestion 21:290–296

Deschner EE, Winawer SJ, Katz S, Katzka I, Kahn E (1983) Proliferative defects in ulcerative colitis patients. Cancer Invest 1:41–47

Eastwood GL, Quimby GF (1982) Effect of chronic aspirin ingestion on epithelial proliferation in rat fundus, antrum and duodenum. Gastroenterology 82:852–856

Fich A, Arber N, Sestieri M, Zajicek G, Rachmilewitz D (1985) Effect of misoprostol and cimetidine on gastric cell labeling index. Gastroenterology 89:57–61

Gilbertson TJ, Stryd RP, Brunden MN, Christianson CA, Rush BD (1984) Changes in thymidine uptake in the gastrointestinal tract of the rat following treatment with 16,16-dimethyl PGE_2. Prostaglandins 27:887–897

Halsey DL, Girard PK, Kuo JF, Blackshear PJ (1987) Protein kinase C in fibroblasts, characteristics of its intracellular location during growth and after exposure to phorbol esters and other mitogens. J Biol Chem 262:2234–2243

Halter LF, Meyrat P, Fritsche R, Muller O, Lentze MJ, Koelz HR (1984) Both topical and systemic treatments with 16,16-dimethyl prostaglandin E_2 are trophic to rat gastric mucosa. Scand J Gastroenterol 19:[Suppl 101]:47–53

Jackson JH, Schranfstatter IU, Hyslop PA, Vosbeck K, Sauerheber R, Weitzman SA, Cochrane CG (1987) Role of oxidants in DNA damage; hydroxyl radical mediates the synergistic DNA damaging effects of asbestos and cigarette smoke. J Clin Invest 80:1090–1095

Jacobs LR (1983) Effect of short-term dietary fat on cell growth in rat gastrointestinal mucosa and pancreas. Am J Clin Nutr 37:361–367

Kensler TW, Bush DM, Kozumbo WJ (1983) Inhibition of tumor promotion by a biomimetic superoxide dismutase. Science 221:75–77

Kragballe K, Desjarlais L, Voorhees JJ (1985) Leukotrienes B4, C4 and D4 stimulate DNA synthesis in cultured human epidermal keratinocytes. Br J Dermatol 113:43–52

Kukreja RC, Kontos HA, Hess ML, Ellis EF (1986) PGH synthase and lipoxygenase generate superoxide in the presence of NADH or NADPH. Circ Res 59:612–619

Kuwayama H, Eastwood GL (1985) Effects of water immersion restraint stress and chronic indomethacin ingestion on gastric antral and fundic epithelial proliferation. Gastroenterology 88:362–365

Lilius EM, Laakso S (1982) A sensitive lipoxygenase assay based on chemiluminescence. Anal Biochem 119:135–141

Lipkin M (1973) Proliferation and differentiation of gastrointestinal cells. Phys Rev 53:891–912

Lipkin M (1974) Phase 1 and phase 2 proliferative lesions of colinic epithelial cells in diseases leading to colonic cancer. Cancer 34:878–888

Lipkin M, Newmark H (1985) Effect of added dietary calcium on colonic epithelial cell proliferation in subjects at high risk for familial colonic cancer. N Engl J Med 313:1381–1384

Lipkin M, Blattner WE, Fraumeni JF, Lynch HT, Deschner E, Winawer S (1983) Tritiated thymidine labeling distribution as a marker for hereditary predisposition to colon cancer. Cancer Res 43:1899–1904

Lipkin M, Uehara K, Winawer S, Sauchey Z, Bauer C, Phillips R, Lynch HT, Blattner WA, Fraumeni FJ (1985) Seventh Day Adventist vegetarians have a quiescent proliferative activity in colonic mucosa. Cancer Lett 26:139–144

Marnett LJ, Wlodawer P, Samuelsson B (1974) Light emmision during the action of prostaglandin synthesis. Biochem Biophys Res Commun 60:1286–1294

Metzger U, Meier J, Uhlschmid G, Weihe H (1984) Influence of various prostaglandin synthesis inhibitors on DMH induced rat colon cancer. Dis Colon Rectum 27:366–369

Moody ICS, Hassan HM (1982) Mutagenicity of oxygen free radicals. Proc Natl Acad Sci USA 79:2855–2859

Narisawa T, Hermanek P, Habs M, Schmahl D (1984) Reduction of carcinogenicity of N-nitrosomethylurea by indomethacin and failure of resuming effect of prostaglandin E_2 (PGE_2) against indomethacin. J Cancer Res Clin Oncol 108:239–242

Nishizuka Y, Takai Y, Kishimoto A, Kikkawa U, Kaibuchi K (1984) Phospholipid turnover in hormone actions. Rec Prog Horm Res 40:301–345

Pollard M, Luckert PH (1983) Prolonged antitumor effect of indomethacin on autochthonous intestinal tumors in rats. JNCI 70:1103–1105

Reddy BS, Watanabe K, Weisburger JH, Wynder EL (1977) Promoting effect of bile acids in colon carcinogenesis in germ free and conventional F344 rats. Cancer Res 37:3238–3242

Romano M, Razandi M, Ivey KJ (1987) Taurocholate-induced damage to rat gastric epithelial cells in vitro: role of oxygen derived free radicals. Gastroenterology 90:1117

Setty BNY, Graeber JR, Stuart MJ (1986) Mitogenic effect of 15-HETE on endothelial cells is mediated via phosphatidylinositol turnover and protein kinase C activation. Clin Res 34:470A

Szelenzi I, Vergin H, Schickander H (1986) Gastric mucosal damage and oxygen free radicals. Gastroenterology 89:1655

Takenawa T, Ishitoya J, Nagai Y (1986) Inhibitory effect of prostaglandin E_2, forskolin and dibutyryl cAMP on arachidonic acid release and inositol phospholipid metabolism in guinea pig neutrophils. J Biol Chem 261:1092–1098

Tutgat GNJ, Offerhaus GJA, VanMinnen AJ, Everts V, Henson-Logmans SC, Samson G (1986) Influence of oral 15(R)-15-methyl prostaglandin E_2 on human gastric mucosa: a light microscopic cell kinetic and ultrastructural study. Gastroenterology 90:1111–1120

Tutton PJM, Barkla DH (1980) Influence of prostaglandin analogues on epithelial cell proliferation and xenograft growth. Br J Cancer 41:47–51

Uribe A, Rubio C, Johansson C (1986) Cell kinetics of rat gastrointestinal mucosa. Scand J Gastroenterol 21:246–252

Wargovich MJ, Eng VWS, Newmark HL (1984) Calcium inhibits the damaging and compensatory proliferative effects of fatty acids on mouse colon epithelium. Cancer Lett 23:253–258

Watson SP, McConnell RT, Lapetina EG (1984) The rapid formation of inositol phosphates in human platelets by thrombin is inhibited by prostacyclin. J Biol Chem 259:13, 199–203

Weitzman SA, Weitberg AB, Clark EP, Stossel TP (1985) Phagocytes as carcinogens: malignant transformation produced by human neutrophils. Science 227:1231–1233

Biochemical Changes in Colorectal Carcinogenesis

N. W. Toribara, S. B. Ho, R. S. Bresalier, and Y. S. Kim

Gastrointestinal Research Laboratory, Veterans Administration Medical Center,
4150 Clement St., San Francisco, CA 94121, USA

Contents

Introduction

Technological advances over the past decade have produced a remarkable expansion
in our knowledge of the basic biological processes involved in cell growth and replication. Nevertheless, our understanding of these processes both under normal and

pathological circumstances is far from complete and, in fact, can be considered to be early in its evolution.

Cell replication can be viewed simplistically as a cascade of events beginning with signals at the external cell surface, which are then transmitted via a complicated and poorly understood system of receptors and messengers to the nucleus, where the appropriate genes are expressed (or suppressed). Translation occurs in the cytoplasm, where the gene products are processed and act to effect cell growth and replication. Derangements anywhere in this complex sequence or events (signal transduction, transcription, translation, or post-translational modification of gene products) could cause autonomy from normal control mechanisms, leading to unrestricted cell growth.

Several problems are inherent in studying cancer in general and colon cancer in particular. These should be borne in mind when reading the literature or designing experiments.

Rapid Normal Cell Turnover. The epithelial cells of the normal colonic mucosa turn over rapidly, while those in some colon malignancies may divide at slower rates. Rapid proliferation of cells per se may not indicate neoplasia, and therefore biochemical parameters associated with rapid proliferation must be differentiated from specific changes associated with carcinogenesis.

Changes Caused by Nonspecific Effects of Experimental Carcinogenic Agents. It is often difficult to distinguish changes due to the toxicity of experimental agents from those specific for carcinogenesis. The possible involvement of exogenous (Nelson et al. 1987) or endogenous (Moshier et al. 1986) retroviruses in the etiology of some colonic cancers could make the task of determining specific carcinogenic markers even more difficult.

Limitations of Animal Models. Carcinogenesis is a multistep process which can be simplistically divided into events involving first "initiation" and then "promotion". During initiation, irreversible but not necessarily malignant changes occur as a result of exposure to carcinogenic or genotoxic agents such as chemicals, radiation, or viruses. Promotion involves continued exposure to these or other agents causing, additional changes which can eventually lead to the development of a neoplastic phenotype (Farber 1984). Unfortunately, in humans these events are usually discovered late in their course, at which time the malignant phenotype is already well established. As a result, it is often difficult to identify and study these early events in man, particularly for colonic cancer.

Thus, understanding the experimental models of colon carcinogenesis and their limitations is extremely important. A given carcinogen may, for example, have different effects in different species. Whether the changes seen in experimental models are truly applicable to carcinogenesis in humans must, therefore, be considered. Most of the experiments in colonic carcinogenesis have used either 1,2-dimethylhydrazine (DMH) or its related metabolites azoxymethane and methylazoxymethanol. Although these agents produce a spectrum of neoplastic changes similar to those seen in human colon carcinomas (LaMont and O'Gorman 1978), the relevance of this model to the etiology of human colon cancers must still be considered speculative.

Heterogeneity in Normal Tissues and in Tumors. Most colonic neoplasms arise from epithelial cells; however, the colonic mucosa consists of a variety of cell types, which makes study of any individual cell type difficult. Even with epithelial layer scraping or differential centrifugation it is difficult to obtain pure populations of columnar epithelial, goblet, neuroendocrine, or Paneth's cells for study. Colon cancers often consist of an admixture of normal and neoplastic elements, and there is even heterogeneity in the frankly malignant cell population itself (Brattain et al. 1984).

To complicate matters even further, the properties of the individual cell types are known to vary with microscopic as well as macroscopic location within the colon. For example, only the lower two-thirds of the epithelial lining cells of the colonic crypts undergo cell division. It is therefore not surprising to find that differences in isoenzymes (Balis et al. 1981), DNA repair (Kanagalingam and Balis 1975), relative proportions of sulfo- and sialomucins (Filipe and Branfoot 1974), and binding of lectins to tissue sections (Freeman et al. 1980) are seen when comparing the lower crypt to the surface epithelial cells. The biochemical properties of the colonic epithelial cells also vary with their position along the length of the colon. Differences have been noted in the chemical composition of the mucin in goblet cells (Reid et al. 1975), expression of blood group antigens (Yuan et al. 1985), lectin binding (Shamsuddin and Trump 1981; Bresalier et al. 1985), and in enzyme activities between proximal and distal colon (Freeman et al. 1978).

Phenotypic Drift in Cell Cultures. Due to the difficulties inherent in obtaining and using fresh tumors, much of the research on colonic carcinogenesis has involved the use of cell lines derived from colon cancers. Establishing cell lines from the heterogeneous cell populations present in fresh tumors leads to selection for certain characteristics, depending upon the conditions used. These cell populations are often phenotypically far removed from normal epithelial cells and are subject to changes in their characteristics with increasing passages and variations in culture conditions.

Increased technological sophistication has caused boundaries between what were once considered separate disciplines in the biological sciences to become less distinct. Biochemistry, biophysics, protein chemistry, and genetics have all become integral parts of molecular biology, just as molecular biology itself has become an indispensable part of the biological research armamentarium. Thus, it has become increasingly difficult to discuss a topic as expansive as "biochemical changes in colorectal carcinogenesis" without overlapping other disciplines. We have attempted to limit the overlap with topics covered elsewhere in this text, although this has not always been entirely possible.

The authors have chosen to organize this chapter according to the cellular location of the biochemical changes, i.e., the cell surface, the cytoplasm, or the nucleus, fully realizing that events in one area of the cell will often have consequences elsewhere.

The Cell Surface

Growth-Modifying Factors and Membrane Receptors

The rates of both normal and malignant cell replication are usually subject to some degree of modification by external factors whose actions are mediated through membrane receptors. The presence of receptors for a specific factor on a cell is thought to be necessary, but not sufficient for a cell to be responsive to that factor. Thus, understanding the effects of growth or inhibitory factors often requires characterization of its receptor (including its K_m, receptor density, and effects of inhibitors) in addition to standard measurements of cell replication. Receptor studies are often difficult to interpret and compare, however, due to inter-laboratory variability in assay conditions and definitions for positivity.

Stimulatory and Inhibitory Substances

Malignant cells have long been noted to be relatively autonomous, requiring fewer exogenous growth factors and being less responsive to control mechanisms than their normal counterparts (Sporn and Roberts 1985). The emerging importance of receptors and postreceptor signal transduction as critical control elements in the normal mitogenic pathway provides at least a partial explanation for this autonomy. A number of tumors are known to secrete autocrine polypeptide factors which can act on their cell of origin (via external receptors) in an autostimulatory or autoinhibitory manner. At least four distinct peptide families of autocrine factors are known, each having its own membrane receptor. Two of these, the transforming growth factor (TGF) α and β families, are known to have effects in experimental colon cancer systems. The platelet-derived growth factor (PDGF) and bombesin-like proteins have known autocrine effects in other cancer systems, but as yet there are no reports of effects on colon carcinomas.

The TGF-α-related peptides are structurally similar to, but distinct from, epidermal growth factor (EGF). Their stimulatory actions are thought to be mediated through the EGF receptor. Production of TGF-α-like activity has been reported in several colon carcinoma cell lines by Coffey et al. (1986), although they were unable to demonstrate any significant effect on soft agar growth of these cells. Partial characterization of another colon cancer-derived autocrine growth factor which does not seem to act through the EGF receptor has been reported (Levine et al. 1985).

TGF-β, originally characterized by its ability to stimulate the growth of NIH 3T3 fibroblasts in soft agar, is now known to be a potent inhibitor of growth in many cell lines. TGF-β is produced by several colon cancer cell lines (Coffey et al. 1986), and, in at least one line, inhibits cell replication and induces morphological evidence of differentiation (Hoosein et al. 1987). Other studies have reported tumor inhibitory factors from colon carcinomas which seem to be distinct from TGF-β, although these have not been well characterized (Levine et al. 1985; Hoagland et al. 1986). TGF-β and the other tumor inhibitory factors appear to affect well-differentiated carcinoma cells to a much greater degree than poorly differentiated cells. The discovery of autocrine inhibitory factors has led to the hypothesis that malignant transformation can result not only from excessive production, expression, and action of positive autocrine growth factors, but also from failure of cells to synthesize, express, or respond to the specific negative growth factors which normally control their growth (Sporn and Roberts 1985).

Angiogenin, a 14.4-kilodalton protein originally isolated from the HT-29 human colonic adenocarcinoma cell line, has potent angiogenic effects in chick embryo and rabbit cornea systems (Fett et al. 1985). Although it was initially thought that the primary function of this protein might be to promote neovascularization (a function of particular importance to tumor growth), it now appears that the angiogenin gene is expressed in a number of normal tissues in which its primary role may not be the stimulation of vascular growth (Rybak et al. 1987; Weiner et al. 1987).

The receptors and postreceptor signal transducers can be abnormal in affinity, quantity, or structure, thus possibly generating an abnormal mitogenic signal without the necessity for excessive growth factor levels. Increased expression of the EGF receptor has been found by immunohistochemical staining methods in well-differentiated colon cancer tissue sections and carcinoma cell lines when compared to normal colon and poorly differentiated carcinoma cells (Bradley et al. 1986). The appearance of unusual tumor-associated Lewis-type carbohydrate chains on the EGF receptors of several colon cancer cell lines has been noted (Basu et al. 1987). The *erb*-B oncogene is known to have considerable homology to the transmembrane and cytoplasmic portions of the EGF receptor, but thus far has not been implicated in colon cancer.

Other studies have suggested associations between insulin-like growth factor II (IGF-II), deoxycholic acid (DCA) receptors, and laminin receptors and colon carcinogenesis.

Tricoli et al. (1986) found 3–50-fold elevations of IGF mRNA transcripts in 50%–60% of distal (rectal and rectosigmoid) human colonic adenocarcinomas examined when compared to adjacent histologically normal areas of the colon. The significance of IGF and IGF-receptor abnormalities in human colon cancer is unknown, although one case report suggests that colon cancer-induced insulin receptors were responsible for the intractable hypoglycemia seen in that patient (Stuart et al. 1986).

Summerton et al. (1983) showed that approximately 25% of human colorectal cancers in their series contained specific receptors for DCA. In animal studies, Summerton et al. (1985) showed that azoxymethane-treated rats concomitantly treated with intrarectal instillation of DCA developed significantly more colorectal carcinomas and a higher percentage of tumors positive for DCA receptors than did rats treated with azoxymethane and intrarectal saline. These results are felt to support the theory that DCA acts as a tumor promoter via specific DCA receptors. An in-depth discussion of the role of bile acids in colorectal carcinogenesis will be presented elsewhere in this book (Cohen and Deschner).

Steroid Effects

Significant sex differences have been noted in both the incidence and mortality of colorectal cancer in humans, leading to speculation that sex steroids and/or steroid-related substances may act as tumor promoters, as is well established in the example of breast cancer. Several experimental models of colon carcinogenesis show increased male incidence, which is abolished by castration and restored by administration of androgen to the castrated animals (Moon and Fricks 1977; Tutton and Barkla 1982; Izbicki et al. 1983). In experimental systems such as animal models or tissue culture, direct effects of hormonal manipulations on tumor growth, morphology, and invasive potential can be measured, as well as measurement of receptor status. Clinically the measurement of specific receptor status is used as the major indication of possible hormonal responsiveness of that tumor.

Although initial reports estimated that as many as 70% of human colorectal carcinomas were positive for one or more steroid receptors, it is now generally felt that this percentage is considerably lower. For example, estrogen receptors are demonstrable in less than 10% of colorectal carcinomas (Wobbes et al. 1984; Stebbings et al. 1986) although one small series reported 24% positivity (Odagiri et al. 1984).

Progesterone and androgen receptors have been reported in 40% – 50% of human colonic carcinomas, but are present at similar levels and percentages in normal colonic tissue (d'Istria et al. 1986; Stebbings et al. 1986). No differences in receptor levels were noted regarding sex, age, tumor location, stage, or morphology in these studies although a nonstatistically significant increase in progesterone and androgen receptor positivity was noted in better-differentiated tumors.

Odagiri et al. (1985) studied colonic neoplasms induced by DMH administration to a strain of rats known to exhibit sex differences in incidence of induced colonic neoplasms. They found significant increases in the incidence and concentration of androgen receptors in induced colonic cancers in the male rats when compared to female rats. There were no sex differences in estrogen or progesterone levels in the induced colonic cancers. This was felt to indicate that gonadal hormones, especially androgens, may play a role in tumorigenesis. In contrast, Izbicki et al. (1986) studied azoxymethane-induced colonic tumors and concluded that androgens had mild inhibitory effects on the development of the tumors in their system.

The literature available at this time suggests that steroid dependency plays, at best, a minimal role in the etiology of colorectal cancer, and that endocrine manipulations will not be of particular value as a therapeutic modality.

Retinol- and Retinoic Acid-Binding Proteins

Vitamin A and its synthetic analogues, collectively known as "retinoids", affect epithelial cell differentiation and proliferation. Various investigators have reported that retinoids can suppress malignant phenotypic changes, both *in vivo* and *in vitro* (Sporn et al. 1976; Bertram et al. 1982). The effects of retinoids are thought to be mediated by cellular binding proteins, which act in much the same manner as hormone receptors to modulate transcription rates of various genes (Sani and Banerjee 1983). Two groups have described cellular retinoic acid-binding protein (cRABP) activities in both human colonic adenocarcinomas (62% – 70%) and adjacent, normal-appearing mucosa from the same patient (Sani et al. 1980; Di Fronzo et al. 1987), with no activity reported in normal human colonic mucosa. Similar findings have been reported by Fex et al. (1986) for cellular retinol-binding protein (cRBP), again examining human colonic adenocarcinomas and adjacent, non-involved mucosa from the same patient. Others have reported cRABP activity in a significant number of normal human colonic mucosal specimens, casting some doubt on the clinical significance of these findings. Ong et al. (1978) reported high retinol- (as opposed to retinoic acid) binding protein levels in DMH-induced rat colorectal adenocarcinomas when compared to adjacent, non-involved mucosa or colonic mucosa from control animals. These differences between the results of rat and human investigations may represent interspecies differences or differences in the etiology of the carcinogenic changes.

Adrenergic Factors

A substantial body of evidence suggests that the sympathetic nervous system exerts influences on epithelial cell proliferation, both in normal and malignant conditions. In studies in rat colon treated with DMH (Kennedy et al. 1985), alpha$_1$ receptors appear to mediate inhibitory effects on cell proliferation in normal crypts and adenomas, but a stimulatory effect on carcinomas. Alpha$_2$ receptors appear to mediate a stimulatory effect on normal colonic epithelial cells, but inhibitory effects on adenomas and carcinomas, possibly mediated by inhibition of adenylate cyclase (Paris et al. 1985). Beta receptor stimulation had inhibitory effects on normal crypt cells and adenomas, but no effect on carcinomas. The relevance of these factors in human colorectal carcinomas is not known.

Gut Hormones

Several gut hormones are felt to exert trophic effects on normal cells in the gastrointestinal tract. A number of studies have examined the effects of elevations of gastrin and enteroglucagon in animal models of carcinogenesis. The effect of elevated gastrin levels (produced by either antral exclusion or exogenous administration of pentagastrin) has been to increase the number and/or size of chemically induced or transplanted tumors in mice (Karlin et al. 1985; Winsett et al. 1986). These effects are felt to be mediated by specific, high-affinity gastrin receptors (Singh et al. 1986). In contrast, elevations of enteroglucagon levels induced by massive small bowel resection had no effect on colonic cell turnover or carcinogenesis after azoxymethane treatment and fecal stream diversion (Bristol et al. 1987; Savage et al. 1987).

Cyclic Adenosine Monophosphate

Cyclic nucleotides are second messenger molecules which may play a role in cellular proliferation and differentiation. Cyclic adenosine monophosphate (cAMP) levels have been observed to be reduced in human colon tumors (DeRubertis et al. 1976) and in rat colonic mucosa following treatment with DMH (Stevens and Loven 1980; DeRubertis and Craven 1980). These differences may be due to differences in the rate of cAMP synthesis rather than degradation, since cAMP phosphodiesterase activities and cAMP levels in response to theophylline were similar in normal and cancerous human tissues. In cultured colon tumor cells, increasing intracellular cAMP levels enhances glycoprotein and carcinoembryonic antigen (CEA) synthesis and release (Hwang et al. 1986). The physiological significance of these changes in cyclic nucleotides remains to be determined.

Extracellular Matrix and Secreted Products

The hallmark of a malignant epithelial cell is its ability to invade and proliferate beyond the confines of its basement membrane. It is this invasive ability which, in part, also differentiates the neoplastic cell of an adenoma from the malignant cell of a carcinoma. Defects in the continuity of the basement membrane can be demonstrated by electron microscopy of carcinomas *in situ* and may represent the earliest stages of progression to invasive carcinoma (Liotta 1986). Invasion of the basement membranes of vascular and lymphatic structures and epithelial tissues are also important during metastasis. Basement membranes are composed of type IV collagen, glycoproteins such as laminin and entactin, and heparin sulfate proteoglycans. It has been proposed that tumor cells invade by attaching to components of the basement membrane and tissue stroma via specific receptors, followed by secretion of hydrolytic enzymes which degrade this extracellular matrix. This then allows movement of the tumor cells through localized areas modified by proteolysis (Liotta et al. 1977, 1986).

Many normal and neoplastic cells contain cell surface binding sites for the basement membrane component laminin. Laminin receptors were strongly expressed in one-third of 20 human colonic adenocarcinomas studied immunohistochemically using a monoclonal antibody (MAb) directed against this receptor (Hand et al. 1985). Overall, 75% of colon cancers examined demonstrated some laminin receptor expression. Conversely, benign colonic adenomas did not demonstrate significant laminin receptor expression, with only 20% showing minimal positivity to the MAb.

Type IV collagen constitutes the structural backbone of the basement membrane. A basement membrane collagen-degrading metalloproteinase (type IV collagenase) has been identified in a variety of tumor cell types and appears to correlate with their metastatic potential (Salo et al. 1983; Liotta 1986). Recently secretion of type IV collagenase has been shown to be positively correlated with the metastatic potential of both murine and human colon carcinoma cells (Bresalier et al. 1987 a, b).

A number of other proteases, including thiol proteases, heparinases, and serine proteases such as plasminogen activator (PA), may contribute to tumor cell invasion. Plasmin is a degradative enzyme which may act directly on matrix glycoproteins such as fibronectin or laminin, activate collagenase, or play a role in degrading fibrin deposits around tumor cells. Plasmin, its precursor plasminogen, two plasminogen activators (urokinase, and tissue-type) and two plasmin inhibitors (alpha$_2$-antiplasmin and alpha$_2$-macroglobulin) constitute the plasmin system which has been studied by a number of investigators in relationship to colon cancer. Burtin et al. (1985) histochemically demonstrated plasminogen at the surface of colon cancer cells. Traces of both types of plasminogen activator were found on the tumor cells, with a predominance of urokinase on invasive cells. This group (Burtin et al. 1987) found enhanced expression of the plasmin system, including PA (especially urokinase) in lymph node metastases from colorectal carcinomas. These latter results are at variance with those of Marks et al. (1983), who found the secretion of PA in short-term culture of colon cancer explants to be less in metastases than primary tumors. Others have reported high levels of urokinase but not tissue-type PA in both colorectal cancers and adenomatous polyps when compared with normal colonic mucosa (Gelister et al. 1986). Urokinase levels were highest in tumors demonstrating venous invasion and extensive local and distant spread (Gelister et al. 1987). A correlation between tumor invasiveness and PA activity was also observed in human primary colon carcinomas by Cajot et al. (1986 a); these same tumors, grown as noninvasive subcutaneous xenografts in nude mice, contained very low levels of PA activity. While subcutaneous xenografts of human colon cancers in nude mice were associated with low levels of PA, gastrointestinal xenografts exhibiting invasive growth expressed higher PA activity (Cajot et al. 1986 b). Circumstantial evidence suggests a role, therefore, for urokinase-type PA in tumor invasion by colonic cancers.

Cell Surface Components

Functional Significance of Glycoconjugates

Many of the cell surface alterations on neoplastic cells occur in the composition, structure, and metabolism of glycoproteins and glycolipids. Glycosylation is a major determinant of the conformation, stability, and organization of the proteins of secreted products, membranes, cytoplasm, and extracellular matrix (Hakomori et al. 1984; Olden et al. 1982; Kornfeld and Kornfeld 1981). Altered glycosylation of membrane lipids affects membrane fluidity and may alter receptor and adhesive protein function. The effects of these alterations upon the interaction of the cell with neighboring cells, the cell substratum, and with various ligands such as hormones, infectious agents, toxins, and antibodies are often profound (Hakomori 1981; Yamakawa and Nagai 1978). In addition, cellular glycoconjugates change during fetal development and may modulate cell differentiation and proliferation (Feizi 1985).

Secreted Glycoconjugates – Mucins

Mucins are highly glycosylated, high molecular weight (greater than 10^6 daltons) glycoproteins which represent a major secretory product of the colonic mucosa. Antigenic distinctions between normal and cancer-associated mucins in the colon were first noted over 20 years ago. More recently, Gold and Miller (1978) and Gold et al. (1981) confirmed and extended these observations, demonstrating that colon cancers contain at least two immunochemically distinct species of mucin. Other studies suggest that colon cancer and transitional mucosa accumulate sialomucins which contain reduced side chain O-acetylated sialic acid (Reid et al. 1985). Bara et al. (1984, 1986) have also reported the presence of oncofetal-type mucin structures in human hyperplastic and adenomatous polyps, adenocarcinomas, and experimentally in the precancerous colonic mucosa of rats treated with DMH.

Lectins have been used extensively to study mucins associated with carcinogenesis in the colon. These proteins and glycoproteins recognize specific carbohydrate moieties such as Gal β-1,3GalNAc, which is typically present in the mucin core region and identified by the lectin peanut agglutinin (PNA). The structure recognized by PNA is expressed almost uniformly in the mucin of malignant but not normal colonic tissues (Boland et al. 1982a). In addition, PNA binding sites have been found in mucosa immediately adjacent to cancers and in premalignant, adenomatous polyps (Boland et al. 1982b). The expression of this cancer-associated carbohydrate structure correlates with the relative risk of developing frank malignancies in adenomas. Similarly, PNA has been shown to bind to colonic mucins in experimental animals predisposed to developing colon cancers either genetically or by administration of a carcinogenic agent (Boland and Ahnen 1985; Boland and Clapp 1987). PNA receptors which are present in the mucins of most primary colon cancers may be masked or lost in their metastases (Bresalier et al. 1984).

The lectin *Ulex europeus* agglutinin (UEA-1) recognizes terminal alpha L-fucose-containing structures, similar to blood group H (0) antigen. This lectin binds to glycoconjugates in normal mucosa of the proximal, but not distal colon. The structure recognized by UEA-1 is highly expressed, however, in carcinomas of both the proximal and distal colon, adenomatous polyps, and premalignant mucosa of patients with familial polyposis and in DMH-treated rats (Yonezawa et al. 1982, 1983; Shioda et al. 1987). SDS polyacrylamide gel electrophoresis of colonic extracts confirms the presence of high molecular weight UEA-1-reactive glycoconjugates in carcinomas of the colon (Matsushita et al. 1985; Irimura et al. 1987), but not in normal distal colonic mucosa.

Cell Surface Glycoconjugates

Biochemical Changes

Cultured human colon carcinoma cell lines and organ explants demonstrate reduced glycoprotein synthesis compared to normal or fetal colonic cells (O'Gorman and LaMont 1978; Kim et al. 1979). The glycoproteins produced by cultured cancer cells contain unique high molecular weight, fucosylated glycopeptides (Youakim and Herscovics 1985) and novel oligosaccharides (Kurosaka et al. 1983).

Colon cancer cell lines of differing biological behavior have been shown to produce differing cell surface proteins and glycoproteins. Marks et al. (1983) noted that highly aggressive cell lines have a high content of 45–95 kilodalton glycoproteins, whereas less aggressive cells synthesize primarily higher molecular weight glycoproteins (92–180 kilodalton) on their surface. Sialylation of tumor cell glycoconjugates has also been correlated with metastatic potential. Kijima-Suda et al. (1986) found that inhibition of sialyltransferase activity in a mouse colon carcinoma cell line was associated with reduced metastatic ability.

Biochemical analysis of glycosphingolipids has revealed both quantitative and qualitative changes in malignant and premalignant colonic tissues. Siddiqui et al. (1978) demonstrated qualitative differences in neutral glycosphingolipids, sulfoglycolipids, and gangliosides of human colonic tumor extracts compared to normal adjacent mucosa. They also found unique glycosphingolipids containing Lewis[b] (Le[b]) and blood group A activities in tumor tissue. Premalignant colonic mucosa from DMH-treated rats contain increased globotriaosylceramide and decreased hematoside and globotetraosylceramide compared to untreated controls. These findings correlate with alterations in fluidity of colonic brush border membranes (Brasitus et al. 1986; Dahiya et al. 1987).

Alterations in Carbohydrate Antigens

Hybridoma technology has allowed the production of MAbs which can be used to identify specific cancer-associated carbohydrate epitopes (see Table 1) in glycoproteins and glycolipids. Cancer-associated carbohydrate alterations can be divided into three categories: (a) expression of antigens not normally present in a particular location or individual; (b) deletion of normally expressed antigens; and (c) synthesis of unique carbohydrate epitopes (Hakomori 1985).

Inappropriate Expression. Colon cancers commonly express carbohydrate antigens which are structurally normal, but which are not usually present in normal colon or in a particular location in the colon (see Table 2). For example, cancers and adenomas in the distal colon commonly express blood group A, B, H, or Le[b] antigens,

Table 1. Alterations of carbohydrate antigens in colon cancer. (Adapted from Bloom et al. (in press))

Aberrant antigen expression	
Examples:	A, B, H, Le^b – distal colon
	Le^x – entire colon
	Le^y – entire colon
	Incompatible A and B
Possible mechanisms:	Reactivation of fetal genes
	Synthesis of A- or B-like antigens
	Alterations at enzyme level
	Alterations at gene level
Antigen deletion (may result in precursor accumulation)	
Examples:	A, B, H, Le^b deletion in proximal colon
	T antigen, H precursor accumulation
Possible mechanisms:	Deficiency of glycosyltransferase
	Lack of precursor substance
	Glycosidase digestion of terminal sugars
Neosynthesis	
Examples: Sialylated antigens	– Sialyl Le^x
	– Sialyl Le^a
Fucosylated antigens	– Extended Le^x
	– Extended Le^y
Possible mechanisms:	Activation of "new" glycosyltransferases
	Chain elongation
	Sialylation
	Fucosylation

which are normally absent in this location. This cancer-associated expression recapitulates the pattern found in the distal fetal colon (Wiley et al. 1981; Denk et al. 1974, 1975). Inappropriate expression of Lewis^x (Le^x) and Lewis^y (Le^y) structures commonly occurs in colonic tumors, and both antigens behave as oncodevelopmental antigens in the colon (Shi et al. 1984; Kim et al. 1986; Cordon-Cardo et al. 1986; Abe et al. 1986). The enhanced expression of Le^x in colon cancers appears to be due to altered precursor (Holmes et al. 1987). The Le^y antigen has a decreasing proximal to distal distribution in normal adult colon. However, carcinomas, adenomas, and hyperplastic polyps in the distal colon show strong expression of this antigen.

Another type of inappropriate antigen expression is the presence of blood group substances (BGS) which are incompatible with the individuals' own blood type. Incompatible BGS expression may be due to altered transcriptional or post-translational events resulting in glycosyltransferase substrate specificity changes. Approximately 60% of colon cancers, as well as transitional mucosa and adenomatous polyps, express incompatible BGS (Yuan et al. 1985; Sakamoto et al. 1986; Itzkowitz 1986a). Hyperplastic polyps and fetal tissue, on the other hand, do not display incompatible BGS. These results suggest that incompatible BGS expression is associated with premalignant and malignant transformation in the colon.

Table 2. Carbohydrate antigens

Antigen	Antigenic determinant	Monoclonal antibody	Reference
H	$Gal \xrightarrow{\beta_{1-4/3}} GlcNAc \text{——} R$ $\quad\mid \alpha_{1-2}$ $\quad Fuc$		
A	$GalNAc \xrightarrow{\alpha_{1-3}} Gal \xrightarrow{\beta_{1-4/3}} GlcNAc \text{——} R$ $\quad\mid \alpha_{1-2}$ $\quad Fuc$		
B	$Gal \xrightarrow{\alpha_{1-3}} Gal \xrightarrow{\beta_{1-4/3}} GlcNAc \text{——} R$ $\quad\mid \alpha_{1-2}$ $\quad Fuc$		
Le^a	$Gal \xrightarrow{\beta_{1-3}} GlcNAc \text{——} R$ $\quad\quad\mid \alpha_{1-4}$ $\quad\quad Fuc$		
Sialyl Le^a	$Gal \xrightarrow{\beta_{1-3}} GlcNAc \text{——} R$ $\mid \alpha_{2-3} \quad\mid \alpha_{1-4}$ $NeuAc \quad Fuc$	19–9	Koprowski et al. (1979)
Le^b	$Gal \xrightarrow{\beta_{1-3}} GlcNAc \text{——} R$ $\mid \alpha_{1-2} \quad\mid \alpha_{1-4}$ $Fuc \quad Fuc$		
Le^y	$Gal \xrightarrow{\beta_{1-4}} GlcNAc \text{——} R$ $\mid \alpha_{1-2} \quad\mid \alpha_{1-3}$ $Fuc \quad Fuc$	AH6	Abe et al. (1983)
Extended Le^y	$Gal \xrightarrow{\beta_{1-4}} GlcNAc \xrightarrow{\beta_{1-3}} Gal \xrightarrow{\beta_{1-4}} GlcNAc \text{——} R$ $\mid \alpha_{1-2} \quad\mid \alpha_{1-3}$ $Fuc \quad Fuc$	CC-1 CC-2	Sun et al. (1987)
Trifucosyl Le^y	$Gal \xrightarrow{\beta_{1-4}} GlcNAc \xrightarrow{\beta_{1-3}} Gal \xrightarrow{\beta_{1-4}} GlcNAc \text{——} R$ $\mid \alpha_{1-2} \quad\mid \alpha_{1-3} \quad\quad\quad\mid \alpha_{1-3}$ $Fuc \quad Fuc \quad\quad\quad Fuc$	KH-1	Kaizu et al. (1986)
Le^x	$Gal \xrightarrow{\beta_{1-4}} GlcNAc \text{——} R$ $\quad\quad\mid \alpha_{1-3}$ $\quad\quad Fuc$	SSEA-1	Gooi et al. (1981)
Extended (dimeric) Le^x	$Gal \xrightarrow{\beta_{1-4}} GlcNAc \xrightarrow{\beta_{1-3}} Gal \xrightarrow{\beta_{1-4}} GlcNAc \text{——} R$ $\quad\mid \alpha_{1-3} \quad\quad\quad\mid \alpha_{1-3}$ $\quad Fuc \quad\quad\quad Fuc$	FH4	Fukushi et al. (1984a)
Sialyl Le^x	$Gal \xrightarrow{\beta_{1-4}} GlcNAc \text{——} R$ $\mid \alpha_{2-3} \quad\mid \alpha_{1-3}$ $NeuAc \quad Fuc$	CSLEX1	Fukushima et al. (1984)
Sialyl extended Le^x	$Gal \xrightarrow{\beta_{1-4}} GlcNAc \xrightarrow{\beta_{1-3}} Gal \xrightarrow{\beta_{1-4}} GlcNAc \text{——} R$ $\mid \alpha_{2-3} \quad\mid \alpha_{1-3} \quad\quad\quad\mid \alpha_{1-3}$ $NeuAc \quad Fuc \quad\quad\quad Fuc$	FH6	Fukushi et al. (1984b)
T antigen	$Gal \xrightarrow{\beta_{1-3}} GalNAc \text{——} R$		

Antigen Deletion. Deletion of carbohydrate antigens may occur by incomplete synthesis, resulting from deficiency of a glycosyltransferase or precursor substance, or by the action of glycosidases. Deletion of BGS A, B, H, and Le^b has been demonstrated in proximal colonic tumors, whereas Le^a antigen deletion may occur in tumors throughout the colon (Ernst et al. 1984; Yuan et al. 1985; Sakamoto et al. 1986). The results of several studies suggest that blood group deletions may be related to the biological aggressiveness of the tumor (Ernst et al. 1984; Wiley et al. 1981; Sakamoto et al. 1986). Deletion of BGS often results in the accumulation of precursor substances. The precursor substance H frequently accumulates in colon cancers and adenomatous polyps (Yuan et al. 1985; Itzkowitz et al. 1986a). T antigen, the precursor of the M and N BGS, also accumulates in a high percentage of colon cancers (Boland et al. 1982a; Yuan et al. 1986).

Neosynthesis. Several cell surface glycoconjugates are preferentially expressed by colorectal neoplasms compared to normal colonic mucosa and come under the category of antigen neosynthesis. These unique epitopes are formed by carbohydrate conjugation reactions which include sialylation, fucosylation, and oligosaccharide chain elongation. CA 19-9 is a sialylated Le^a derivative which is present on circulating glycoproteins and cell surface glycolipids in patients with neoplasms of epithelial origin (Magnani et al. 1982, 1983). Sialosyl-Le^a is present in 60%–90% of colorectal cancers (Atkinson et al. 1982; Arends et al. 1983) and adenomatous polyps (Gong et al. 1985). Sialylated derivatives of Le^x antigen (Fukushima et al. 1984) also accumulate in colon cancers. The MAb FH6 recognizes sialyl, difucosyl Le^x (Fukushi et al. 1984b) and appears to be the most cancer specific in histochemical studies. It stains no normal colonic tissue, but reacts with 82% of colorectal cancers, failing to react with several poorly differentiated and colloid carcinomas (Itzkowitz et al. 1986b).

The MAb FH4 recognizes the difucosylated and trifucosylated Le^x determinants (Fukushi et al. 1984a). This antibody, which rarely binds to normal colonic mucosa or hyperplastic polyps, reacts with 94% of colorectal cancers and also binds to adenomatous polyps commensurate with their malignant potential (Itzkowitz et al. 1986b; Yuan et al. 1987).

Extended Le^y determinants recognized by MAb CC-1 and CC-2 (Sun et al. 1987) and trifucosyl Le^y antigens recognized by MAb KH-1 (Kaizu et al. 1986) are more specific for cancer tissue than the simple Le^y antigen. These neosynthesized antigens are rarely present on normal, transitional, or hyperplastic mucosa, but are found on 60%–80% of cancers and 36%–51% of adenomatous polyps (Kim et al. 1986).

Oligosaccharide elongation, sialylation, and polyfucosylation therefore represent aberrant biochemical processing of glycoconjugates in malignant cells. The preferential expression of these antigens by cancerous tissue may be both quantitative and qualitative, but the resulting antigens appear to be sensitive and specific markers of malignant transformation in the colon. The mechanism responsible for these changes may involve the activation of new glycosyltransferases or the modification of enzyme-substrate specificity.

Immunochemical techniques have demonstrated several other tumor-associated glycoconjugates whose epitope specificities have not been completely determined. Among the antigens described in colon cancer are colon-ovarian tumor antigen

Table 3. Glycosyltransferase and glycosidase activities in colon cancer

	Human	Rodent	Reference
Glycosyltransferase			
Galactosyltransferase I	0, −	−	Kim et al. (1974);
Galactosyltransferase II	−	+ [a]	LaMont and Isslebacher
Galactosyltransferase III	−		(1975);
Fucosyltransferase I	−		LaMont et al. (1974);
Fucosyltransferase II	−		Whitehead et al. (1979);
Sialyltransferase I	0	−	Kuhns and Schoentag
Sialyltransferase II	0	−	(1981)
N-Acetylgalactosaminyltransferase	−		
N-Acetylglucosaminyltransferase	−	−	
Glycosidases			
N-Acetylhexosaminidase	i	i	Mian and Cowen (1974);
N-Acetylglucosaminidase	−, 0	+, − [a]	Mian et al. (1979);
N-Acetylgalactosaminidase	0	+, − [a]	Brattain et al. (1977, 1979);
α-Galactosidase	0	0	Kim et al. (1974);
β-Galactosidase	0	+, 0	Freeman et al. (1978)
α-Mannosidase	0	0	
α-Fucosidase		+	

[a] Difference present when compared to normal distal colon only.
+, Increase; −, decrease; 0, no change; i, isoenzyme change.

(COTA), CA50 antigen, α-1-acid glycoprotein, TAG-72 antigen, sialomucins and YPan-1 and SPan-1 antigens. Further studies are needed to determine the structures and biological relevance of these glycoconjugates in colon cancer (for a review see Bloom et al., in press).

Synthetic and Degradative Enzymes

Alterations of glycosyltransferases and glycosidases associated with colon carcinogenesis have been studied using various experimental systems, including homogenized human and rat tissues and epithelial cell cultures (see Table 3).

Decreased glycosyltransferase but not glycosidase activities have been found in human colon cancer extracts when compared to normal mucosa (Kim et al. 1974; Kim and Isaacs 1975). Tumor tissues have a lower carbohydrate content than normal tissue, probably due to decreases in the activities of the mucin-type glycoprotein conjugating enzymes. Decreases in α-2-fucosyltransferase (H enzyme) in blood group A, B, and H patients, and N-acetyl-galactosaminyltransferase (A enzyme) in blood group A patients have been found in colonic tumors compared to normal tissue (Kuhns and Schoentag 1981). These decreases in glycosyltransferase activity may result in incomplete glycoprotein oligosaccharide synthesis and contribute to altered blood group expression in colonic neoplasms.

Glycosyltransferase activities depend to some extent upon the enzyme source. Whitehead et al. (1979) compared the activities of six glycosyltransferases and three glycosidases in cultured human fetal colonocytes, cultured human colon carcinoma cells, and surgically obtained human colon cancer and adjacent normal mucosal specimens. Tumor tissue demonstrated the lowest specific activities of these enzymes, whereas cultured carcinoma cells had the highest levels of two galactosyltransferases. Activities of the mucin biosynthetic enzymes showed considerably more variation between colon cancer cell lines in this study than was found in surgical colon cancer specimens by Kim et al. (1974). Qualitative changes in glycosyltransferases have been identified in cultured colon cancer cell lines. Thin-layer isoelectric focusing of the most abundant glycosyltransferase (galactosyltransferase I) obtained from colon tumor cell lines shows that each cell line has a unique galactosyltransferase isoenzyme pattern which cannot be attributed to culture confluence, growth conditions, blood type, or passage number (Whitehead et al. 1979). Unique galactosyltransferase isoenzymes have also been reported in the sera of patients (Weiser et al. 1976) and animal models (Podolsky et al. 1977).

Changes in the synthetic and degradative enzymes for glycoconjugates occur in premalignant and malignant colonic mucosa of rats treated with DMH. DMH-treated, but nonmalignant colonic mucosa contains significant increases in carbohydrate content and galactosyltransferase activity compared to that of normal, untreated animals (Freeman et al. 1978). DMH-induced colonic tumors generally contain decreased glycosyltransferase activities (LaMont et al. 1974; Freeman et al. 1978). Glycosidase activities in DMH-induced colonic tumors are variable, both increases and decreases having been reported (Mian and Cowen 1974; Freeman et al. 1978). The finding of lower glycosyltransferase activity in experimental DMH-induced colonic tumors is similar to the decrease found in human tumors. Glycosidase activities in experimentally induced colonic neoplasms differ from those in man, however, suggesting that chronic DMH toxicity or interspecies differences may need to be considered in interpreting these results.

Qualitative differences in β-hexosaminidase isoenzymes have been documented in both experimental and human cancers. DMH-induced tumors contain hexosaminidase enzymes with different kinetic properties and altered isoenzyme patterns compared to control colons (Mian et al. 1979; Brattain et al. 1979). Brattain et al. (1977) demonstrated that human colon cancer extracts contain a higher proportion of β-hexosaminidase B than β-hexosaminidase A, opposite to the ratio found in normal colonic mucosa. No kinetic differences were found between the enzymes from normal and malignant tissues. In contrast, β-hexosaminidase ratios in different cultured human colon cancer cells were variable (Tsao et al. 1979). These isoenzyme differences and their relationship to the biological behavior or glycoconjugate expression of these cell lines are unclear.

The Cytoplasm

Intermediary Metabolism

Malignant cells are characterized by quantitative and qualitative changes in the expression of enzymes involved in carbohydrate, protein, nucleic acid, polyamine, and other metabolic pathways (see Table 4). Many of these changes are common to various types of malignancies and may confer selective advantage for the growth of the malignant cell (Weber 1977).

Table 4. Changes in enzyme activities associated with colon cancer

	Human	Rodent	Reference
Nucleic acid metabolism			
Pyrimidine (Synthetic)			
Thymidine kinase	+	+	Weber et al.
CTP synthetase	+	+	1978, 1980;
OMP decarboxylase	+	+	Ballis et al. 1981
Uridine kinase	+	+	
Uracil phosphoribosyl transferase	+	+	
Orotate phosphoribosyl transferase	+	+	
(Degradative)			
Uridine phosphorylase	−	−	
Dihydrothymine dehydrogenase		−	
Purine (Synthetic)			
Glutamine PRPP amidotransferase		+	
(Degradative)			
Xanthine oxidase		−	
Adenosine deaminase	i	i	
Carbohydrate metabolism			
Glycolytic			
Pyruvate kinase	+	+	Weber et al.
Hexokinase	+		1978, 1980;
Lactate dehydrogenase	+, i		Langvad 1968;
Phosphofructokinase	0		McGinty et al. 1973;
Synthetic			Shonk et al. 1965
UDPG pyrophosphorylase	−		
Fructose 1,6-diphosphatase	0		
Glycerol phosphate dehydrogenase	−		
Pentose phosphate shunt			
Glucose-6-phosphate dehydrogenase	+	0	
Transaldolase	+	0	
6-phosphogluconate dehydrogenase	+	−	
Protein metabolism			
(Nonessential amino acid synthesis)			
Pyrroline-5-carboxylate reductase	+		Herzfeld and
Phosphoserine phosphatase	+		Greengard 1980
(Collagen synthesis)			
Peptidyl proline hydroxylase	+		
Mitochondrial and peroxisomal enzymes			
Succinic dehydrogenase	−		Sun et al. 1981;
Monoamine oxidase	−		McGinty et al. 1973;
Cytochrome oxidase	−		Wattenberg 1959
Urate oxidase	+		

+, Increase; −, decrease; 0, no change; i, isoenzyme change.

Oxidative Metabolism

Decreases in oxidative respiration and glycerol phosphate cycle activity have been associated with colon carcinoma. Histochemical studies demonstrate reduced activities of aminopeptidase, nonspecific esterase, cytochrome oxidase, succinate dehydrogenase, monoamine oxidase, and acid phosphatase in hyperplastic polyps, adenomas, and carcinomas compared to normal colonic tissue (Czernobilsky and Tsou 1968; Nachlas and Hannibal 1961). McGinty et al. (1973) found that small carcinomas which have a reduction in all five of the above enzymes are more likely to be associated with nodal metastases than tumors with reductions in only one or two enzymes. It is possible that decreased levels of oxidative enzymes are related to more rapid growth in neoplastic tissues. Using biochemical analysis, Sun et al. (1981) confirmed that the activities of cytochrome oxidase, succinic dehydrogenase and monoamine oxidase are decreased in colon carcinomas. Other oxygen-consuming enzymes in peroxisomes are variably changed; urate oxidase is increased and catalase decreased. In carcinomas, monamine oxidase is decreased more than other mitochondrial enzymes, suggesting a qualitative change in the outer mitochondrial membrane.

Glucose Metabolism

Warburg (1956) found that rapidly growing tumor cells exhibit increased aerobic glycolysis and decreased respiration. This pattern of altered carbohydrate metabolism (which favors glycolysis over gluconeogenesis) has been confirmed in a variety of cancerous tissues (Weber 1977), including those of the colon. Glycolytic enzyme activities in colorectal cancer homogenates are approximately two-fold greater overall than those in homogenates of normal colonic tissue. The activity of phosphofructokinase (the rate-limiting glycolytic enzyme), however, remains at control values (Shonk et al. 1965; Weber et al. 1980).

The capacity of malignant tissues to divert carbohydrate substrates into alternative pathways is limited. The activity of fructose 1,6-diphosphatase, a key enzyme in gluconeogenesis, is essentially unchanged in malignant compared to normal tissue, while glycerolphosphate dehydrogenase, which catalyzes the initial steps of triacylglycerol formation, is consistently decreased in colon cancer (Shonk et al. 1965). In contrast, the pentose phosphate biosynthetic enzymes, glucose-6-phosphate dehydrogenase, 6-phosphoglucose dehydrogenase, and transaldolase, are increased by 2.6-, 1.5-, and 1.8-fold, respectively, in human colon cancer tissue (Weber et al. 1980). These quantitative changes may reflect channeling of substrate into the pentose phosphate pathway to increase the formation of precursors of purine and pyrimidine synthesis.

Qualitative alterations in glycolytic enzymes also occur in colon cancer tissue. Langvad (1968) analyzed the isoenzyme pattern of lactate dehydrogenase (LDH) in colon carcinoma and samples of histologically normal colon at varying distances from the tumors. In malignant tissue and transitional mucosa, the activities of the isoenzymes LDH 4 and LDH 5 were relatively increased. This isoenzyme shift may contribute to the high capacity for anaerobic glycolysis in malignant tissue.

In normal colon, glycogen levels in the epithelium are low. In contrast, colonic tumors demonstrate large accumulations of glycogen. Altered glycogen metabolism in cultured colon carcinoma cells is linked to growth rate, with glycogen accumulation increasing as cells pass from exponential to stationary growth phase. Rousset et al. (1984) found that in cultured HT-29 colon tumor cells, glycogen is synthesized by the glucose-6-phosphate-dependent, phosphorylated form of glycogen synthetase in contrast to normal tissue. It is possible that this enzyme remains activated by the high concentrations of glucose-6-phosphate found in the tumor cells. Glycogen synthetase activity decreases as cell division decreases, whereas glycogen phosphorylase activity is positively correlated with growth rate. The modifications of glycogen metabolism which are associated with colonic carcinomas may, in turn, affect the glycosylation of cellular components such as glycoproteins and glycolipids, which are also known to be altered in colonic neoplasms.

Several groups have demonstrated that glucose metabolism plays a role in the differentiation of some human colon carcinoma cell lines. In the absence of glucose, HT-29 and CaCo-2 cells exhibit a differentiated enterocytic phenotype, with apical villi and brush border enzymes. When grown in the presence of glucose, HT-29 cells lose these differentiated features, whereas CaCo-2 cells do not (Zweibaum et al. 1985). Wice et al. (1985) found that undifferentiated HT-29 cells accumulate uridine diphosphate (UDP)-N-acetylhexosamines, while differentiated HT-29 and CaCo-2 cells grown in glucose free media maintain low concentrations of UDP-N-acetylhexosamine. These results suggest that changes in the glycosylation of proteins by altered nucleotide-sugar precursors may play a key role in the inability of cancer cells to differentiate.

Protein Synthesis

The selective impairment of protein and DNA synthesis by sodium cyanate in various animal tumors without impairment of protein synthesis in normal tissues illustrates a qualitative change in tumor cell protein synthesis. Intraperitoneal sodium cyanate decreases the incorporation of ^{3}H-amino acids into cytoplasmic and nuclear protein fractions of DMH-induced colonic neoplasms in the rat compared to nonneoplastic colonic epithelial tissue (Allfrey et al. 1977). Conversion of sodium cyanate to an active metabolite by cytochrome P450 may be necessary for this protein inhibitory effect. In at least one carcinoma cell culture system, this sensitivity to sodium cyanate is reversed by exposing the cells to sodium butyrate, a putative differentiating agent (Boffa et al. 1981). The mechanism of protein inhibition in malignant cells by the sodium cyanate metabolite is unknown, although some evidence suggests that it may involve alterations of cellular mRNA synthesis and the initiation of protein synthesis (Lazarus and Panasci 1987).

Alterations in enzyme activities found in neoplasms are often also seen in the corresponding fetal tissue. Herzfeld and Greengard (1980) compared the activities of enzymes involved in DNA, collagen, amino acid, and glucose metabolism in homogenates of human fetal colonic mucosa, nonneoplastic adult colon, and colon carcinoma. Carcinomas and fetal colonic mucosa both demonstrate increases of thymidine kinase, peptidyl proline hydroxylase, phosphoserine phosphatase, ornithine transcarbamylase, γ-glutamyl transpeptidase, and ornithine aminotransferase when compared to nonneoplastic adult colon. However, colon carcinoma differs from fetal colon and benign adult colon by containing elevated hexokinase, glucose-6-phosphate dehydrogenase, and pyrroline-5-carboxylate reductase activities.

Polyamine Metabolism

One enzyme which has been the subject of considerable discussion and study in the colon cancer literature over the past few years has been ornithine decarboxylase

(ODC). This enzyme catalyzes the conversion of ornithine to putrescine, the rate-limiting step in the biosynthetic pathway for polyamines (putrescine, spermidine, and spermine). Polyamines are highly regulated and are present in significant amounts in virtually all higher eukaryotic cells, which suggests that these compounds have considerable biological importance despite the lack of knowledge regarding their physiological functions. Investigators utilizing α-difluoromethylornithine (DFMO), which is a specific, irreversible inhibitor of ODC, have shown that the polyamines are integrally involved in cell replication. Since a comprehensive review of these studies is beyond the scope of this chapter, only the points pertinent to colon cancer will be discussed. Interested readers are referred to recent general reviews on the polyamines by Pegg and McCann (1982), Russell (1983), Morris and Marton (1981), and Tempero (1986).

Early studies noted the short half-life of the key enzymes in the polyamine biosynthesis and degradative pathways (less than 1 h) and the association of polyamine levels with traverse of cells through the cell cycle. It has only been recently, with the development of specific inhibitors such as DFMO, that inhibition of polyamine synthesis has been shown in many cell systems to also inhibit cell proliferation and differentiation (Pegg and McCann 1982), possibly through effects on microfilaments prior to cell division (Sunkara et al. 1979).

Early reports by Kingsnorth et al. (1983 a, b) indicated that low levels of DFMO inhibited cell replication in cultured human colon cancer cells and reduced DMH-induced colonic tumor formation in mice. Shortly thereafter, a series of studies reported that ODC levels were elevated in human adenomas and adenocarcinomas when compared to uninvolved mucosal specimens from the same patients (Rozhin et al. 1984; LaMurglia et al. 1986, Herrera-Ornelas et al. 1987; Moorehead et al. 1987). In addition, these groups reported that ODC activity in histologically normal-appearing mucosa from patients with colon cancer was elevated above levels in normal controls. In conjunction with the findings of increased DNA content and synthetic rate in normal-appearing mucosa of patients with colon neoplasms, these studies support the view that increased proliferative activity is an obligatory step in the progression to colon cancer. Significant elevations of ODC have been observed in the histologically normal mucosa of patients with familial polyposis when compared to normal controls (Luk et al. 1987) as well as reports of increased ODC levels in conditions favoring the development of experimental colon cancer (Takano et al. 1981; Luk et al. 1986; Hamilton and Luk 1987). These results suggest that ODC levels could serve as a marker of neoplastic potential in the colonic epithelium of certain patient populations.

Several reports indicating that colonic cancer cells might be selectively sensitive to ODC inhibition by DFMO (Kingsnorth et al. 1983 b; Tutton and Barkla 1986), DFMO + cyclosporine A (Saydjari et al. 1987), or prostaglandin E_2 inhibitors (Narisawa et al. 1985), have led to speculation that ODC inhibitors might be clinically useful in antineoplastic drug therapy. Although phase I trials of a combination of human leukocyte interferon and DFMO were not particularly successful against colon cancer (Talpaz et al. 1986), phase II trials of DFMO alone are still ongoing in patients with metastatic colon cancer (Abeloff et al. 1986).

Cytoskeleton

Cytoskeletal elements are essential for determining cellular morphology, migration, and division (Geiger et al. 1984; Mooseker 1985). Abnormalities in the cytoskeleton could contribute to the development of a malignant phenotype by altering contact inhibition, invasiveness, signal transduction, or chromosome segregation during mitosis.

Cytoskeletal proteins are divided into three groups based on their size: (a) microfilaments – 6 nm in diameter (actin, myosin); (b) intermediate filaments – 10 nm in diameter (cytokeratins, vimentin, desmin, neurofilaments, and glial fibrillary acidic protein); (c) microtubules – 25 nm in diameter (tubulin).

Polyclonal and monoclonal antibodies have provided most of the information concerning the cytoskeletal patterns of normal and malignant cells (Chen et al. 1985).

The microfilament actin is prominently expressed in colon cancers and appears to undergo complex modification during carcinogenesis. Actin has been shown to be apically distributed in cells from both primary tumors and metastases (Yeger et al. 1986). Friedman et al. (1984, 1985) studied the actin pattern of normal cultured colonic epithelial, adenoma, and carcinoma cells from the general population and epithelial and adenoma cells from the colons of familial polyposis patients. Carcinomas had the fewest actin filaments and adenomas the most. Actin content was intermediate in nonneoplastic epithelia, with familial polyposis epithelium containing fewer actin filaments than nonpolyposis control epithelial cells.

Cytokeratins are the major intermediate filament proteins in epithelial cells. The type of cytokeratin present depends on the tissue of origin and stage of differentiation (Cooper et al. 1985). In normal colonic epithelial cells, cytokeratins are expressed in the middle and upper portions of the crypt with no expression in the proliferative compartments of the lower crypt (Chesa et al. 1986). Tubular adenomas and hyperplastic polyps demonstrate only sparse areas of cytokeratin staining. In contrast, prominent cytokeratin staining is seen throughout the glands of villous adenomas, the adenomas and histologically normal mucosa of patients with familial polyposis, and in colon carcinomas. This suggests that cytokeratin alterations may be useful in distinguishing colonic mucosal lesions at high risk for malignant transformation from those at low risk.

Microtubule abnormalities have been associated with the development of aneuploidy in other systems, but have not been reported in colonic neoplasms.

Nuclear and DNA Changes

Enzymes in the DNA Synthetic Pathway

A number of changes have been noted in enzymes involved in metabolism of DNA precursors. Although some of these changes are reported to involve specific neoplasia-related isoenzyme forms, the majority of the changes appear to be associated with generally increased DNA synthetic activity.

Purine Metabolism

Adenosine deaminase (ADA) is an enzyme which catalyzes the deamination of adenosine as well as several adenosine analogues, most notably adenine arabinoside (ara-A). Trotta and Balis (1977) found unique isoenzymes of ADA in experimentally induced colon carcinomas in rats and in surgically resected specimens from human colonic carcinomas when compared to corresponding normal colon in the respective species. Ten Kate et al. (1986) studied ADA-complexing protein (which binds two ADA molecules into a dimeric form) in colonic carcinomas using immunohistochemical techniques and found that a membranous distribution pattern seemed to be correlated with the degree of differentiation of the tumor.

Weber et al. (1978) studied the nucleotide synthetic pathways in DMH-induced colon tumors in the mouse and noted that the activity of glutamine phosphoribosyl pyrophosphate (PRPP) amidotransferase, one of the enzymes involved in purine biosynthesis, increased seven-fold, while the enzyme catalyzing the rate-limiting step in purine catabolism, xanthine oxidase, was decreased to 7% of its normal value. It thus appears that in this system, carcinogenesis is accompanied by reciprocal changes in synthetic and catabolic enzyme activities.

Pyrimidine Metabolism

Thymidine kinase (TK) catalyzes the first step in the salvage pathway (the formation of deoxythymidine monophosphate (dTMP) by phosphorylation of thymidine). TK has been studied by several groups. Herzfeld and Greengard (1980) found a five-fold increase in TK activity in human colonic adenocarcinomas when compared to normal colon. Sakamoto et al. (1985) confirmed and extended this observation, noting that TK activities were also elevated approximately 1.6-fold in adenomatous polyps when compared to normal human colon. In addition, they isolated two TK isoenzyme forms, one of which was elevated in both polyps and adenocarcinomas, and a second which was elevated only in the adenocarcinomas and accounted for most of the TK activity in those samples. The same pattern of TK activity has been found in DMH-induced colonic carcinomas in rats (Sakamoto et al. 1987). This latter study also showed a 3.3-fold increase in thymidylate synthetase activity (the enzyme responsible for the de novo synthesis of dTMP). However, Dutrillaux and Muleris (1986) report a decrease in thymidylate synthetase activity in human colon carcinomas.

The activities of other enzymes in the pyrimidine biosynthetic pathway have also been shown to increase during carcinogenesis. Cytidine triphosphate (CTP) synthetase (9.3-fold), uracil phosphoribosyltransferase (6.0-fold), and orotidine monophosphate (OMP) decarboxylase (8.6-fold) all increase in experimentally induced colon carcinomas, while the activities of the pyrimidine catabolic enzymes, uridine phosphorylase and dihydrothymine dehydrogenase decrease when compared to normal colon (Weber et al. 1978).

Dutrillaux and Muleris (1986) suggest that the DNA precursor biosynthetic enzyme changes seen in colon carcinomas are not due to general induction or suppression resulting from increased replicative activity, but due to specific chromosomal deletions or rearrangements affecting the loci of the different enzymes.

Deoxyribonucleic Acid

Genetic Abnormalities

Since carcinogenesis involves the acquisition of heritable traits in the transformed cells, it is logical that changes must occur at the DNA level. Many of these changes are at a genomic level and may be accessible to molecular biological investigations. A number of chromosomal abnormalities are known to be associated with colon cancer. A considerable body of information is accumulating on the role of oncogenes in the pathogenesis of colon cancer, particularly regarding point mutations of the K-*ras* gene (Bos et al. 1987; Forrester et al. 1987). Oncogenes will be covered in depth elsewhere in this text (James and Sikora).

Recently Bodmer et al. (1987) have reported finding a chromosome 5 deletion (mapping near bands 5q21–q22) which is associated with certain autosomally dominant cases of familial adenomatous polyposis (FAP). Solomon et al. (1987) extended this work to nonfamilial colorectal carcinomas and found that at least 23% of the 45 heterogeneous colon tumors examined showed partial or complete loss of an allele at the FAP locus. Several other groups have reported abnormalities of chromosomes 1, 7, 8, 12, 14, and 17 in colon cancer (Becher et al. 1983; Levin and Reichman 1986; Reichman et al. 1981; Paraskeva et al. 1984; Fearon et al. 1987). However, only the 17p somatic loss in colon cancers reported by Fearon et al. (1987) appears to affect a significant percentage of tumors. The isolation and cloning of the FAP and 17p genes and elucidation of the mechanism of action of their gene products should have exciting and far-reaching effects on our understanding of colorectal carcinogenesis and strategies for its prevention and therapy.

Cellular DNA Content

Histological studies have suggested for many years that carcinomas often have an increased number of cells with abnormal DNA content. However, the advent of fluorescence-activated cell sorting (FACS) has allowed rapid, accurate measurement of cellular DNA content without the effort needed for more "classical" and laborious histochemical techniques. Techniques have been developed to measure the nuclear DNA content in fresh tumor or paraffin-embedded tissue from samples as small as endoscopic pinch biopsies (Petersen 1985; Hedley et al. 1983; McKinley et al. 1985).

The DNA content of the epithelial cells appears to increase as the cells proceed through the initiation and promotion phases of carcinogenesis, paralleling the changes in the DNA synthetic enzymes discussed above. Administration of DMH (Suzuki and Umehara 1986) and azoxymethane (Matthews and Cooke 1986) to rats led to increased DNA content in histologically normal-appearing colon as well as overtly neoplastic lesions. This is felt to be due to the increasing number of dividing cells at progressively higher positions in the colonic crypts which is known to accompany experimentally induced carcinogenesis. Such changes have also been described in the histologically normal-appearing mucosa of patients with colonic tumors (Suzuki et al. 1985). These studies suggest that one of the early steps in initiation is increased proliferative activity. Later steps in the progression to a frankly malignant phenotype may be facilitated by carcinogen-induced reductions in the capacity of the colonic epithelium to effect DNA repair (Kanagalingam and Balis 1975).

Most of the studies utilizing flow cytometry agree that aneuploidy (having an abnormal number of chromosomes, not an exact multiple of the haploid number) is present in about 60% of colorectal cancers arising in the general population (Armitage et al. 1985; Melamed et al. 1986; Goh and Jass 1986), although certain subpopulations such as colorectal carcinomas in ulcerative colitis patients (Fozard et al. 1986) and in patients having synchronous adenomas (Quirke et al. 1986) appear to have a somewhat lower rate of aneuploidy (approximately 30%). Aneuploidy is significantly associated with the degree of dysplasia exhibited by benign colonic adenomas. Aneuploidy was present in 4% of histologically mildly dysplastic, 18% of moderately dysplastic, and 36% of severely dysplastic adenomas (Goh and Jass 1986). However, no correlation was found between the histologic degree of differentiation of adenocarcinomas and aneuploidy in this study.

The prognostic significance of finding aneuploidy in a given tumor is not clear. Armitage et al. (1985) found a 19% 5-year survival rate in patients having aneuploid colorectal cancers compared to a rate of 43% in patients having diploid cancers. Quirke et al. (1987) similarly found a significant positive predictive value for aneuploidy in colorectal cancers, particularly when combined with a high level of cell proliferation. On the other hand, Melamed et al. (1986) found no difference in 3-year survival rates between aneuploid and diploid colon cancers. Finan et al. (1986) also failed to find a significant difference in survival between aneuploid and diploid colon carcinomas, although they studied only advanced malignancies with known metastases.

Thus, the suggestion by some groups (Kokal et al. 1986) that flow cytometric DNA analysis be used as a routine part of the preoperative evaluation would appear premature at this time (Koss and Greenbaum 1986).

Nuclear Proteins

Several studies have found changes in nonhistone nuclear proteins. Increases in nuclear levels of antigens with molecular weights of approximately 34000 and 105000 in humans (Bauer et al. 1986) and 44000 and 62000 in DMH-induced carcinomas in rats (Boffa and Allfrey 1977) have been described. Decreases in levels of two nonhistone nuclear proteins (molecular weight approximately 15000) during carcinogenesis have also been reported (Boffa et al. 1980). Chakrabarty et al. (1985) noted differences in the ^{32}P-labeled phosphorylation/dephosphorylation patterns of certain nuclear proteins between aggressive and non-aggressive subpopulations of colonic tumors, although the silver-stained, two-dimensional electrophoretic patterns of these proteins remained essentially the same. These antigens may represent nuclear oncogene products although data on this is not available at this time.

Concluding Perspectives

A wide array of alterations in cellular biochemical processes have been associated with colorectal cancer. Malignant colonic cells secrete autocrine factors which affect their own growth, and proteases which aid in invasion of the extracellular matrix.

Changes in cell surface receptors, proteins, and glycoproteins affect the cell – cell and substratum interactions of these cancer cells. Abnormalities in cytoplasmic and nuclear processes and cytoskeletal elements affect cell growth and replication and contribute to the malignant phenotype.

The majority of reports concerning these events are descriptive, recording observed differences between normal and malignant colonocytes. In order to understand fully how the various changes described above result in malignancy will now require a coordinated multidisciplinary effort to examine their functional significance.

References

Abe K, McKibbin JM, Hakomori S (1983) The monoclonal antibody directed to difucosylated type 2 chain (Fucα1 → 2 Galβ1 → 4 [Fucα1 → 3] GlcNAc; Y determinant). J Biol Chem 258: 11 793–11 797

Abe K, Hakomori S, Ohshiba S (1986) Differential expression of difucosyl type 2 chain (Le^y) defined by monoclonal antibody AH6 in different locations of colonic epithelia, various histological types of colonic polyps, and adenocarcinomas. Cancer Res 46:2639–2644

Abeloff MD, Rosen ST, Luk GD, Baylin SB, Zeltzman M, Sjoerdsma A (1986) Phase II trials of α-difluoromethylornithine, an inhibitor of polyamine synthesis, in advanced small cell lung cancer and colon cancer. Cancer Treat Rep 70:843–845

Allfrey VG, Boffa LC, Vidali G (1977) Selective inhibition with sodium cyanate of protein synthesis in colon cancer cells. Cancer 40:2692–2698

Arends JW, Verstynen C, Bosman FT, Hilgers J, Steplewski Z (1983) Distribution of monoclonal antibody-defined monosialoganglioside in normal and cancerous human tissues: an immunoperoxidase study. Hybridoma 2:219–229

Armitage NC, Robins RA, Evans DF, Turner DR, Baldwin RW, Hardcastle JD (1985) The influence of tumour cell DNA abnormalities on survival in colorectal cancer. Br J Surg 72:828–830

Atkinson BF, Ernst CS, Herlyn M, Steplewski Z, Sears HF, Koprowski H (1982) Gastrointestinal cancer-associated antigen in immunoperoxidase assay. Cancer Res 42:4820–4823

Balis ME, Higgins PJ, Salser JS (1981) Enzymes of normal, premalignant, and malignant colonic cells. In: Bruce WR, Correa P, Lipkin M, Tannenbaum SR, Wilkins TD (eds) Banbury report no 7: Gastrointestinal cancer: endogenous factors. Cold Spring Harbor, New York, pp 129–139

Bara J, Nardelli J, Gadenne C, Prade M, Bertin P (1984) Differences in the expression of mucus-associated antigens between proximal and distal human colon adenocarcinomas. Br J Cancer 49:495–501

Bara J, Gautier R, Daher N, Zaghouani H, Decaens C (1986) Monoclonal antibodies against oncofetal mucin M1 antigens associated with precancerous colonic mucosae. Cancer Res 46:3983–3989

Basu A, Murthy U, Rodeck U, Herlyn M, Mattes L, Das M (1987) Presence of tumor-associated antigens in epidermal growth factor receptors from different human carcinomas. Cancer Res 47:2531–2536

Bauer KD, Clevenger CV, Endow RK, Murad T, Epstein AL, Scarpelli DG (1986) Simultaneous nuclear antigen and DNA content quantitation using paraffin-embedded colonic tissue and multiparameter flow cytometry. Cancer Res 46:2428–2434

Becher R, Gibas Z, Sandberg AA (1983) Involvement of chromosomes 7 and 12 in large bowel cancer: trisomy 7 and 12q-. Cancer Genet Cytogenet 8:329–332

Bertram JS, Mordan LJ, Domanska-Janik K, Bernacki RJ (1982) Inhibition of in vitro neoplastic transformation by retinoids. In: Arnott MS, Van Eys J, Wang YM (eds) Molecular interrelations of nutrition and cancer. Raven, New York, pp 315–335

Bloom EJ, Itzkowitz SH, Kim YS (in press) Carbohydrate tumor markers in colon cancer and polyps. In: Moyer MP, Posk GH (eds) Colon cancer cells. Academic, New York

Bodmer WF, Bailey CJ, Bodmer J, Bussey HJR, Ellis A, Gorman P, Lucibello FC, Murday VA, Rider SH, Scambler P, Sheer D, Solomon E, Spurr NK (1987) Localization of the gene for familial adenomatous polyposis on chromosome 5. Nature 328:614–616

Boffa LC, Allfrey VG (1977) Changes in chromosomal proteins in colon cancer. Cancer 40:2584–2591

Boffa LC, Diwan BA, Gruss R, Allfrey VG (1980) Differences in colonic nuclear proteins of two mouse strains with different susceptibilities to 1,2-dimethylhydrazine-induced carcinogenesis. Cancer Res 40:1774–1780

Boffa LC, Kozak S, Allfrey VG (1981) Activation of sodium cyanate for selective inhibition of protein synthesis in cultured tumor cells. Cancer Res 41:60–66

Boland CR, Ahnen DJ (1985) The binding of lesions to goblet cell mucin in premalignant colonic epithelium of the CF-1 mouse. Gastroenterology 89:127–137

Boland CR, Clapp NK (1987) Glycoconjugates in the colon of new world monkeys with spontaneous colitis. Gastroenterology 92:625–634

Boland CR, Montgomery CK, Kim YS (1982a) Alterations in human colonic mucin occurring with cellular differentiation and malignant transformation. Proc Natl Acad Sci USA 79:2051–2055

Boland CR, Montgomery CK, Kim YS (1982b) A cancer-associated mucin alteration in benign colonic polyps. Gastroenterology 82:664–672

Bos JL, Fearon ER, Hamilton SR, Verlaan-de Vries M, van Boom JH, van der Eb AJ, Vogelstein B (1987) Prevalence of ras gene mutations in human colorectal cancers. Nature 327:293–297

Bradley SJ, Garfinkle G, Walker E, Salem R, Chen LB, Steele G (1986) Increased expression of the epidermal growth factor receptor on human colon carcinoma cells. Arch Surg 121:1242–1247

Brasitus TA, Dudeja PK, Dahiya R (1986) Premalignant alteration in the lipid composition and fluidity of colonic brush border membranes of rats administered 1,2-dimethylhydrazine. J Clin Invest 77:831–840

Brattain MG, Kimball PM, Pretlow TG (1977) β-hexosaminidase isoenzymes in human colonic carcinoma. Cancer Res 37:731–735

Brattain MG, Green C, Kimball PM, Marks M, Khaled M (1979) Isoenzymes of β-hexosaminidase from normal and colonic carcinoma. Cancer Res 39:4083–4090

Brattain MG, Levine AE, Chakrabarty S, Yeoman LC, Willson JK, Long B (1984) Heterogeneity of human colon carcinoma. Cancer Metastasis Rev 3:177–191

Bresalier RS, Boland CR, Kim YS (1984) Characteristics of colorectal carcinoma cells with high metastatic potential. Gastroenterology 87:115–122

Bresalier RS, Boland CR, Kim YS (1985) Regional differences in normal and cancer-associated glycoconjugates of the human colon. J Natl Cancer Inst 75:249–260

Bresalier RS, Hujanen ES, Raper SE, Roll FJ, Itzkowitz SH, Martin GR, Kim YS (1987a) An animal model for colon cancer metastasis: establishment and characterization of murine cell lines with enhanced liver-metastasizing ability. Cancer Res 47:1398–1406

Bresalier RS, Raper SE, Hujanen ES, Kim YS (1987b) A new animal model for human colon cancer metastasis. Int J Cancer 39:625–630

Bristol JB, Ghatei MA, Smith JHF, Bloom SR, Williamson RCN (1987) Elevated plasma enteroglucagon alone fails to alter distal colonic carcinogenesis in rats. Gastroenterology 92:617–624

Burtin P, Chavanel G, Andre J (1985) The plasmin system in human colonic tumors: an immunofluorescence study. Int J Cancer 35:307–314

Burtin P, Chavanel G, Andre-Bougaran J, Gentile A (1987) The plasmin system in human adenocarcinomas and their metastases. A comparative immunofluorescence study. Int J Cancer 39:170–178

Cajot J-F, Sordat B, Kruithof E, Bachman F (1986a) Human primary colon carcinomas xenografted into nude mice. I. Characterization of plasminogen activators expressed by primary tumors and their xenografts. J Natl Cancer Inst 77:703–712

Cajot J-F, Sordat B, Bachman F (1986b) Human primary colon carcinomas xenografted into nude mice. II. Modulation of tumor plasminogen activator activity by the host tissue environment. J Natl Cancer Inst 77:1099–1107

Chakrabarty S, Jan Y, Miller CA, Brattain MG (1985) Selective nuclear protein phosphorylation/dephosphorylation in subpopulations of human colonic carcinoma cells. Cancer Lett 28:291–297

Chen LB, Rosenberg S, Nadakavukaren KK, Walker ES, Shepherd EL, Steele GD (1985) The cytoskeleton. In: Springer TA (ed) Hybridoma technology and the biosciences and medicine. Plenum, New York, pp 251–268

Chesa PG, Rettig WJ, Melamed MR (1986) Expression of cytokeratins in normal and neoplastic colonic epithelial cells. Implications for cellular differentiation and carcinogenic. Am J Surg Pathol 10:829–835

Coffey RJ, Shipley GD, Moses HL (1986) Production of transforming growth factors by human colon cancer lines. Cancer Res 46:1164–1169

Cooper D, Schermer A, Sun T-T (1985) Classification of human epithelia and their neoplasms using monoclonal antibodies to keratins: strategies, applications, and limitations. Lab Invest 52:243–256

Cordon-Cardo C, Lloyd KO, Sakamoto J, McGroarty ME, Old LJ, Melamed MR (1986) Immunohistologic expression of blood group antigens in normal human gastrointestinal tract and colonic carcinoma. Int J Cancer 37:667–676

Czernobilsky B, Tsou KC (1968) Adenocarcinoma, adenomas and polyps of the colon. Cancer 21:165–177

Dahiya R, Dudeja PK, Brasitus TA (1987) Premalignant alterations in the glycosphingolipid composition of colonic epithelial cells of rats treated with 1,2-dimethylhydrazine. Cancer Res 47:1031–1035

Denk H, Holzner JH, Obiditsch-Mayr I (1975) Epithelial blood group antigens in colon polyps. I. Morphologic distribution and relationship to differentiation. J Natl Cancer Inst 54:1313–1317

Denk H, Tappeiner G, Holzner JH (1974) Blood group substances as carcinofetal antigens in carcinomas of the distal colon. Eur J Cancer 10:487–490

DeRubertis FR, Chayoth R, Field JB (1976) The content and metabolism of cyclic adenosine 3′,5′-monophosphate and cyclic guanosine 3′,5′-monophosphate in adenocarcinoma of the human colon. J Clin Invest 57:641–649

DeRubertis FR, Craven PA (1980) Early alterations in rat colonic mucosal cyclic nucleotide metabolism and protein kinase activity induced by 1,2-dimethylhydrazine. Cancer Res 40:4589–4598

DiFronzo G, Cappelletti V, Miodini P, Bertario L, Ravasi G (1987) Role of cellular retinoic acid binding protein (cRABP) in patients with large bowel cancer. Cancer Detect Prev 10:327–333

d'Istria M, Fasano S, Catuogno F, Gaeta F, Bucci L, Benassal G, Mazzeo F, Delrio G (1986) Androgen and progesterone receptors in colonic and rectal cancers. Dis Colon Rectum 29:263–265

Dutrillaux B, Muleris M (1986) Induction of increased salvage pathways of nucleotide synthesis by dosage effect due to chromosome imbalances may be fundamental in carcinogenesis: the example of colorectal carcinoma. Ann Genet (Paris) 29:11–15

Ernst C, Thurin J, Atkinson B, Wurzel H, Herlyn M, Stromberg N, Cevin C, Koprowski H (1984) Monoclonal antibody localization of A and B isoantigens in normal and malignant fixed human tissues. Am J Pathol 117:451–461

Farber E (1984) Pre-cancerous steps in carcinogenesis. Biochim Biophys Acta 738:171–180

Fearon ER, Hamilton SR, Vogelstein B (1987) Clonal analysis of human colorectal tumors. Science 238:193–197

Feizi T (1985) Demonstration by monoclonal antibodies that carbohydrate structures of glyco-proteins and glycolipids are oncodevelopmental antigens. Nature 314:53–57

Fett JW, Strydom DJ, Lobb RR, Alderman EM, Bethune JL, Riordan JF, Vallee BL (1985) Isolation and characterization of angiogenin, an angiogenic protein from human carcinoma cells. Biochemistry 24:5480–5486

Fex G, Ekelund G, Leandoer L, Sternby NH (1986) Cellular retinol-binding protein (CRBP) in human colorectal adenocarcinoma. Br J Cancer 53:687–690

Filipe MI, Branfoot AC (1974) Abnormal patterns of mucus secretion in apparently normal mucosa of large intestine with carcinoma. Cancer 34:282–290

Finan PJ, Quirke P, Dixon MF, Dyson JED, Giles GR, Bird CC (1986) Is DNA aneuploidy a good prognostic indicator in patients with advanced colorectal cancer? Br J Cancer 54:327–330

Forrester K, Almoguera C, Han K, Grizzle WE, Perucho M (1987) Detection of high incidence of K-*ras* oncogenes during human colon tumorigenesis. Nature 327:298–303

Fozard JBJ, Quirke P, Dixon MF, Giles GR, Bird CC (1986) DNA aneuploidy in ulcerative colitis. Gut 27:1414–1418

Freeman HJ, Kim Y, Kim YS (1978) Glycoprotein metabolism in normal proximal and distal rat colon and changes associated with 1,2-dimethylhydrazine-induced colonic neoplasia. Cancer Res 38:3385–3390

Freeman HJ, Lotan R, Kim YS (1980) Application of lectins for detection of goblet cell glycoconjugate differences in proximal and distal colon of the rat. Lab Invest 42:405–412

Friedman E, Verderame M, Lipkin M, Pollack R (1985) Altered actin cytoskeletal patterns in two premalignant stages in human colon carcinoma development. Cancer Res 45:3236–3242

Friedman E, Verderame M, Winawer S, Pollack R (1984) Actin cytoskeletal organization loss in the benign-to-malignant tumor transition in cultured human colonic epithelial cells. Cancer Res 44:3040–3050

Fukushi Y, Hakomori S, Nudelman E, Cochran N (1984a) Novel fucolipids accumulating in human adenocarcinoma. II. Selective isolation of hybridoma antibodies that differentially recognize mono-, di-, and trifucosylated type 2 chain. J Biol Chem 259:4681–4685

Fukushi Y, Nudelman E, Levery SB, Rauvala H, Hakomori S (1984b) Novel fucolipids accumulating in human adenocarcinoma. III. A hybridoma antibody (FH6) defining a human cancer-associated difucoganglioside ($VI^3NeuAcV^3III^3Fuc_2nLc_6$). J Biol Chem 259:10511–10517

Fukushima K, Hirota M, Terasaki PI, Wakisaka A, Togashi H, Chia D, Suyama N, Fukushi Y, Nudelman E, Hakomori S (1984) Characterization of sialosylated Lewis^x a new tumor associated antigen. Cancer Res 44:5279–5285

Geiger B, Kreis TE, Gigi O, Schmid E, Mittnacht S, Jorcano JL, von Bassewitz DB, Franke WW (1984) Dynamic rearrangements of cytokeratins in living cells. In: Levine AJ, Vande Wonde GF, Topp WC, Watson JD (eds) Cancer cells, the transformed phenotype. Cold Spring Harbor, New York, pp 201–215

Gelister JSK, Mahmoud M, Gaffney PJ, Boulos PB (1986) Plasminogen activators in human colorectal neoplasia. Br Med J 293:728–731

Gelister JSK, Jass JR, Mahmoud M, Gaffney PJ, Boulos PB (1987) Role of urokinase in colorectal neoplasia. Br J Surg 74:460–463

Goh HS, Jass JR (1986) DNA content and the adenoma-carcinoma sequence in the colorectum. J Clin Pathol 39:387–392

Gold DV, Miller F (1978) Comparison of human colonic mucoprotein antigen from normal and neoplastic mucosa. Cancer Res 38:3204–3211

Gold DV, Shochat D, Miller F (1981) Protease digestion of colonic mucin: evidence for the existence of two immunochemically distinct mucins. J Biol Chem 256:6354–6358

Gong E, Hirohashi S, Shimosato Y, Watanabe M, Ino Y, Teshima S, Kodaira S (1985) Expression of carbohydrate antigen 19-9 and stage specific embryonic antigen 1 in nontumorous and tumorous epithelia of the human colon and rectum. J Natl Cancer Inst 75:447–454

Gooi HC, Feizi T, Kapadia A, Knowles BB, Solter D, Evans MJ (1981) Stage specific embryonic antigen involves $\alpha1 \rightarrow 3$ fucosylated type 2 blood group chains. Nature 292:156–158

Hakomori S (1981) Glycosphingolipids in cellular interaction, differentiation, and oncogenesis. Annu Rev Biochem 50:733–764

Hakomori S (1985) Aberrant glycosylation in cancer cell membranes as focused on glycolipids overview and perspectives. Cancer Res 45:2405–2414

Hakomori S, Fukuda M, Sekiguchi K, Carter WG (1984) Chemistry and function of pericellular and intercellular glycoproteins: fibronectin, laminin and other matrix components. In: Piez K, Reddi AH (eds) Extracellular matrix biochemistry. Elsevier/North-Holland Biomedical, Amsterdam, pp 229–275

Hamilton SR, Luk GD (1987) Induction of colonic mucosal ornithine decarboxylase activity by chronic dietary ethanol consumption in rats. Gastroenterology 92:1423

Hand PH, Thor A, Schlom J, Rao CN, Liotta L (1985) Expression of laminin receptor in normal and carcinomatous human tissues as defined by a monoclonal antibody. Cancer Res 45:2713–2719

Hedley DW, Friedlander ML, Taylor IW, Rugg CA, Musgrove E (1983) Method for analysis of cellular DNA content in paraffin-embedded pathological material using flow cytometry. J Histochem Cytochem 31:1333–1335

Herrera-Ornelas L, Porter C, Pera P, Greco W, Petrelli NJ, Mittelman A (1987) A comparison of ornithine decarboxylase and S-adenosylmethionine decarboxylase activity in human large bowel mucosa, polyps, and colorectal adenocarcinoma. J Surg Res 42:56–60

Herzfeld A, Greengard O (1980) Enzyme activities in human fetal and neoplastic tissues. Cancer 46:2047–2054

Hoagland JG, Scoggin S, Giavazzi R, Campbell D, Kanellopoulos K, Jessup JM (1986) Tumor-derived suppressor factors (TDSFs) in normal and neoplastic colon and rectum. J Surg Res 40:467–474

Holmes EH, Ostrander GK, Clausen H, Graem N (1987) Oncofetal expression of Le^x carbohydrate antigens in human colonic adenocarcinomas. Regulation through type 2 core chain synthesis rather than fucosylation. J Biol Chem 262:11331–11338

Hoosein NM, Brattain DE, McKnight MK, Levine AE, Brattain MG (1987) Characterization of the inhibitory effects of transforming growth factor-β on a human colon carcinoma cell line. Cancer Res 47:2950–2954

Hwang WI, Sack TL, Kim YS (1986) Effects of cyclic adenosine 3′,5′-monophosphate upon glycoprotein and carcinoembryonic antigen synthesis and release by human colon cancer cells. Cancer Res 46:3371–3374

Irimura T, Ota DM, Cleary KR (1987) *Ulex europeus* agglutinin-I-reactive high molecular weight glycoproteins of adenocarcinoma of distal colon and rectum and their possible relationship with metastatic potential. Cancer Res 47:881–889

Itzkowitz SH, Yuan M, Ferrell LD, Palekar A, Kim YS (1986a) Cancer-associated alterations of blood group antigen expression in human colorectal polyps. Cancer Res 46:5976–5984

Itzkowitz SH, Yuan M, Fukushi Y, Palekar A, Phelps PC, Shamsuddin AM, Trump BF, Hakamori S, Kim YS (1986b) Lewis^x- and sialylated Lewis^x-related antigen expression in human malignant and nonmalignant colonic tissues. Cancer Res 46:2627–2632

Izbicki JR, Schmitz R, Kamran D, Izbicki W (1983) Androgens as promoters of colon carcinogenesis. Cancer Detect Prev 6:355–362

Izbicki JR, Wambach G, Hamilton SR, Harnisch E, Hogenschurz R, Izbicki W, Kusche J (1986) Androgen receptors in experimentally induced colon carcinogenesis. J Cancer Res Clin Oncol 112:39–46

Kaizu T, Levery SB, Nudelman E, Stenkamp RE, Hakomori S (1986) Novel fucolipids of human adenocarcinoma: monoclonal antibody specific for trifucosyl Le^y (III^{3}FucV^{3}FucVI^{2}FucnLc$_6$) and a possible three-dimensional epitope structure. J Biol Chem 261:11254–11258

Kanagalingam K, Balis ME (1975) In vivo repair of rat intestinal DNA damage by alkylating agents. Cancer 36:2364–2372

Karlin DA, McBath M, Jones RD, Elwyn KE, Romsdahl MM (1985) Hypergastrinemia and colorectal carcinogenesis in the rat. Cancer Lett 29:73–78

Kennedy MFG, Tutton PJM, Barkla DH (1985) Adrenergic factors regulating cell division in the colonic crypt epithelium during carcinogenesis and in colonic adenoma and adenocarcinoma. Br J Cancer 52:383–390

Kijima-Suda I, Miyamoto Y, Toyoshima S, Itoh M, Osawa T (1986) Inhibition of experimental pulmonary metastasis of mouse colon adenocarcinoma 26 sublines by a sialic acid: nucleoside conjugate having sialyltransferase inhibiting activity. Cancer Res 46:858–862

Kim YS, Isaacs R (1975) Glycoprotein metabolism in inflammatory and neoplastic diseases of the human colon. Cancer Res 35:2092–2097

Kim YS, Isaacs R, Perdomo JM (1974) Alterations of membrane glycopeptides in human colonic adenocarcinoma. Proc Natl Acad Sci USA 71:4869–4873

Kim YS, Whitehead JS, Perdomo J (1979) Glycoproteins of cultured epithelial cells from human colonic adenocarcinoma and fetal intestine. Eur J Cancer 15:725–735

Kim YS, Yuan M, Itzkowitz SH, Sun Q, Kaizu T, Palekar A, Trump BF, Hakomori S (1986) Expression of Le^y and extended Le^y blood groups-related antigens in human malignant, premalignant and nonmalignant colonic tissues. Cancer Res 46:5985–5992

Kingsnorth AN, King WW, Diekema KA, McCann PP, Ross JS, Malt RA (1983a) Inhibition of ornithine decarboxylase with 2-difluoromethylornithine: reduced incidence of dimethylhydrazine-induced colon tumors in mice. Cancer Res 43:2545–2549

Kingsnorth AN, Russell WE, McCann PP, Diekema KA, Malt RA (1983b) Effects of
    α-difluoromethylornithine and 5-fluorouracil on the proliferation of a human colon adeno-
    carcinoma cell line. Cancer Res 43:4035–4038
Kokal W, Sheibani K, Terz J, Horoda JR (1986) Tumor DNA content in the prognosis of
    colorectal carcinoma. JAMA 255:3123–3127
Koprowski H, Steplewski Z, Mitchell K, Herlyn M, Herlyn D, Fuhrer P (1979) Colorectal
    carcinoma antigens detected by hybridoma antibodies. Somatic Cell Genet 5:957–971
Kornfeld R, Kornfeld S (1981) Structure of glycoproteins and their oligosaccharide units. In:
    Lennary WJ (ed) The biochemistry of glycoproteins and proteoglycans. Plenum, New York,
    pp 1–34
Koss LG, Greenbaum E (1986) Measuring DNA in human cancer. JAMA 255:3158–3159
Kuhns WS, Schoentag R (1981) Carcinoma-related alterations of glycosyltransferases in human
    tissue. Cancer Res 41:2767–2772
Kurosaka A, Nakajima H, Funakoshi I, Matsuyama M, Nagayo T, Yamashina I (1983) Struc-
    ture of the major oligosaccharides from a human rectal adenocarcinoma glycoprotein. J Biol
    Chem 258:11 594–11 598
LaMont JT, Isselbacher KJ (1975) Alterations in glycosyltransferase activity in human colon
    cancer. J Natl Cancer Inst 54:53–56
LaMont JT, O'Gorman TA (1978) Experimental colon cancer. Gastroenterology 75:1157–1169
LaMont JT, Weiser MM, Isselbacher KJ (1974) Cell surface glycosyltransferase activity in
    normal and neoplastic intestinal epithelium of the rat. Cancer Res 34:3225–3228
LaMurglia GM, Lacaine R, Malt RA (1986) High ornithine decarboxylase activity and poly-
    amine levels in human colorectal neoplasia. Ann Surg 204:89–93
Langvad E (1968) Lactate dehydrogenese isoenzyme patterns in the tumor bearing colon. Int J
    Cancer 3:17–29
Lazarus P, Panasci LC (1987) Mechanism of decrease of protein synthesis by sodium cyanate
    in murine P388 leukemia cells. Cancer Res 47:5102–5107
Levin B, Reichmann A (1986) Chromosomes and large bowel tumors. Cancer Genet Cytogenet
    19:159–162
Levine AE, McRae LJ, Hamilton DA, Brattain DE, Yeoman LC, Brattain MG (1985) Identi-
    fication of endogenous inhibitory growth factors from a human colon carcinoma cell line.
    Cancer Res 45:2248–2254
Liotta LA (1986) Tumor invasion and metastasis – role of the extracellular matrix: Rhoads
    memorial lecture. Cancer Res 46:1–7
Liotta LA, Kleinerman J, Catanzara P, Gynbrandt D (1977) Degradation of basement mem-
    brane by murine tumor cells. J Natl Cancer Inst 58:1427–1439
Luk GD, Hamilton SR, Yang P, Smith JA, O'Ceallaigh D, McAvinchey D, Hyland J (1986)
    Kinetic changes in mucosal ornithine decarboxylase activity during azoxymethane-induced
    colonic carcinogenesis in the rat. Cancer Res 46:4449–4452
Luk GD, Silverman AL, Giardiello FM (1987) Biochemical markers in patients with familial
    colonic neoplasia. Semin Surg Oncol 3:126–132
Magnani JL, Nilsson B, Brockhaus M, Zopf D, Steplewski Z, Koprowski H, Ginsburg V (1982)
    A monoclonal antibody-defined antigen associated with gastrointestinal cancer is a ganglio-
    side containing sialylated lacto-N-fucopentaose II. J Biol Chem 257:14 365–14 369
Magnani JL, Steplewski Z, Koprowski H, Ginsburg V (1983) Identification of the gastro-
    intestinal and pancreatic associated antigen detected by monoclonal antibody 19-9 in the sera
    of patients as a mucin. Cancer Res 43:5489–5492
Marks ME, Danbury BH, Miller CA, Brattain MG (1983) Cell surface proteins and glycopro-
    teins from biologically different human colon carcinoma cell lines. J Natl Cancer Inst
    71:663–771
Matsushita Y, Yonezawa S, Nakamura T, Shimizu S, Ozawa M, Muramatsu T, Sato E (1985)
    Carcinoma-specific Ulex europaeus agglutinin-I binding glycoproteins of human colorectal
    carcinoma and its relation to carcinoembryonic antigen. J Natl Cancer Inst 75:219–226
Matthews J, Cooke T (1986) Changes in crypt cell DNA content during experimental colonic
    carcinogenesis. Br J Cancer 53:787–791
McGinty F, Delides G, Harrison D (1973) The significance of enzyme histochemical patterns in
    carcinoma of the large intestine in man. Gut 14:502–505
McKinley M, Budman D, Caccese W, Weissman G, Scheidt N, Kahn E, Bronzo R (1985)

Evaluation of colonic neoplasia by flow cytometry of endoscopic biopsies. Am J Gastroenterol 80:47–49

Melamed MR, Enker WE, Banner P, Janov AJ, Kessler G, Darzynkiewicz Z (1986) Flow cytometry of colorectal carcinoma with three-year follow-up. Dis Colon Rectum 29:184–186

Mian N, Cowen DM (1974) Glycosidases in normal and dimethylhydrazine-treated rats and mice with special reference to the colonic tumors. Br J Cancer 29:438–446

Mian N, Herries DG, Cowen DM, Batte EA (1979) The multiple forms and kinetic properties of the N-acetyl-β-D-hexosaminidases from colonic tumors and mucosa of rats treated with 1,2-dimethylhydrazine. Biochem J 177:319–330

Moon RC, Fricks CM (1977) Influence of gonadal hormones and age on 1,2-dimethylhydrazine-induced colon carcinogenesis. Cancer 40:2502–2508

Moorehead RJ, Hoper M, McKelvey ST (1987) Assessment of ornithine decarboxylase activity in rectal mucosa as a marker of colorectal adenomas and carcinomas. Br J Surg 74:364–365

Mooseker MS (1985) Organization, chemistry and assembly of the cytoskeletal apparatus of the intestinal brush border. Annu Rev Cell Biol 1:209–241

Morris DR, Marton LJ (eds) (1981) Polyamines in biology and medicine. Dekker, New York

Moshier JA, Luk GD, Huang RCC (1986) mRNA from human colon tumor and mucosa related to the *pol* gene of an endogenous A-type retrovirus. Biochem Biophys Res Commun 139:1071–1077

Nachlas MN, Hannibal MJ (1961) Histochemical observations of the polyp-carcinoma sequence. Surg Gynecol Obstet 112:534–542

Narisawa T, Hosaka S, Niwa M (1985) Prostaglandin E_2 counteracts the inhibition by indomethacin of rat colon ornithine decarboxylase induction by deoxycholic acid. Jpn J Cancer Res 76:338–344

Nelson RL, Wilson W, Samelson SL, Khoobyarian N (1987) The interaction of retrovirus and chemical carcinogen in experimental colon carcinogenesis. Surgery 101:172–175

Odagiri E, Jibiki K, Demura R, Shinozaki H, Nakamura S, Demura H, Suzuki H (1984) Steroid receptors and the distribution of IR-carcinoembryonic antigen in colon cancer. Dis Colon Rectum 27:787–791

Odagiri E, Jibiki K, Kato Y, Nakamura S, Oda S-I, Demura R, Demura H (1985) Steroid receptors in dimethylhydrazine-induced colon carcinogenesis. Cancer 56:2627–2634

O'Gorman TA, LaMont JT (1978) Glycoprotein synthesis and secretion in human colon cancers and normal colonic mucosa. Cancer Res 38:2784–2789

Olden K, Parnet JB, White SL (1982) Carbohydrate moieties of glycoproteins, a reevaluation of their function. Biochim Biophys Acta 650:209–232

Ong DE, Markert C, Chiu J-F (1978) Cellular binding proteins for vitamin A in colorectal adenocarcinoma of rat. Cancer Res 38:4422–4426

Paraskeva C, Buckle BG, Sheer D, Wigley CB (1984) The isolation and characterization of colorectal epithelial cell lines at different stages in malignant transformation from familial polyposis coli patients. Int J Cancer 34:49–56

Paris H, Bouscarel B, Cortinovis C, Murat JC (1985) Growth-related variation of α-adrenergic receptivity in the HT 29 adenocarcinoma cell-line from human colon. FEBS Lett 184:82–86

Pegg AE, McCann PP (1982) Polyamine metabolism and function. Am J Physiol 243:C212–C221

Petersen SE (1985) Flow cytometry of human colorectal tumors: nuclear isolation by detergent technique. Cytometry 6:452–460

Podolsky DK, Weiser MM, Westwood JC, Gammon M (1977) Cancer-associated serum galactosyltransferase activity. J Biol Chem 252:1807–1813

Quirke P, Fozard JBJ, Dixon MF, Dyson JED, Giles GR, Bird CC (1986) DNA aneuploidy in colorectal adenomas. Br J Cancer 53:477–481

Quirke P, Dixon MF, Clayden AD, Durdey P, Dyson JED, Williams NS, Bird CC (1987) Prognostic significance of DNA aneuploidy and cell proliferation in rectal adenocarcinomas. J Pathol 151:285–291

Reichmann A, Martin P, Levin B (1981) Chromosomal banding patterns in human large bowel cancer. Int J Cancer 28:431–440

Reid PE, Culling CFA, Dunn WL, Ramey CW, Clay MG (1975) Differences in chemical composition between the epithelial glycoproteins of the upper and lower halves of rat colon. Can J Biochem 53:1328–1332

Reid PE, Owen DA, Dunn WL, Ramey CW, Lazosky, Clay MG (1985) Chemical and histochemical studies of normal and diseased human gastrointestinal tract. III. Changes in the histochemical and chemical properties of the epithelial glycoproteins in the mucosa close to colonic tumors. Histochem J 17:171–181

Rousset M, Paris H, Chevalier G, Terrain B, Murat J-C, Zweibaum A (1984) Growth-related enzymatic control of glycogen metabolism in cultured human tumor cells. Cancer Res 44:154–160

Rozhin J, Wilson PS, Bull AW, Nigro ND (1984) Ornithine decarboxylase activity in the rat and human colon. Cancer Res 44:3226–3230

Russell DH (1983) Clinical relevance of polyamines. CRC Crit Rev Clin Lab Sci 18:261–311

Rybak SM, Fett JW, Yao Q-Z, Vallee BL (1987) Angiogenin mRNA in human tumor and normal cells. Biochem Biophys Res Commun 146:1240–1248

Sakamoto J, Furukawa K, Cordon-Cardo C, Yin BWT, Rettig WJ, Oettgen HF, Old LJ, Lloyd KO (1986) Expression of Lewis[a], Lewis[b], X and Y blood group antigens in human colonic tumors and normal tissue and in human tumor-derived cell lines. Cancer Res 46:1553–1561

Sakamoto S, Kuwa K, Tsukada K, Sagara T, Kasahara N, Okamoto R (1987) Relative activities of thymidylate synthetase and thymidine kinase in 1,2-dimethylhydrazine-induced colon carcinomas in rats. Carcinogenesis 8:405–408

Sakamoto S, Sagara T, Iwama T, Kawasaki T, Okamoto R (1985) Increased activities of thymidine kinase isozymes in human colon polyp and carcinoma. Carcinogenesis 6:917–919

Salo T, Liotta LA, Trggvason K (1983) Purification and characterization of a murine basement membrane collagen-degrading enzyme secreted by metastatic tumor cells. J Biol Chem 258:3058–3063

Sani BP, Banerjee CK (1983) Cellular receptor mediation of the action of retinoic acid. In: Meyskens FL, Prasad KN (eds) Modulation and mediation of cancer by vitamins. Karger, Basel, pp 153–161

Sani BP, Banerjee CK, Peckham JC (1980) The presence of binding proteins for retinoic acid and dihydrotestosterone in murine and human colon tumors. Cancer 46:2421–2429

Savage AP, Matthews JL, Ghatei MA, Cooke T, Bloom SR (1987) Enteroglucagon and experimental intestinal carcinogenesis in the rat. Gut 28:33–39

Saydjari R, Townsend CM, Barranco SC, Thompson JC (1987) Effects of cyclosporine and α-difluoromethylornithine on the growth of mouse colon cancer in vitro. Life Sci 40:359–366

Shamsuddin AKM, Trump BF (1981) Colon epithelium. I. Light microscopic, histochemical, and ultrastructural features of normal colon epithelium of male Fischer 344 rats. J Natl Cancer Inst 66:375–388

Shi ZR, McIntyre LJ, Knowles BB, Solter D, Kim YS (1984) Expression of a carbohydrate differentiation antigen stage specific embryonic antigen 1 in human colonic adenocarcinoma. Cancer Res 44:1142–1147

Shioda Y, Brown WR, Ahnen AJ (1987) Serial observations of colonic carcinogenis in the rat. Premalignant mucosa binds *Ulex europeus* agglutinin. Gastroenterology 92:1–12

Shonk CE, Arison RN, Koven BJ, Majima H, Boxer GE (1965) Enzyme patterns in human tissues. III. Glycolytic enzymes in normal and malignant tissues of the colon and rectum. Cancer Res 25:206–213

Siddiqui B, Whitehead JS, Kim YS (1978) Glycosphingolipids in human colonic adenocarcinoma. J Biol Chem 253:2168–2175

Singh P, Walker JP, Townsend CM, Thompson JC (1986) Role of gastrin and gastrin receptors on the growth of a transplantable mouse colon carcinoma (MC-26) in BALB/c mice. Cancer Res 46:1612–1616

Solomon E, Voss R, Hall V, Bodmer WF, Jass JR, Jeffreys AJ, Lucibello FC, Patel I, Rider SH (1987) Chromosome 5 allele loss in human colorectal carcinomas. Nature 328:616–619

Sporn MB, Roberts AB (1985) Autocrine growth factors and cancer. Nature 313:745–747

Sporn MB, Dunlop NM, Newton DL, Smith JM (1976) Prevention of chemical carcinogenesis by vitamin A and its synthetic analogs (retinoids). Fed Proc 35:1332–1338

Stebbings WSL, Farthing MJG, Vinson GP, Northover JMA, Wood RFM (1986) Androgen receptors in rectal and colonic cancer. Dis Colon Rectum 29:95–98

Stevens RH, Loven DP (1980) Intracellular adenosine and guanosine 3′,5′-cyclic monophosphate concentrations in rat small and large bowel following a single and multiple exposure to 1,2-dimethylhydrazine. Cancer Lett 9:151–159

Stuart CA, Prince MJ, Peters EJ, Smith FE, Townsend CM, Poffenbarger PL (1986) Insulin receptor proliferation: a mechanism for tumor-associated hypoglycemia. J Clin Endocrinol Metab 63:879–885

Summerton J, Flynn M, Cooke T, Taylor I (1983) Bile acid receptors in colorectal cancer. Br J Surg 70:549–551

Summerton J, Goeting N, Trotter GA, Taylor I (1985) Effect of deoxycholic acid on the tumour incidence, distribution, and receptor status of colorectal cancer in the rat model. Digestion 31:77–81

Sun AS, Sepkowitz K, Geller SA (1981) A study of some mitochondrial and peroxisomal enzymes in human colonic adenocarcinoma. Lab Invest 44:13–17

Sun Q, Siddiqui B, Nudelman E, Hakomori S, Ho JJL, Kim YS (1987) New murine monoclonal antibodies to a human colonic cancer-associated glycolipid, extended difucosylated Le^y glycolipid. Cancer J 1:213–221

Sunkara PS, Rao PN, Nishioka K, Brinkley BR (1979) Role of polyamines in cytokinesis of mammalian cells. Exp Cell Res 119:63–68

Suzuki H, Umehara N (1986) Early mucosal changes in dimethylhdrazine-induced colonic carcinogenesis in rats. Jpn J Surg 16:140–143

Suzuki H, Honda E, Matsumoto K, Iriyama K (1985) Tissue CEA determination and cytophotometric DNA analysis of colorectal mucosa in patients with colorectal cancer. Jpn J Surg 15:449–454

Takano S, Matsushima M, Erturk E, Bryan GT (1981) Early induction of rat colonic epithelial ornithine and S-adenosyl-L-methionine decarboxylase activities by N-methyl-N'-nitro-N-nitrosoguanidine or bile salts. Cancer Res 41:624–628

Talpaz M, Plager C, Quesada J, Benjamin R, Kantarjian H, Gutterman J (1986) Difluoromethylornithine and leukocyte interferon: a phase I study in cancer patients. Eur J Cancer Clin Oncol 22:685–689

Tempero M (1986) Bile acids, ornithine decarboxylase, and cell proliferation in colon cancer: a review. Dig Dis 4:49–56

Ten Kate J, Van Den Ingh HFGM, Khan PM, Bosman FT (1986) Adenosine deaminase complexing protein (ADCP) immunoreactivity in colorectal adenocarcinoma. Int J Cancer 37:479–485

Tricoli JV, Rall LB, Karakousis CP, Herrera L, Petrelli NJ, Bell GI, Shows TB (1986) Enhanced levels of insulin-like growth factor messenger RNA in human colon carcinomas and liposarcomas. Cancer Res 46:6169–6173

Trotta PP, Balis ME (1977) Enzyme variants in normal and neoplastic intestinal mucosa. Cancer 40:2592–2599

Tsao D, Freeman HJ, Kim YS (1979) β-Hexosaminidase isoenzymes in tissues, cultured cells, and media from human fetal intestine and colonic adenocarcinoma. Cancer Res 39:3405–3410

Tutton PJM, Barkla DH (1982) The influence of androgens, antiandrogens, and castration on cell proliferation in the jejunal and colonic crypt epithelia, and in dimethylhydrazine-induced adenocarcinoma of rat colon. Virchows Arch [B] 38:351–355

Tutton PJM, Barkla DH (1986) Comparison of the effects of an ornithine decarboxylase inhibitor on the intestinal epithelium and on intestinal tumors. Cancer Res 46:6091–6094

Warburg O (1956) On the origin of cancer cells. Science 123:309–314

Wattenberg LW (1959) A histochemical study of five oxidative enzymes in carcinoma of the large intestine in man. Am J Pathol 35:113–137

Weber G (1977) Enzymology of cancer cells. N Engl J Med 296:486–493

Weber G, Kizaki H, Tzeng D, Shiotani T, Olah E (1978) Colon tumor: enzymology of the neoplastic program. Life Sci 23:729–736

Weber G, Lui MS, Takeda E, Denton JE (1980) Enzymology of human colon tumors. Life Sci 27:793–799

Weiner HL, Weiner LH, Swain JL (1987) Tissue distribution and developmental expression of the messenger RNA encoding angiogenin. Science 237:280–282

Weiser MM, Podolsky DK, Isselbacher KJ (1976) Cancer-associated isoenzyme of serum galactosyltransferase. Proc Natl Acad Sci USA 73:1319–1327

Whitehead JS, Fearney FJ, Kim YS (1979) Glycosyltransferase and glycosidase activities in cultured human fetal and colonic adenocarcinoma cell lines. Cancer Res 39:1259–1263

Wice BM, Trugnan G, Pinto M, Rousset M, Chevalier G, Dussaulx E, Lacroix B, Zweibaum A (1985) The intracellular accumulation of UDP-*N*-adenylhexosamine is concomitant with the mobility of human colon cancer cells to differentiate. J Biol Chem 260:139–146

Wiley EL, Mendelsohn G, Eggleston JC (1981) Distribution of carcinoembryonic antigens and blood group substances in adenocarcinoma of the colon. Lab Invest 44:507–513

Winsett OE, Townsend CM, Glass EJ, Rae-Venter B, Thompson JC (1986) Gastrin stimulates growth of colon cancer. Surgery 99:302–307

Wobbes T, Beex LV, Koenders AM (1984) Estrogen and progestin receptors in colonic cancer? Dis Colon Rectum 27:591–592

Yamakawa T, Nagai Y (1978) Glycolipids at the cell surface and their biological significance. Trends Biochem Sci 3:128–131

Yeger H, Baumal R, Kahn HJ, Duwe G, Phillips MJ (1986) The use of cytoskeletal characteristics of tumor cells for the diagnosis of colon and breast adenocarcinomas. Am J Clin Pathol 86:697–705

Yonezawa S, Nakamura T, Tanaka S, Sato E (1982) Glycoconjugate with *Ulex europaeus* agglutinin-1-binding sites in normal mucosa, adenoma, and carcinoma of the human large bowel. J Natl Cancer Inst 69:777–785

Yonezawa S, Nakamura T, Tanaka S, Moruta K, Nishi M, Sato E (1983) Binding of *Ulex europaeus* agglutinin 1 in polyposis coli: comparative study with solitary adenocarcinoma in the sigmoid colon and rectum. J Natl Cancer Inst 71:19–24

Youakim A, Herscovics A (1985) Cell surface glycopeptides from human intestinal epithelial cell lines derived from normal colon and colon adenocarcinomas. Cancer Res 45:5505–5511

Yuan M, Itzkowitz SH, Boland CR, Kim YD, Tomita JT, Polekas A, Bennington JL, Trump BJ, Kim YS (1986) Comparison of T-antigen expression in normal, premalignant, and malignant human colonic tissue using lectin and antibody immunohistochemistry. Cancer Res 46:4841–4847

Yuan M, Itzkowitz SH, Ferrell LD, Fukushi Y, Palekar A, Hakomori S, Kim YS (1987) Expression of Lewis[x] and sialylated Lewis[x] antigens in human colorectal polyps. J Natl Cancer Inst 78:479–488

Yuan M, Itzkowitz SH, Palekar A, Shamsuddin AM, Phelps PC, Trump BF, Kim YS (1985) Distribution of blood group antigens A, B, H, Lewis[a], and Lewis[b] in human normal, fetal, and malignant colonic tissue. Cancer Res 45:4499–4511

Zweibaum A, Pinto M, Chevalier G, Dussaulx E, Triadau N, Lacroix B, Haffen K, Brun J-L, Rousset M (1985) Enterocytic differentiation of a subpopulation of the human colon tumor cell line HT-29 selected for growth in sugar-free medium and its inhibition by glucose. J Cell Physiol 122:21–29

Inhibitors of Colorectal Carcinogenesis: Experimental and Therapeutic Aspects

N. D. Nigro and A. W. Bull Jr

Wayne State University, School of Medicine, Clinical Laboratories, 645 Mullett Street, Detroit, MI 48226, USA

Contents

Introduction

Evidence from epidemiological, clinical, and laboratory studies including animal experiments suggests that cancer develops from a complex, multistage interaction between genetic and environmental factors. In colorectal cancer, the environmental component of the process, which is diet, contributes more to cancer formation than the inheritance factor in most people (Doll 1980). The diet contains a large number of compounds that affect the carcinogenic process in some manner, and it is their combined effect that determines the degree of cancer risk from dietary factors. Since the identification and elimination of the carcinogens that initiate colon cancer formation appear to be difficult, the current emphasis in research on prevention is focused mainly on ways to alter the carcinogenic process. While a complete interruption of the process is desirable, it is not essential because simply slowing its progression enough so that clinical cancer does not develop during the normal span of life would also prevent cancer morbidity and mortality.

Quantitatively the ingredients of the diet can be divided into two classes, sometimes referred to as "macro- and microconstituents". Both classes contain substances that

Table 1. Inhibitors of intestinal carcinogenesis

Natural	Synthetic
Selenium	Phenols
Calcium	Disulfiram
Plant sterols	Prostaglandin inhibitors
Vitamins	Difluoromethylornithine
Diallyl sulfide	
Protease inhibitors	
Isocyanates	

affect carcinogenesis. However, this discussion is limited to those present in relatively small amounts (microconstituents). It is further restricted to those that inhibit cancer development in the colon. Since the colon is the most distal part of the digestive tract and since it has a slowly moving, highly bacterial content, dietary factors act on the carcinogenic process in an indirect and complex manner. This makes intervention more difficult than in tissues where the action is more direct. However, this area of research has become more productive recently, and it appears that acceptable diets can include enough inhibitors to overcome the enhancement factors thus reducing cancer risk. If the effect is strong enough, it would lower the incidence of colorectal cancer in countries where the disease is common, as it is in the United States.

Inhibitors can be grouped according to the time in the carcinogenic process at which they act, to their chemical class, or to their mode of action (Wattenberg 1983). Most inhibitors to be discussed in this chapter affect carcinogenesis after the initiation event, but at least one is known to affect initiation only, and others may act on more than one phase of the process. Furthermore, the mechanism of action of most inhibitors is poorly understood. Consequently, it is difficult to classify them satisfactorily, so we have elected to review inhibitors according to whether they occur naturally in the diet or are synthetic chemicals or drugs (Table 1).

Natural Inhibitors

Selenium

Shamberger and Willis (1971) were among the first to suggest the possibility that cancer mortality rates have an inverse association with the amount of selenium (Se) in the water and plants or with the level of selenium in banked blood in different regions of the United States. In a recent review, Clark (1985) concluded that the evidence supporting this hypothesis that decreased selenium status in humans is positively associated with cancer mortality is increasing. It is particularly evident in breast and colorectal cancer. Human intervention trials are in progress to test the effectiveness of selenium supplementation in the prevention of cancer (Clark and Combs 1986).

Selenium occurs naturally in several different forms in water, soil, and in food grown in that soil. Inorganic selenium is present as selenide (S^{2-}), selenite (SeO_3^{2-}), and selenate (SeO_4^{2-}). The organic forms of selenium of major importance in carcinogenesis are selenomethionine and selenocysteine which are analogues of the sulfur-containing amino acids (Buell 1983). Different forms of selenium have been used in investigations related to cancer, but the inorganic species has been used in most animal experiments.

Many animal studies show that selenium-supplemented diets inhibit cancer in several organs including the colon. However, the amount required is far in excess of that needed to maintain adequate nutrition, which in the rat is about 0.25 ppm. For example, Jacobs et al. (1977) found that the addition of 4.0 ppm selenite in the drinking water of rats fed a normal diet reduced the incidence of dimethylhydrazine (DMH) -induced colon tumors from 87% to 40%, and the tumor frequency from 2.6 to 0.73 per rat. Later, Soullier et al. (1981) showed that the addition of selenite (8.0 ppm) to the drinking water of rats fed a high-fat diet reduced the number of azoxymethane (AOM) -induced colon tumors from 6.5 to 3.1 per rat. The inhibition occurred almost exclusively in the proximal half of the colon where the concentration of selenium in the tissue was greatest. Although no gross toxic effect was observed in these animals, others have reported selenium toxicity at levels as low as 8 ppm in rats (Jacobs and Frost 1981).

The mechanism of selenium inhibition of tumorigenesis is unknown. The effect is not organ specific, suggesting that it is a generalized systemic mechanism. The dominant theory is that since selenium is an essential component of glutathione peroxidase, it acts by protecting the cell against oxidative damage (Lane and Medina 1983). However, Le Boeuf and Hoekstra (1985) have shown that selenium in high concentrations depresses cell proliferation in general through a decrease in protein synthesis. Whatever the mechanism, it is clear that the inhibitory effect of selenium in the animal model occurs only when it is given in amounts in excess of that required for adequate nutrition.

In humans, the daily requirement for selenium is not known precisely, but a range of 50–200 µg is suggested by the National Research Council (1980). Current evidence from all sources indicates that higher levels are needed to prevent cancer (Levander and Morris 1984). Supplements of at least 300 µg per day have been suggested for use in human chemoprevention trials. Larger amounts may be necessary, especially for people who have a high cancer risk (Clark and Combs 1986).

Studies are needed to determine the optimal dose of selenium which can be used safely in the general population and further, the amount required to prevent colorectal cancer for those at high risk.

Calcium

There is evidence that calcium may inhibit cancer in general and colorectal cancer specifically. Newmark et al. (1984) at the Ludwig Institute for Cancer Research in Toronto proposed a hypothesis which was based on the findings of a number of shot-term studies. These studies showed that the toxic and potentially promoting effect of increased concentrations of free fatty acids and bile acids in the colon can be inhibited by the presence of ionized calcium. They suggested a mechanism of action which is based on the formation of insoluble calcium soaps from the free acids. Later,

Lipkin and Newmark (1985) showed that calcium supplementation did affect colonic epithelial cell proliferation in humans. In the study, consumption of a supplement of 1.25 g $CaCO_3$ per day for 2–3 months reduced the high rate of colonic cell proliferation in people at high risk for colon cancer to the rate in those at low risk.

The inhibition of intestinal carcinogᵉnesis by dietary calcium has been studied in several animal models. In a series of experiments from the Ludwig Institute and from our laboratory in cooperation with the Ludwig Institute, supplements of $CaHPO_4$ yielding 0.1% or 1.0% calcium were given to animals fed 3% or 30% beef tallow (Bull et al. 1987). In all diets the CA:P ratio was 1:1. Two different strains of rats and two doses of AOM were used. In both studies, high calcium supplementation did not inhibit intestinal tumorigenesis in animals consuming either the high- or low-fat diets. However, a recent study reported that a supplement of calcium (1.0% vs. 0.5%) reduced the incidence of DMH-induced colon tumors from 86% in the low-calcium group to 53% in the high-calcium group (Pence and Buddingh 1987). This effect was observed only in rats consuming a 20% corn oil diet. No effect was seen in animals fed 5% corn oil diets or those supplemented with vitamin D_3 plus calcium. More studies are required to determine whether calcium does in fact inhibit intestinal tumorigenesis.

Plant Sterols

Vegetables are rich in plant sterols, especially beta-sitosterol, campesterol, and stigmasterol which together comprise about 20% of sterols in our diet (Subbish 1971). These sterols are known to prevent the absorption of cholesterol thereby reducing serum cholesterol in rats and in humans. Furthermore, vegetarians have a lower incidence of colorectal cancer than the general population living in the same area. This may be due in part to the sterol content of vegetables.

Raicht et al. (1980) studied the effect of beta-sitosterol on colon tumor formation in rats treated with the direct-acting carcinogen, N-methyl-N-nitrosourea. The addition of a 0.2% beta-sitosterol supplement to the diet inhibited both the incidence and the frequency of colon tumors compared to rats without the supplement. The incidence was reduced to 33% from 50% and the number of tumors per rat to 0.44 from 1.1 in controls. Although the total number of tumors was dramatically reduced, the number of invasive carcinomas was the same in the treated as in the control animals. The author concluded that beta-sitosterol may prevent adenoma formation, but may not prevent the transition from adenoma to carcinoma. In a follow-up study, Deschner et al. (1982) investigated the effect of dietary supplementation with beta-sitosterol on colonic epithelial cell proliferation in rats both with and without carcinogen treatment. They found that the plant sterol slowed cell proliferation in the colon in both situations, suggesting a mechanism for reduced expression of neoplastic formation.

Vitamins

Some vitamins appear to inhibit cancer when they are given in amounts greater than that required for maintenance of general health or as supplements to eliminate a deficiency (Bertram et al. 1987). Much of the evidence is epidemiological, although in vitro and animal experiments are supportive, especially for vitamin A. Deficiency of this vitamin increases susceptibility of animals to induced cancer in several organs including the colon. The natural and synthetic forms of the vitamin affect the growth and differentiation of cells in general. Epidemiological studies have shown a relationship between vitamin A intake or its serum levels and cancer incidence in several organs including the colon. Animal studies using synthetic forms, such as 13-*cis*-retinoic acid among others, have not shown a significant inhibitory effect on chemically induced intestinal cancer. Furthermore, in large doses, these compounds are toxic. On the other hand, the carotenoids, especially beta-carotene found in fruit and vegetables, appear to have a cancer-protective effect. Again, the evidence is mainly epidemiological, and it is not certain that the carotenoids in the food are responsible for the observed effect.

Deficiency of vitamin C is associated with cancers of the stomach, esophagus, larynx, and cervix. It is thought that these associations occur because vitamin C inhibits the formation of nitrosamines. However, there is no evidence epidemiologically or in the laboratory that there is an association with colorectal cancer. In one report, vitamin E, an antioxidant, has been shown to be inhibitory in chemically induced colon cancer in mice (Cook and McNamara 1980). It acts by blocking membrane autoxidation and may function synergistically with selenium. These observations regarding vitamin E are provocative but the evidence that it reduces risk of cancer in humans remains conjectural. In summary, the evidence that any of the vitamins has an inhibitory effect in intestinal carcinogenesis is minimal, certainly not nearly as strong as it is for cancers of the upper gastrointestinal tract, bladder, breast, and lung.

Miscellaneous Natural Inhibitors

Diallyl sulfide (DAS) is a major component of garlic oil. Wargovich and Goldberg (1985) did experiments suggesting that DAS affects either the metabolic activation or the distribution of the intestinal carcinogen DMH. When DAS was given to mice prior to the administration of the carcinogen, it effectively inhibited intestinal carcinogenesis (Wargovich 1987). These results suggest that such compounds in garlic and onions may add an inhibitory effect to the diet.

Naturally occurring protease inhibitors such as the Bowman-Birk inhibitor (BBI) are present in soybeans. There has been one report on its effect in intestinal tumorigenesis in mice (Weed et al. 1985). Male CDI mice were given 0.5% BBI in the diet and treated with DMH. Tumor incidence was reduced from 24% in the controls to 0% in the treated group. The animals had no evidence of pancreatic toxicity, but other studies using similar levels of protease inhibitors report a toxic effect in the pancreas.

Sodium cyanate has been reported by Wattenberg (1984) to inhibit DMH-induced colon tumors when added to the diet and given after carcinogen administration. The compound was studied because of its structural relationship to several naturally occurring inhibitors present in cruciferous vegetables such as broccoli, cabbage, and Brussels sprouts. The mechanism of inhibition is unknown.

Synthetic Inhibitors

Phenols

Phenols constitute a diverse class of compounds which have been reported to possess carcinogenic inhibitory properties. These compounds occur naturally in plants, and large amounts of synthetic phenols are consumed by humans as food additives. In general, phenols act as antioxidants and can inhibit carcinogenesis by scavenging of active metabolites, by the inhibition of metabolic activation, or by the induction of enzymes involved in the detoxification of xenobiotics.

There are two synthetic phenolic antioxidants which are of special importance with respect to human exposure. Butylated hydroxyanisole (BHA) and butylated hydroxy-toluene (BHT) are widely used as food additives. It has been estimated that in the United States the human consumption of these compounds is on the order of several milligrams per day. Both BHA and BHT are potent inhibitors of polycyclic aromatic hydrocarbon-induced tumorigenesis in several organs in animals. However, the results in the colon are inconclusive (Wattenberg 1985).

BHT, when given in the diet (6600 ppm) to male F-344 rats, inhibited the incidence and frequency of AOM-induced intestinal tumors (Weisburger et al. 1977). The effect was obtained only when BHT was given concurrently with AOM. Barbolt and Abraham (1977) performed a similar experiment using BHT in DMH-induced colon tumors in Sprague-Dawley rats. There was no inhibition of tumorigenesis in the latter study. Reddy et al. (1983) showed in another experiment that CF1 mice given BHA concurrently with a carcinogen developed a lower tumor incidence and frequency than the control animals.

The results from the above experiments suggest that the phenolic antioxidants BHA and BHT may inhibit some aspect of carcinogen activation. However, the binding of radiolabeled DMH to DNA was not decreased by feeding rats diets containing 0.66% of either antioxidant. Therefore, some other aspect of the initiation process or possibly an early event in promotion must have been affected by the compounds (Bull et al. 1981).

Disulfiram

The ingestion of disulfiram was shown by Wattenberg (1975) to have a strong inhibitory effect on intestinal carcinogenesis in mice given DMH. The effect of disulfiram on the metabolism of DMH was studied by Fiala et al. (1977). DMH is activated by conversion, in sequence, to azomethane, AOM, methylazoxymethanol, and finally to the ultimate carcinogen, methyldiazonium ion. Fiala et al. (1977) found that disulfiram was a potent inhibitor of the conversion of DMH to azomethane. Subsequently Nigro and Campbell (1978) showed that disulfiram was a potent inhibitor of AOM-induced tumorigenesis in rats, which suggests that the drug also blocks metabolic activation at another point in the pathway.

Prostaglandins

There is evidence to suggest that tumor initiation, promotion, and metastasis may require prostaglandin biosynthesis for their development (Honn et al. 1981). Therefore, it is reasonable to consider the possibility that the inhibition of prostaglandin production may have an influence on tumorigenesis. Aspirin and indomethacin, both nonsteroidal anti-inflammatory drugs, are known to reduce the formation of prostaglandins. Kudo et al. (1980) investigated the effect of indomethacin on chemically induced colon cancer in rats. The drug was administered intrarectally for a short time after tumors were known to have developed and it inhibited their growth. The author concluded that indomethacin may have therapeutic value. Narisawa et al. (1978), working in the same laboratory, continued the studies giving the drug intraperitoneally three times a week at varying intervals during a 36-week course of study. They confirmed the finding that early administration of indomethacin inhibited colonic tumor growth, while later treatment reduced the size of tumors that had already developed. In another experiment, Narisawa et al. (1981) found that the drug was effective when given orally in the drinking water. Pollard and Luckert (1983) did a similar study and obtained the same results. Later Pollard et al. (1983) examined the effect of a new, less toxic prostaglandin synthesis inhibitor, piroxicam, and found that it also inhibited the growth of colon tumors in rats. The findings of these studies suggest that nonsteroidal anti-inflammatory agents may be useful as inhibitors and as adjunct therapy for colorectal cancer. More studies are required to find an effective drug with even less toxicity.

Difluoromethylornithine

Cell proliferation is the hallmark of tumorigenesis. Polyamine levels and polyamine-synthetic enzyme activities are high in proliferating normal cells and in cells undergoing neoplastic change. Ornithine decarboxylase (ODC) activity, the rate-limiting enzyme in polyamine biosynthesis, is increased above normal levels in neoplastic tissue (Luk et al. 1986). Difluoromethylornithine (DFMO) is an enzyme-activated irreversible inhibitor of ODC activity and it has been shown to inhibit tumor growth in several organ systems. Kingsnorth et al. (1983) studied the effect of 1% DFMO in the drinking water on DMH-induced colon tumors in mice. He found that DFMO reduced colon polyamine levels and the incidence of colon tumors. Rozhin et al. (1984) found that DFMO (0.01%−1.0%) in the drinking water inhibited intestinal tumor formation in a dose-dependent manner in the AOM rat tumor model. The reduction in tumorigenesis was accompanied by a similar inhibition of deoxycholate-induced ODC activity. This suggests that inhibitors of ODC make good candidates for the inhibition of carcinogenesis. DFMO is a potentially useful compound for this purpose since it is effective and relatively nontoxic.

Use of Combinations of Inhibitors

In the animal model it seems that there is no single natural inhibitor effective enough in the colon that, when added to the diet, would reduce risk to any significant extent.

Synthetic chemicals and drugs have been identified that are more potent inhibitors, but at effective levels most may be too toxic for use in the prevention of colorectal cancer in humans. This does not rule out their possible use in people at high cancer risk. A possible solution to the problem of inadequate effect or of toxicity is the use of combinations of several inhibitors given in nontoxic amounts that singly are ineffective but together exert a significant inhibitory effect.

There are illustrations of this approach in several tumor models. In intestinal cancer, Nigro et al. (1982) showed that small amounts of selenium, 13-*cis*-retinoic acid, and beta-sitosterol added to the drinking water or diet of rats injected with AOM had little or no inhibitory effect when given alone or in combinations of two, but when all three were given together there was nearly a 50% reduction in the average number of intestinal tumors per rat. In a second, more recent study, the authors used combinations of DFMO with piroxicam or fish oil (Nigro et al. 1986). The combination of a low dose of DFMO (0.05%) and a low dose of piroxicam (65 mg/kg diet) reduced colon tumor formation much more than either one alone, whereas the combination of DFMO and fish oil was not more effective than DFMO alone.

Studies such as these suggest that the addition of several inhibitors to the diet is currently the most practical method for reducing colorectal cancer risk. More work needs to be done to find the best combination of agents. Recent advances in our knowledge of the effect of some of the macronutrients, especially fat, suggest that a combination of changes in the macro- and micronutrient components of the diet could reduce cancer risk effectively without altering our current diets too drastically. Thus, appropriate guidelines could be developed that would permit enjoyable eating and good compliance.

Implications for Therapy

The possibilities that inhibitors may play a role in the therapy of colorectal cancer are substantial, but the subject is only in the early stages of development. Even appropriate alterations of the diet may help reduce cancer progression and recurrence in patients who have had successful primary therapy. Better communication and cooperation between researchers and clinicians is needed to take full advantage of some of the new knowledge developed in the field of carcinogenesis to help patients who already have cancer. The following are illustrations of compounds that may be useful as adjunct therapy for colorectal cancer.

The animal studies on the effect of prostaglandin inhibitors indicate that nonsteroidal anti-inflammatory drugs are effective in reducing the number and size of intestinal tumors. Based on this information, Waddell and Loughry (1983) treated a few familial polyposis patients with sulindac. One patient with multiple colonic polyps was treated for 1 year and the polyps disappeared. Three other patients who had polyps in the rectal stump (colon had already been removed) were successfully treated with the drug. Studies have been done using DFMO in combination with chemotherapeutic agents in other organ systems in animals with encouraging results. Tutton and Barkla (1986) have shown in animals that the drug suppresses cell proliferation more effectively in neoplastic tissue than in normal colon mucosa. Sunkara and Rosenberger (1987) did an animal study showing that DFMO inhibited pulmonary metastases in mice implanted with Lewis lung carcinoma. Phase I and II clinical trials have also been done (Abeloff et al. 1984, 1986). The Phase I study showed the drug to be well tolerated, but the Phase II trial did not show a significant therapeutic effect against advanced colon cancer. However, the combination of DFMO and other cancer drugs is currently under investigation.

Conclusion

The carcinogenic process in the colon is difficult to suppress so it is not surprising that the number of possible microconstituent inhibitors identified so far is quite small. The possibilities, based primarily on epidemiological data, include vitamins A, C, and E, the carotenoids, selenium, calcium, and some chemicals found in fruit and vegetables, such as diallyl sulfide. None alone or in combination appear to be potent enough to prevent colorectal cancer in people who eat a high-fat, low-fiber diet. Therefore, other dietary changes are required to reduce the incidence of this type of cancer. Naturally, removal of the carcinogen would be the best way to prevent the disease, but it is not likely to be possible in the near future. Consequently, there must be some alteration in the major dietary components (fat and fiber) to help reduce cancer risk. This need only be modest in amount since the addition of more fruit and vegetables that contain specific inhibitors would add enough suppressive effect to reduce the incidence of colorectal cancer in the general population. On the other hand, people who have a significant inheritance factor may require an additional supplement of inhibitors, perhaps including a synthetic compound.

Continued research is required to determine more clearly the effectiveness of the microconstituent dietary inhibitors that have been reviewed and to identify new ones. Epidemiological studies that focus on this aspect of cancer prevention are the best approach to the discovery of new potential inhibitors. Animal studies are useful for confirmation and for the elucidation of possible mechanisms of action. Finally, human intervention trials are required to demonstrate effectiveness in humans. A few such studies are in progress and no doubt more will be initiated in the near future (Bertram et al. 1987).

Inhibitors of carcinogenesis, especially the synthetic compounds may also be of value in the treatment of the disease. It is reasonable to expect that substances which slow cell proliferation and/or induce differentiation may have an inhibitory effect on the disease process itself. Preliminary investigations on their use as adjunctive therapy in animals and in humans are encouraging.

References

Abeloff MD, Slavik M, Luk GD, Griffin CA, Hermann J, Blanc O, Sjoersdma A, Baylin SB (1984) Phase I trial and pharmacokinetic studies of alpha-difluoromethylornithine – an inhibitor of polyamine biosynthesis. J Clin Oncol 2:124–130

Abeloff MD, Rosen ST, Luk GD, Baylin SB, Zeltzman M, Sjoersdma A (1986) Phase II trials of alpha-difluoromethylornithine, an inhibitor of polyamine synthesis, on advanced small cell lung cancer and colon cancer. Cancer Treat Rep 70:843–845

Barbolt TA, Abraham R (1977) Experientia 35:257–258

Bertram JS, Kolonel LN, Meyskens FL (1987) Rational and strategies for chemoprevention of cancer in humans. Cancer Res 47:3012–3031

Buell DN (1983) Potential hazards of selenium as a chemopreventive agent. Semin Oncol 10:311–321

Bull AW, Burd AD, Nigro ND (1981) Effect of inhibitors of tumorigenesis on the formation of O^6-methylguanine in the colon of 1,2-dimethylhydrazine-treated rats. Cancer Res 41:4938–4941

Bull AW, Bird RP, Bruce RW, Nigro ND, Medine A (1987) Effect of calcium on azoxymethane-induced intestinal tumors in rats. Gastroenterology 92:1332

Clark LC (1985) The epidemiology of selenium and cancer. Fed Proc 44:2584–2589

Clark LC, Combs GF (1986) Selenium compounds and the prevention of cancer: research needs and public health implications. J Nutr 116:170–173

Cook MG, McNamara P (1980) Effect of dietary vitamin E on dimethylhydrazine-induced colonic tumors in mice. Cancer Res 40:1329–1331

Deschner EE, Cohen BI, Raicht RF (1982) The kinetics of the protective effect of beta-sitosterol against MNU-induced colonic neoplasia. J Cancer Res Clin Oncol 103:49–54

Doll R (1980) The epidemiology of cancer. Cancer 45:2475–2485

Fiala ES, Bobotas G, Kulakis C, Wattenberg LW, Weisberger JH (1977) Effects of disulfiram and related compounds on the metabolism in vivo of the colon carcinogen, 1,2-dimethylhydrazine. Biochem Pharmacol 26:1763–1968

Honn KV, Bockman RS, Marnett LJ (1981) Prostaglandins and cancer: a review of tumor initiation through tumor metastases. Prostaglandins 21:833–864

Jacobs M, Forst C (19819 Toxicological effects of sodium selenite in Swiss mice. J Toxicol Environ Health 8:587–598

Jacobs MM, Jansson B, Griffin AC (1977) Inhibitory effects of selenium on 1,2-dimethyl-hydrazine and methylazoxymethanol acetate induction of colon tumors. Cancer Lett 2:133–138

Kingsnorth AN, King WWK, Diekma KA, McCann PP, Ross JS, Malt RA (1983) Inhibition of ornithine decarboxylase with 2-difluoromethyl-ornithine: reduced incidence of dimethylhydrazine-induced colon tumors in mice. Cancer Res 43:2545–2549

Kudo T, Narisawa T, Abo S (1980) Antitumor activity of indomethacin on methylazoxymethanol-induced large bowel tumors in rats. Gann 71:260–264

Lane HW, Medina D (1983). Selenium concentration and glutathione peroxidase activity in normal and neoplastic development of the mouse mammary gland. Cancer Res 43:1558–1561

LeBouef RA, Hoekstra WG (1985) Changes in cellular glutathione levels: possible relation to selenium-mediated anticarcinogenesis. Fed Proc 44:2563–2567

Levander OA, Morris VC (1984) Dietary selenium levels needed to maintain balance in North American adults consuming self-selected diets. Am J Clin Nutr 39:809–815

Lipkin M, Newmark HL (1985) Effect of added dietary calcium on colonic epithelial cell proliferation in subjects at high risk for familial colonic cancer. N Engl J Med 313:1381–1384

Luk GD, Hamilton SR, Yang P, Smith JA, O'Ceallaigh DO, McAvinchey D, Hyland J (1986) Kinetic changes in mucosal ornithine decarboxylase activity during azoxymethane-induced colonic carcinogenesis in the rat. Cancer Res 46:4449–4452

Narisawa T, Kono K, Yamaguchi T, Takahashi T (1978) Cancer chemotherapy using autochthonous large bowel cancer in rats. Gann 69:431–435

Narisawa T, Sato M, Tani M, Kudo T, Takahashi T, Goto A (1981) Inhibition of development of methylnitrosourea-induced rat colon tumors by indomethacin treatment. Cancer Res 41:1954–1957

National Research Council (1980) Recommended dietary allowances, 9th edn. National Academy Press, Washington DC

Newmark HL, Wargovich MJ, Bruce WR (1984) Colon cancer and dietary fat, phosphate, and calcium: a hypothesis. JNCI 72:1323–1325

Nigro ND, Campbell RL (1978) Inhibition of azoxymethane-induced intestinal cancer by disulfiram. Cancer Lett 5:91–95

Nigro ND, Bull AW, Wilson PS, Soullier BK, Alousi MA (1982) Combined inhibitors of carcinogenesis: effect on azoxymethane-induced intestinal cancer in rats. JNCI 69:103–107

Nigro ND, Bull AW, Boyd ME (1986) Inhibition of intestinal carcinogenesis in rats: effect of difluoromethylornithine with piroxicam or fish oil. JNCI 77:1309–1313

Pence B, Buddingh F (1987) Inhibition of dietary fat promotion of colon carcinogenesis by supplemental calcium or vitamin D. Proc Am Assoc Cancer Res 28:154

Pollard M, Luckert PH (1983) Prolonged antitumor effect of indomethacin on autochthonous intestinal tumors in rats. JNCI 70:1103–1105

Pollard M, Luckert PH, Schmidt MA (1983) The suppressive effect of piroxicam on autochthonous intestinal tumors in the rat. Cancer Lett 21:57–61

Raicht RF, Cohen BI, Fazzini EP, Sarwal AN, Takahashi M (1980) Protective effect of plant sterols against chemically induced colon tumors. Cancer Res 40:403–405

Reddy BS, Maeura Y, Weisburger JH (1983) Effect of various levels of dietary butylated hydroxyanisole on methylazoxymethanol acetate-induced colon carcinogenesis in CF1 mice. JNCI 71:1299–1305

Rozhin J, Wilson PS, Bull AW, Nigro ND (1984) Ornithine decarboxylase activity in the rat and human colon. Cancer Res 44:3226–3230

Shamberger RJ, Willis CE (1971) Selenium distribution and human cancer mortality. CRC Crit Rev Clin Lab Sci 2:211–221

Soullier BK, Wilson PS, Nigro ND (1981) Effect of selenium on azoxymethane-induced intestinal cancer in rats fed high fat diet. Cancer Lett 12:343–348

Subbish R (1971) Significance of dietary plant sterols in man and experimental animals. Mayo Clin Proc 46:549–559

Sunkara PS, Rosenberger AL (1987) Antimetastastic activity of DL-alpha-difluoromethylornithine, an inhibitor of polyamine biosynthesis, in mice. Cancer Res 47:933–935

Tutton PJM, Barkla DH (1986) Comparison of the effects of an ornithine decarboxylaxe inhibitor on the intestinal epithelium and on intestinal tumors. Cancer Res 46:6091–6094

Waddell WR, Loughry RW (1983) Sulindac for polyposis of the colon. J Surg Oncol 24:83–87

Wargovich MJ (1987) Diallyl sulfide, a flavor component of garlic (*Allium sativum*), inhibits dimethylhydrazine-induced colon cancer. Carcinogenesis 8:1239–1241

Wargovich MJ, Goldberg MT (1985) Diallyl sulfide: a naturally occurring thioether that inhibits carcinogen-induced nuclear damage to colon epithelial cells in vivo. Mutat Res 143:127–129

Wattenberg LW (1975) Inhibition of dimethylhydrazine-induced neoplasia of the large intestine by disulfiram. JNCI 54:1005–1006

Wattenberg LW (1983) Inhibition of neoplasia by minor dietary constituents. Cancer Res (Suppl) 43:2448s–2453s

Wattenberg LW (1984) Inhibition of carcinogen-induced neoplasia by sodium cyanate, tert-butyl isocyanate, and benzyl isothiocyanate administered subsequent to carcinogen exposure. Cancer Res 41:2991–2994

Wattenberg LW (1985) Chemoprevention of cancer. Cancer Res 45:1–8

Weed HG, McGandy RB, Kennedy AR (1985) Protection against dimethylhydrazine-induced adenomatous tumors of the mouse colon by the dietary addition of an extract of soybeans containing the Bowman-Birk protease inhibitor. Carcinogenesis 8:1239–1241

Weisburger EK, Evarts RP, Wenk ML (1977) Inhibitory effect of butylated hydroxytoluene (BHT) on intestinal carcinogenesis in rats by azoxymethane. Food Cosmet Toxicol 15:139–141

Oncogenes in Colorectal Cancer

N. James and K. Sikora

Department of Clinical Oncology, Royal Postgraduate Medical School, Hammersmith Hospital, Ducane Road, London W12 0HS, UK

Contents

Introduction

Carcinogenesis is a multistage process known to involve changes at the genetic level. Over the last decade it has become possible to identify precisely some of the genes involved in this process. These are called "oncogenes". Intriguingly, similar DNA sequences are present in species as diverse as yeast, Drosophila and man. This high degree of conservation across vast reaches of evolutionary time would appear to indicate a role of fundamental importance in normal cellular function. Thus, it is not surprising that abnormalities affecting these genes have serious consequences. An "oncogene" can be defined as a gene whose changed expression or altered product is essential to the production or maintenance of the malignant state.

Terminology

The original evidence for specific genes having a role in carcinogenesis came from the RNA tumour viruses. These possess only three genes: two coding for structural proteins and a third for reverse transcriptase, the enzyme that produces a DNA copy of the virus allowing its incorporation into the host DNA (Bishop and Warmus 1982). The additional substitution of a fourth gene gives these viruses the ability to rapidly induce tumours in vivo and also to transform cells in vitro (transformed cells lose contact inhibition and pile up on the plates instead of forming a monolayer). The transforming sequences within the genetic material of the viral gene were termed "viral oncogenes" (v-onc). Subsequently, it was shown that the v-oncs share common sequences with cellular genes which were thus termed "cellular oncogenes" (c-onc) (Weinberg 1982).

This raises the chicken and egg problem of which came first. Do these viruses cause cancer or have they hijacked cellular genes involved in growth control? Several factors indicate the latter explanation. Viruses carrying v-oncs reproduce less efficiently than normal viruses. The extensive involvement of c-oncs in normal cellular growth and differentiation indicates the likely origin of oncogenes. V-oncs are probably as essential to the virus as malaria is to the mosquito. Cellular oncogenes in fact do not usually possess transforming potential in their native state and are termed "proto-oncogenes" to distinguish them from genes with the ability to transform (Table 1).

How Oncogenes Work

The control of cell growth and development is a multilayered processes, as outlined in Fig. 1. Oncogenes have been shown to be involved at each level of this process, and it can be seen easily that alterations to this finely balanced system could result in unregulated cell growth transformation.

Table 1. Some examples of oncogenes, their location on human chromosomes and their function

Oncogene	Species of retrovirus origin	Tumour	Human gene	Function of product
v-*src*	Chicken	Sarcoma	c-*src*	Tyrosine kinase
v-*ras*	Rat	Sarcoma	c-*ras*	GTP binding protein
v-*myc*	Chicken	Leukaemia	c-*myc*	Nuclear binding protein
v-*fes*	Cat	Sarcoma	c-*fes*	Tyrosine kinase
v-*sis*	Monkey	Sarcoma	c-*sis*	GF
v-*erbB*	Chicken	Erythroblastosis	c-*erbB*	EGFR
v-*myb*	Chicken	Myeloblastosis	c-*myb*	Nuclear binding protein
v-*fms*	Cat	Sarcoma	c-*fms*	GFR
v-*abl*	Mouse	Leukaemia	c-*abl*	Tyrosine kinase
v-*fos*	Mouse	Osteosarcoma	c-*fos*	Nuclear binding protein

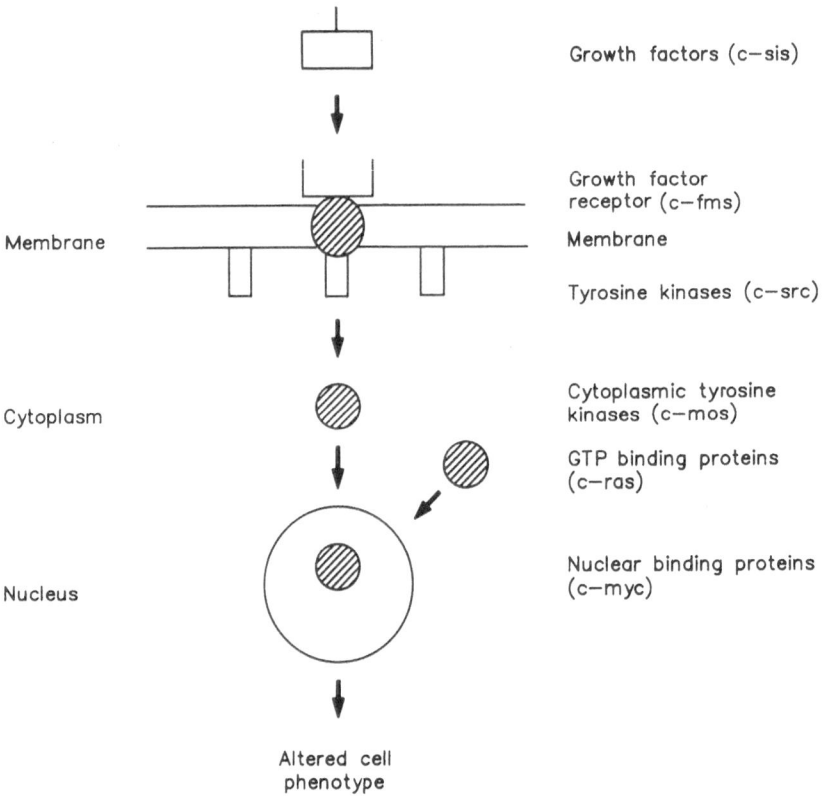

Growth factors (c-sis)

Growth factor
receptor (c-fms)

Membrane

Tyrosine kinases (c-src)

Cytoplasmic tyrosine
kinases (c-mos)

GTP binding proteins
(c-ras)

Nuclear binding proteins
(c-myc)

Membrane

Cytoplasm

Nucleus

Altered cell
phenotype

Fig. 1. The network of control of cell growth. (From Sikora 1986)

Growth Factors

Growth factors (GFs) are the extracellular proteins that act as growth modulators. They have several properties that indicate an involvement in carcinogenesis. Some GFs will transform normal cells in vitro. Conversely, in some systems, the induction of cell transformation can result in an increased production of GFs. The observation that these factors can both initiate and be a product of transformation suggests the possibility of self-perpetuating positive feedback loops with unregulated cell division as the consequence. This phenomenon, termed "autocrine secretion", has been implicated in various situations involving rapid growth, such as wound repair, embryogenesis, as well as malignant transformation. Examples of GFs involved in transformation include lymphokines, such as interleukin 2 and bombesin. Interleukin 2, also known as "T cell growth factor", is able to trigger T lymphocyte proliferation (M. Malkovsky and P. M. Sondel, to be published). The latter has been shown clearly to be a self-stimulating GF for cell lines derived from small cell carcinoma of the bronchus. In both these systems, the maintenance of the transformed state depends on the presence of the factor. Both transformation and GF stimulation result in similar biochemical changes, such as increased tyrosine phosphorylation and altered cellular lipid metabolism. One human oncogene, c-*sis,* has been shown to have sequence homology with a known GF, platelet-derived growth factor (PDGF) (Waterfield et al. 1983).

Growth Factor Receptors

There are several possible modes of involvement of oncogenes at the level of the cell surface receptor. The presence of the appropriate GF switches the receptor on with the resultant increase in tyrosine kinase activity within the cell, stimulating the other transmembrane section. The kinase is also regulated by an internal regulatory region allowing responses to intracellular events. The consequences of the increased kinase activity are at present unknown, but such activities are the hallmark of transformed cells.

There are several ways in which the GF receptor (GFR) may be altered to produce unregulated tyrosine kinase activity. For example, the external receptor may be altered to a permanently "on" position. An example of this is c-*erb*B which codes the cellular receptor for epidermal growth factor (EGF). The equivalent viral gene, v-*erb*B codes the receptor with a truncated external domain. In addition, there are alterations in the regulatory domain internally. It can thus be postulated that transformation requires alteration within the external domain leaving the receptor in the "on" position together with removal of internal regulatory influence, allowing the maintenance of the activated state. However, no examples of truncated receptors have yet been discovered in human malignancies with abnormal expression of GFRs, such as breast and bladder carcinomas. A second possibility would be alterations in the kinase region itself to produce an enzyme with permanently high activity. A possible example of this type of change is the c-*fms* oncogene which codes the receptor for the colony stimulating factor of CSF1 (Sherr et al. 1983). The transforming viral gene v-*fms* possesses enhanced kinase activity compared with its cellular counterpart. A third explanation of the role of GFRs in transformation is that increased expression of normal gene product is sufficient to bring about the necessary changes, a model which fits observations in breast and bladder carcinomas.

Intracellular Messengers

The best candidate for oncogene involvement at this level is the *ras* family of genes. The gene products have structural similarities to proteins termed "G-" and "N-proteins" which control adenylate cyclase activity. *Ras*-coded products have also been shown to have GTPase activity. The main interest in this area of research centres on the intracellular functions of the 21-kilodalton protein coded by the *ras* gene termed "p21 ras" (Der and Cooper 1983). A non-proliferative signal transduction role based on the GTPase activity of p21 and modulated by an as yet uncharacterised protein has been suggested. The effect of specific mutations on p21 GTP-binding and its relevance to transformation is also under investigation.

Nuclear Effectors

Several oncogenes of possible clinical importance, such as *myc, myb* and *fos*, code for nuclear associated proteins (Evan and Hancock 1986). At present their precise localisation and function are unknown. A working hypothesis would be that these oncogenes may be involved in control of gene expression.

Clinical Correlates

It is clear that oncogenes are involved at crucial points in the cell cycle. For the oncogene hypothesis to be true, it is necessary to demonstrate that oncogene products are essential for the production and maintenance of the transformed state in actual malignancies. Several ways have been postulated in which proto-oncogenes (the normal cellular gene) may be converted into transforming oncogenes. Firstly, the normal gene may be abnormally expressed either by interference with its control region (termed "promoter insertion" which is known to occur in experimental models) or by transposition to an abnormal site where its expression is unregulated. Secondly, the gene may be duplicated (termed "amplification") resulting in larger quantities of mRNA production simply because of the larger number of gene copies. Thirdly, the gene itself may be altered with production of an abnormal product with transforming potential. These mechanisms are not mutually exclusive.

To look for oncogene activity, there are several lines of attack. The DNA can be examined for multiple copies or abnormal forms of suspected oncogenes. The mRNA can be analysed for abnormal transcripts or for inappropriate quantities of a normal transcript. Thirdly, the protein products of oncogenes can be looked for, again in either inappropriate forms or quantities. Finally, the putative oncogenes can be "implanted" into suitable cell cultures to look for transforming potential – this is termed a "transfection assay".

Abnormal Expression of a Normal Gene Product

An example of this mechanism occurs in Burkitt's lymphoma in which the c-*myc* gene is translocated from chromosome 8 to chromosome 2, 14 or 22. It is of great interest that the *myc* locus is translocated to the regions of these genes coding for immunoglobulin components – highly transcribed genes in the stem cell of the tumour, the B lymphocyte. The translocated gene is transcribed at significant but variable levels further supporting a role for *myc* in this tumour (Hamlyn and Rabbits 1983).

Multiple Gene Copies – Gene Amplification

The best example of this phenomenon is the amplification of N-*myc* in untreated neuroblastoma. The oncogene c-*myc* is a normal cellular gene. In 1984 a variant form was found in human neuroblastoma cell lines and termed "N-*myc*". Subsequent studies showed that N-*myc* could transform other cell lines under certain conditions. Multiple copies – up to 300 – of N-*myc* are found in clinical specimens in many cases. Of great interest is the observation that amplification of N-*myc* was associated with shorter progression-free survival, advanced stage and tendency to metastasise; in short, N-*myc* amplification correlates with more aggressive disease (Brodeur et al. 1985).

Amplification of both c-*myc* and N-*myc* is also found in small cell lung cancer. However, the correlation with prognosis is not so clear-cut, and thus other factors apart from gene copy number must also be important.

Abnormal Genes

The Philadelphia (Ph′) chromosome is found in the majority of patients with chronic myelocytic leukaemia (CML) and is characterised by the translocation of the c-*abl* oncogene on chromosome 9 to the breakpoint cluster region (*ber*) of chromosome 22 to produce a chimeric *bcr-abl* gene (Gale and Cannani 1985). This gene codes for a protein with enhanced tyrosine kinase activity – a hallmark of oncogenic activity. Recently, it has been shown that Ph′-negative patients have abnormalities in their *bcr* gene and that hybrid *bcr-abl* mRNA is detectable in these patients, providing evidence of a uniform molecular abnormality in this apparently heterogenous group.

Clinical Potential

The discovery of oncogenes and the development of suitable assays for clinical use has led to a greater understanding of malignant disease. We are now beginning to evaluate their diagnostic and therapeutic potential (Table 2).

Diagnosis

Monoclonal antibodies directed against oncogenes or their products may prove to be of value as a diagnostic tool. Released oncogene products could be useful tumour markers either for scanning, diagnostic or follow-up purposes. Immunocytochemical techniques have already shown potential in a variety of malignancies including breast and cervical carcinomas, and monoclonal antibodies linked to radionuclides have

Table 2. Clinical potential of oncogenes

Diagnosis	Prognosis
Tumour markers	EGFR in breast cancer
Immunocytochemistry	*ras* expression in breast cancer
Tumour localisation	n-*myc* amplification in neuroblastoma
Cancer risk prediction	
	Therapy
	Monoclonal antibodies to oncogene products
	Drugs interacting with oncogene products

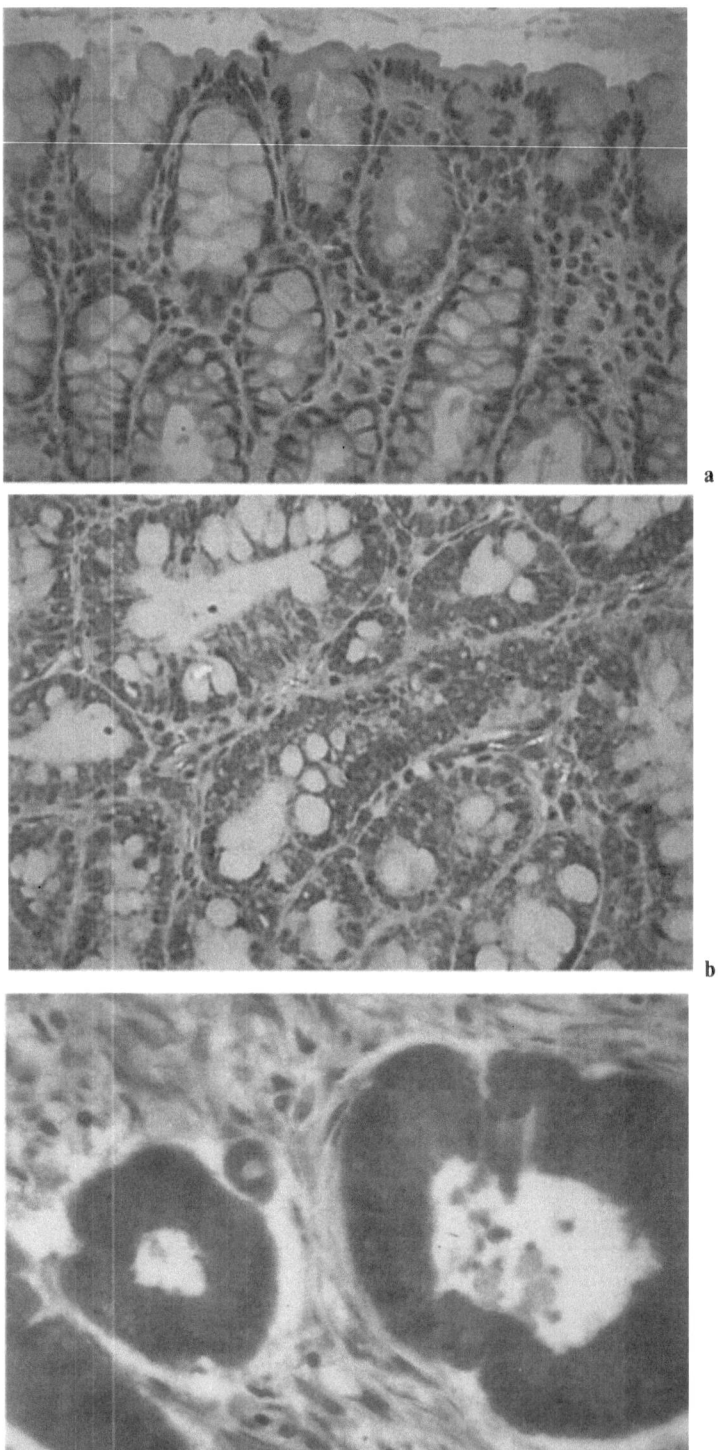

a

b

c

been used to localise tumours accurately (Sikora 1986). Finally, patients at high risk of developing a malignancy could have their DNA probed for high-risk genes – for example, the gene for familial polyposis coli – providing an accurate risk assessment before the development of clinical disease.

Prognosis

The association of N-*myc* amplification and prognosis in neuroblastoma has already been mentioned. A potentially more important association occurs in breast cancer between the expression of the EGFR and prognosis. Recent studies have shown that the EGFR status of the primary tumour is the most important single variable for predicting relapse-free and overall survival (Sainsbury et al. 1985). Amplification of a closely associated oncogene c-*erb* B-2 correlates with a poor prognosis and may be detected by immunohistological means (Venter et al. 1987). Over-expression of the *ras* gene is associated with lymph node metastases in breast cancer. The study of oncogene expression may thus allow the accurate identification of poor-prognosis tumours. This may be of great value in selecting which patients will benefit from more aggressive treatment, a particular problem in breast cancer with its extremely variable natural history.

Treatment

The discovery of a novel set of growth control proteins provides new targets for antineoplastic agents. Possible approaches include the use of monoclonal antibodies directed against oncogene products linked to either a cell toxin or suitable radionuclide. In the longer term, compounds interacting with oncogene products may provide a new generation of chemotherapeutic drugs. Currently, inhibitors of surface receptors, tyrosine kinases and the GTPase activity of the *ras* gene are under intense investigation.

Colorectal Carcinoma and c-*ras*

Activation of the c-*ras* oncogene, which is situated on chromosome 12 in humans, has been demonstrated in colonic carcinomas (Spandidos and Kerr 1984) (Fig. 2). Such activation is manifested either by gene over-expression, yielding high levels of a normal protein p21 (molecular weight 21 000) or by the synthesis of an altered protein (mutant p21) in which glycine is substituted by valine or glutamine at positions 12 or 61. Moreover, it has been shown that microinjections of both mutant p21 and exces-

Fig. 2a–c. c-*ras* expression in colorectal carcinoma: a normal colon; b morphologically normal colon adjacent to resected colorectal carcinoma showing enhanced c-*ras* expression detected by a monoclonal antibody; c well-differentiated adenocarcinoma of the colon showing increased c-*ras* expression

sive amounts of normal p21 into NIH 3T3 cells (a mouse fibroblast cell line) induce morphological transformation and stimulate quiescent cells to enter the S-phase of the cell cycle. Transient reversion of the *ras* oncogene-induced cell transformation has been demonstrated by microinjection of anti-p21 monoclonal antibodies. These findings support the concept that the *ras* oncogene acts directly through its protein product.

We have studied the distribution pattern of p21 at the resection margins of patients undergoing potentially "curative" excision of colorectal carcinomas (N. Habib, N. Markham, K. Sikora, to be published). This study was performed in order to determine if there is any correlation between the degree of oncogene expression and the subsequent development of tumour recurrence. The hypothesis of this investigation was based on the possibility that oncogene over-expression may reflect the neoplastic cellular transformation prior to tumour establishment. Therefore, we speculated that over-expression of *ras* oncogene at the resection margin in patients undergoing potentially curative surgery may identify those patients who are at risk of developing tumour recurrence.

We found over-production of *ras* oncogene product in 15 of 18 patients who developed subsequent tumour recurrence and in three of 12 patients who are alive with no recurrence (mean follow-up 14 months), P less than 0.01. Such studies show how oncogene over-expression may be useful in identifying patients at risk of developing tumour recurrence as it reflects the multistage carcinogenic process at a molecular level.

Colorectal Carcinoma and c-*myc*

The c-*myc* oncogene has been implicated in the processes of normal cell proliferation and differentiation. Elevated levels of c-*myc* mRNA and its gene product (p62^{c-myc}) have been detected in a variety of solid tumours and cultured cell lines. Its precise role in normal cell function and in neoplastic transformation and progression has yet to be elucidated. We have used a monoclonal antibody, raised by peptide immunisation, to determine the distribution by immunoperoxidase staining of the c-*myc* oncogene product in archival specimens of colonic polyps and carcinomas (Stewart et al. 1986). Samples from 42 patients with colon carcinoma, 24 with benign polyps and 15 normal colon biopsies were examined. Normal colon revealed maximal staining in the mid-zone of the crypts, corresponding to the zone of differentiation and maturation. The staining was predominantly cytoplasmic. Adenomatous polyps revealed the most intense pattern of staining in areas of dysplastic change. Colonic tumours showed a wide range of staining. Well-differentiated tumours contained more cytoplasmic p62^{c-myc} than poorly differentiated tumours. These findings suggest that the c-*myc* oncogene product may play an important role in the evolution of colonic neoplasia.

Familial Polyposis and Colorectal Cancer

Recently, the gene responsible for familial adenomatous polyposis (also known as "familial polyposis coli") has been located in a small section of chromosome 5. Blood was taken from a series of family members who suffered from this disease and DNA extracted from their lymphocytes. A range of probes were used to look for genetic linkage between the disease and restriction fragment length polymorphism (Bodmer et al. 1987). One probe, C11P11, was found to link deletions to specific segment of chromosome 5. It can thus be deduced that the loss of gene function at this site is a key step in the generation of adenomas. A further study evaluated the role of this gene in the development of sporadic colorectal carcinoma in 45 patients (Solomon et al. 1987). It was found that at least 20% of patients had tumours in which one of the alleles on the long arm of chromosome 5 was lost, again suggesting that becoming recessive to this gene may well be a critical step in the development of colorectal cancer. The exact relationship between adenoma and carcinoma is not clear. No doubt in the near future this gene will be cloned and its protein product identified. In this way, the genetic basis of both adenomatous polyposis and the much bigger clinical problem – colorectal cancer – may be clarified.

Conclusions

Oncogenes have provided a fascinating insight into the mechanisms by which cell growth is controlled. Abnormalities in this process appear to be of major importance in the generation of malignant disease. However, the study of oncogene abnormalities has so far generated a lot of interesting association, but, with a few exceptions such as the EGFR studies, little of direct relevance to clinical medicine – a situation analogous to that seen with HLA association. At present, no oncogene abnormality seems to be obligatory for carcinogenesis. Could oncogene abnormalities just be epiphenomena or can the apparent gaps be filled by alternative oncogenes as yet undiscovered? The area holds fascinating promise for future research.

References

Bishop JM, Warmus H (1982) Functions and origins of retroviral transforming genes in RNA tumour viruses. In: Weiss RA, Teich N, Warmus H, Coffin J (eds) RNA tumor viruses: molecular biology of tumor viruses. Cold Spring Harbor, New York, pp 999–1108

Bodmer WF, Bailey CJ, Bodmer J et al. (1987) Localisation of the gene for familial adenomatous polyposis and chromosome 5. Nature 328:614–616

Brodeur GM, Seeger RC, Schwab M et al. (1985) Amplification of n-*myc* and untreated human neuroblastomas correlates with advanced disease state. Science 231:1121–1124

Der CJ, Cooper GM (1983) Altered gene products are associated with activation of cellular *ras* K genes in human lung and colon carcinomas. Cell 32:201–208

Evan G, Hancock DC (1986) Studies on the interaction of the human c-*myc* protein with cell nuclei. Cell 43:253–261

Gale RP, Cannani E (1985) The molecular biology of chronic myeloginous leukaemia. Br J Haematol 60:395–408

Hamlyn PH, Rabbits TH (1983) Translocation joint c-*myc* and immunoglobulin gamma 1 genes in a Burkitt lymphoma. Nature 304:135–139

Sainsbury JRC, Farndon JR, Sherbert GV et al. (1985) Epidermal growth factor receptors and oestrogen receptors in human breast cancer. Lancet 1:364–366

Sherr CJ, Rettenmeyer CW, Saccar et al. (1983) The c-*fms* proto-oncogene product is related to the receptor for the mononuclear phagocyte growth factor, CSF1. Cell 41:665–667

Sikora K, Evan G, Stewart J, Watson J (1985) Detection of the c-*myc* oncogene product of testicular cancer. Br J Cancer 82:171–176

Solomon E, Voss R, Hall V et al. (1987) Chromosome 5 allele loss in human colorectal carcinomas. Nature 328:616–618

Spandidos DA, Kerr IB (1984) Elevated expression of the human ras oncogene family in pre-malignant and malignant tumours of the colorectum. Br J Cancer 49:681–688

Stewart J, Evan G, Watson J, Sikora A (1986) Detection of the c-*myc* oncogene product in colonic polyps and carcinomas. Br J Cancer 53:1–6

Venter DJ, Tuzi NL, Kumar S, Gullick WJ (1987) Over expression of the c-*erb*B2 oncoprotein in human breast carcinomas. Lancet 2:69–72

Waterfield MD, Scrace GT, Whittle N et al. (1983) Platelet derived growth factor structurally related to the putative transforming protein p28 sis of Simian sarcoma virus. Nature 304:35–39

Weinberg RA (1982) Fewer and fewer oncogenes. Cell 30:3–4

Morphology of Colorectal Cancer

Histogenesis of Colorectal Carcinoma

K. C. Liu and N. A. Wright

Department of Histopathology, Royal Postgraduate Medical School, Hammersmith Hospital, Du Cane Road, London W12 0HS, UK

Contents

Introduction

Colonic cancer, a disease whose incidence increases with rising affluence, is the most common gastrointestinal malignancy throughout the western world. In the UK alone, there approximat 16000 deaths each year. The overall situation can be better appreciated from the detailed description given in the first section of this book.

There has been intensive research into cell growth and histogenesis of the development of colonic carcinogenesis. Studies involving animal models, e.g. DMH (1,2-dimethylhydrazine) in rats and mice, have yielded much information. The question which has to be asked is whether the results obtained using an animal model can be applied to the situation in man. Some researchers have compared the human and animal results (Spjut 1972; Ahnen 1985). Spjut concluded that there were similarities in both morphology and distribution between the two systems; he also claimed that the adenomas and carcinomas in rats and man resembled one another to the point of being indistinguishable. In Ahnen's review, the pathological features of DMH-induced colonic tumours were considered to span the entire spectrum of tumours seen in human colon, from tubular adenomas through polypoid and sessile carcinomas to mucinous adenocarcinomas (Newberne and Rogers 1973; Sunter et al. 1978; Wiebecke et al. 1973). The study of cell kinetics of colonic epithelium showed an analogous change in proliferative compartments in both animal and human colon (Wiebecke et al. 1973; Maskens 1976). There is also similar colonic mucin synthesis in human and animal neoplasia (Filipe 1975). However, there are areas of disagreement, and one of these is whether the adenoma is the precancerous lesion. This will be discussed in the latter part of this review.

Animal Studies – the DMH Model

The acute and chronic changes caused by DMH in the mucosa of the colon are described in this volume by Simanowski: here we would like to give an account of the evolution of dysplasia and neoplasia in such models.

Evolution of Dysplasia and Neoplasia

Some authors consider that colonic tumours arise from the epithelium of morphologically normal looking crypts (Pozharisski 1975). Most, however, authors agree that dysplasia and atypia arise from an established neoplasm – the adenoma. Detailed accounts of morphological changes can be found in several papers (Wiebecke et al. 1973; Chang 1978, 1980; Sunter et al. 1981).

The changes noted comprise altered patterns of cell differentiation and filling of the crypt with abnormal, basophilic cells which have hyperchromatic nuclei. Chang pointed to an abnormal looking crypt, among a group of hyperplastic crypts, which contained stratified cuboidal cells with large nuclei as the starting point of such changes.

Based on all the observations, a two-stage hypothesis of tumour morphogenesis was suggested (Richards 1977; Chang 1978, 1980):

1. Hyperplastic crypts become repopulated with transformed cells, which may be modified stem cells. They migrate or behave similarly to non-neoplastic proliferating epithelial cells, but undergo partially defective differentiation or no differentiation into cell lineages. They continue to grow and eject the normal population.
2. With the accumulation of transformed stem cells, a proliferative focus form, in effect a small adenoma.

These small adenomas share many features with the minute lesions of familial polyposis coli (Lane and Lev 1963). While the upper part of the crypt grows continuously, the basal crypt degenerates. If a tumour arises from such an adenoma, the lesion will be pleoclonal; as the initial lesion is a monocryptal adenoma, and colonic crypts are themselves clonal, the lesion has arisen from any one of up to 700 cells.

Most of the colonic neoplasms exhibit a relatively small and well differentiated tubular adenoma. The most invasive and least differentiated carcinomas with signet-ring cells originate as a very invasive mucosal lesion with no in situ precursor stage (Wiebecke et al. 1973; Pozharisski 1975; Sunter 1980). In order to classify the carcinomas, according to their apparent origin, Sunter et al. (1978) studied 378 tumours, 26% of which were adenomas. Tumours defined as adenomas were those which were tubular or tubulovillous in structure, well differentiated with no sign of invasion through muscularis mucosae, and macroscopically appeared as sessile or preduncu-lated mucosal polyps. The carcinomas were divided into three groups as follows:

Group 1 (16%): resembling adenomas macroscopically, but showing invasion through muscularis mucosae.

Group 2 (40%): moderately differentiated adenocarcinomas, growing as an ulcerated polyp or plague, with a peripheral rim of adenomatous tissue, probably from residual non-invasive neoplasm.

Group 3 (18%): a heterogeneous group, all poorly differentiated, with a variety of appearances, infiltrating bowel widely and frequently showing signs of metastasis.

Most of the adenomas and group 1 carcinomas are confined to the distal half of the colon. Group 2 is more widely distributed. The poorly differentiated group 3 carcinomas are concentrated at the proximal end, but sparing the proximal 10%.

Adenoma – Carcinoma Sequence

It was suggested by the work of Morson (1978) and others that neoplasms arise from non-invasive adenoma; this will be discussed in the section below on colonic cancer in man. Several authors reported that this sequence does not occur in the rat model of colonic cancer, using DMH (Spjut 1972; Ward 1974; Maskens 1976; Pozharisski et al. 1979). They found no invasion through muscularis mucosae from adenomas (Spjut 1972). Similar observations were reported in mouse models, induced tumours being found in flat mucosae without polyp formation (Thurnherr et al. 1973). Wright (1984) highlighted the misconception that colonic adenomas must be polypoid; sessile adenomas are well recognized in human pathology (Muto et al. 1985).

In case of Maskens' study (1976), although polypoid adenomas were not observed, focal areas of atypia that resembled flat adenomas were seen. Maskens also claimed that DMH-induced carcinomas do not go through a benign polyp stage; rather, these lesions are merely non-invasive, are not benign and are not always polypoid. On the other hand, many workers (Wiebecke et al. 1973; Haase et al. 1973; Chang 1978; Sunter et al. 1978) have consistent results showing the progression from benign adenomas to polypoid adenocarcinomas in both mice and rats. In Sunter's study (Sunter et al. 1978), the distribution of group 1 carcinomas and adenomas suggested the two were associated, and the increase in group 2 carcinoma with the duration of DMH treatment indicated a process of continuous cancer formation. As many as 55% of carcinomas from DMH rats originated in adenomas, but there were also carcinomas that did not arise from adenomas. In group 3 tumours, agreeing with other reports (Wiebecke et al. 1973), de novo carcinomas appear with only hyperplastic mucosae and no adenomatous changes.

Colonic Neoplasms in Man

Various methods have been employed to elucidate the exact development of colonic cancer in man. Examination of large bowels at autopsy and of surgical specimens and regular screening of high-risk groups (those families suffering from familial polyposis) are a few of the methods used. Using organ culture techniques, isolated colonic mucosa has also been studied. It is interesting to note that specific changes occur during the long latent period of development from a hyperplastic lesion to an invasive carcinoma. Day and Morson (1978) followed non-invasive adenomas for 13 years before an invasive event occurred.

Cell Proliferation Studies of Colonic Neoplasms and Surrounding Mucosae

In human mucosae maintained in organ culture, various carcinogens (DMH, methylazoxymethanol, N-methyl-N'-nitrosoguanidine) were used. They all inhibited DNA synthesis (Mak et al. 1979). As in the animal studies, adenomas did seem to arise from the upper part of the crypt. Valdes-Depera and Beckfield (1957) suggested that tubular adenomas arose in the superficial portion of the rectal crypt. This has been supported by detailed autoradiography studies of small lesions in patients with polyposis coli (Cole and McKalen 1963). Lipkin (1974) and Deschner and Lipkin (1975) also showed that the cell proliferative zone was prominent at the top of rectal crypts in small adenomas of polyposis coli and also within the normal-looking rectal crypts. All these findings supported an origin of adenomas from the upper crypt surface. Besides the shift of the proliferative zone, there is also an increase in its size (Wiebecke et al. 1974; Terpstra et al. 1987). Cell proliferative rate also increased along the entire colon; this included the normal mucosa of patients with colonic neoplasms (Bleiberg et al. 1985).

Here we should consider some results from cell kinetic studies. In general, colonic carcinomas appear to grow very slowly, having an average doubling time of 600 days (Welin et al. 1963). Adenomas appear to grow even more slowly (Day and Morson 1978). For early carcinoma, Stragand et al. (1980) performed an animal study which included transplantation of tumours onto nude mice. There seemed to be an initial period of rapid growth with a high growth fraction and low cell loss. As the tumours grew, however, the doubling time increased from 6.8 days to 13.7 days.

The thymidine labelling indices are very variable, with reports ranging from 2.25% to 42% (Bleiberg et al. 1972; Ota et al. 1985). In very advanced carcinomas, metaphase arrest techniques involving injection of vincristine and biopsy were used to measure the potential doubling time (t_{PD}) of such tumours (Camplejohn et al. 1973). The t_{PD} was greater in tumours than in the normal mucosa, 192 h compared with 82 h. The growth fractions were found to be 0.13–0.25, with a rate of cell loss of 0.99. This may be due to the sheer volume of the tumours, which could not have an efficient blood supply.

Overall Pathway of Colonic Cancer Development

Colonic epithelial cells begin to develop some characteristics of malignancy while they still look normal, passing through specific phases. Lipkin (1974) suggested a two-phase process:

1. A proliferative lesion develops: there is no suppression of DNA synthesis, and no retention or accumulation of abnormal cells in the crypt occurs at this stage.
2. A proliferative lesion is established and cells develop properties which enable them to be retained in mucosae in increasing numbers.

The evidence suggests that most malignant tumours develop from non-invasive adenomas; the de novo carcinomas occur in ulcerative colitis. The adenomas show several patterns of differentiation: tubular, villous and mixed tubulovillous. Tubular and tubulovillous differentiation are predominant (Muto et al. 1975; Morson et al. 1983). The incidence of malignancy has been reported to be proportional to the amount of villous component present (Appel et al. 1977), but this has been disputed (Galandiuk et al. 1987). The presence of multiple adenomas, family history of colorectal cancer and the size and degree of dyplasia play an important part in determining the invasive potential of adenomas (Muto et al. 1975; Morson et al. 1983, Eide 1986; Galandiuk et al. 1987).

A mechanism for a dysplasia–carcinoma sequence has been suggested by Morson et al. (1983). Depending on their genotypes, those with an autosomal recessive gene are more sensitive to the "adenogenic" effect of some environmental factors. Most adenomas remain small, but some increase in size and develop into carcinomas. While most of the tumours go through the adenoma stage before they become carcinomas, a very small proportion – the de novo carcinomas – do not. Those developed in ulcerative colitis are thought to be of this category.

Histogenesis of Colonic Carcinomas

There are many types of polyps, and most authors accept that only neoplastic polyps have malignant potential, though some disagree (Goldman et al. 1970; Potet and Soullard 1971; Gebbers and Laissue 1986; Bengoechea et al. 1987).

Duke (1947) suggested that tubular adenomas arose through proliferation and lateral expansion in the basal proliferative zone of the rectal crypts, while villous adenomas arose from surface proliferation. However, other experimental findings (Valdes-Depera and Beckfield 1957; Cole and McKalen 1963; Lipkin 1974; Deschner and Lipkin 1975), suggested that the proliferative zone was high up in the rectal crypts.

By means of serial sectioning of minute adenomas in familial polyposis coli (Nakamura and Kino 1984), buds of single-gland adenomas were found to originate from the normal proliferation zone of normal crypts, growing out onto the lamina propria and forming the single-gland adenomas in the upper part of the mucosa.

This supported a previous view concerning the location of the proliferative zone (Nakamura et al. 1978), namely that there is no expansion or shift in the normal colon mucosae before and after development of adenomas.

Maskens (1979) suggested that new adenomatous glands were produced in addition to and between existing normal crypts, including a downward invagination of surface epithelium. He proposed the following sequence of events:

1. Cells continue to synthesize DNA while migrating upward.
2. DNA-synthesizing cells accumulate on the mucosal surface, with infolding of surface epithelium between existing crypts.
3. The development of new crypts results either from infolding or branching of adenomatous glands.
4. Neoplastic glands accumulate in the upper part of the mucosae, producing the specific shape of polyps.

All these steps are based on one assumption, namely that the DNA-synthesizing cells have a greater tendency to adhere to the surface basement membrane than do the differentiated cells.

Other mucosal changes occur adjacent to adenomas. In one study (Urbanski et al. 1986) 984 colonic polyps were investigated. In additional to adenomatous mucosae, three different mucosal patterns were recognized – transitional, eosinophilic and hyperplastic. There was strong association between eosinophilic and transitional mucosae and hyperplastic mucosae. The authors suggested a sequence of transitional mucosae turning into eosinophilic mucosae before the formation of the adenomas. This may represent a fertile ground for the development of adenomatous transformation. In another study (Lanza et al. 1985), hyperplastic changes were observed in the immediate vicinity or at the base of adenomas which were more extensive and frequent with larger adenomas. Sialomucin was also predominantly present. The authors suggested that mucosal hyperplasia may be a local change parallel or secondary to tumour development. Such secretory changes were more frequent in the left colon, confirming earlier findings (Greaves et al. 1980; Filipe et al. 1980).

As the large adenomas with severe dysplasia are concentrated in the sigmoid colon and rectum (Falterman et al. 1974; Konishi and Morson 1982), these findings again confirmed the association of such changes with malignancy.

Adenoma – Carcinoma Sequence

The existence of an adenoma–carcinoma sequence has been supported by evidence from many sources, much of it circumstantial. The problem in such studies is that detailed examination of adenoma and carcinoma is limited to one point in time. Therefore in human studies most of the results are obtained from epidemiological analysis.

Morson et al. (1983) stated two circumstances supporting the existence of such a sequence:

1. One third of all operation specimens of colorectal cancer contain one or more adenomas in addition to the carcinoma: 7% of the patients involved develop secondary or metachronous tumour in the remaining bowel.
2. Among patients having synchronous carcinomas, excluding those with familial polyposis coli and ulcerative colitis, 75% have associated adenomas (Heald and Bussey 1975).

A further piece of evidence for the adenoma–carcinoma sequence is the similarity of distribution displayed by adenomas and carcinomas (Helwig 1959; Fitts 1961; Enterline et al. 1962). Of the 1500 adenomas in Fitts' study, 2.5% were found to be invasive, and 61 of Enterline's 1700 tubular adenomas had foci of invasion through muscularis mucosae.

Spratt et al. (1958) and Ekelund (1963), however, come to the opposite conclusion about the distribution. In patients having both adenomas and carcinomas, the adenomas were sited more distally than the carcinomas in the right colon. In Spratt's study, 43 of 425 tubular adenomas showed "cytological malignancy", but only one showed stalk invasion. Horn (1971) observed 325 colonic carcinomas, and found no evidence of a residual adenoma. These authors concluded that colonic carcinomas arise as minute infiltrating adenocarcinomas in non-adenomatous mucosae. Spratt also denied the presence of residual adenomatous lesion in quite advanced adenocarcinomas. This observation can be explained, as once invasive growth is established, destruction of overlying adenomas will surely occur, confirmed by Morson (1966).

The age distribution of adenomas and carcinomas seemed to support the existence of the adenoma–carcinoma sequence. Results from screening indicated that the incidence of carcinomas peaked 7 years later than adenomas. Morson (1976) followed up three patients with adenomas who developed carcinomas at the same sites 5–13 years later. In patients with polyposis coli an average age difference of 12 years between adenomas and carcinomas occurs (Morson 1978).

Conclusion

Many experiments have been performed in order to find out the sequence of events culminating in the formation of invasive tumours. The detailed animal studies mostly agree that dysplasia and atypia arise as adenomas. Some studies, however, come to the conclusion that tumours arise from the epithelia of morphologically normal crypts. This disagreement may be settled if a common concept of what constitutes an adenoma can be reached and the concept of flat adenoma can be accepted.

In human studies, most of the evidence seems to be in favour of existence of the adenoma–carcinoma sequence. Strong evidence to the contrary will have to be presented if it is to be disproved.

References

Ahnen DJ (1985) Are animal models of colon cancer relevant to human disease? Dig Dis Sci 30 [Suppl]:103S–106S

Appel MF, Spjut HJ, Estrada RG (1977) The significance of villous component in colonic polyps. Am J Surg 134:770–771

Bengoechea O, Martinez-Penuela JM, Larrinaga B, Valerdi J, Borda F (1987) Hyperplastic polyposis of the colorectum and adenocarcinoma in a 24 year old man. Am J Surg Pathol 11:323–327

Bleiberg H, Mainguet P, Galand P (1972) Cell renewal in familial polyposis: comparison between polyps and adjacent mucosa. Gastroenterology 63:240–245

Bleiberg H, Buyse M, Galand P (1985) Cell kinetic indicators of premalignant stages of colorectal cancer. Cancer 56:124–129

Camplejohn RS, Bone G, Aherne WA (1973) Cell proliferation in rectal mucosa. A stathmokinetic study. Eur J Cancer 9:577–581

Chang WWL (1978) Histogenesis of symmetrical 1,2-dimethylhydrasine induced neoplasms of the colon in the mouse. JNCI 60:1405–1418

Chang WWL (1980) Pathogenesis and biological behaviour of 1,2-dimethylhydrazine-induced colonic neoplasms in the mouse. In: Appleton DR, Sunter JP, Watson AJ (eds) Cell proliferation in the gastrointestinal tract. Pitman Medical, London, pp 278–297

Cole JW, McKalen A (1961) Observations of cell renewal in human rectal mucosa in vivo with thymidine ^{3}H. Gastroenterology 41:122–125

Cole JW, McKalen A (1963) Studies on the morphogenesis of adenomatous polyps in the human colon. Cancer 16:998–1002

Day DW, Morson BC (1978) The adenoma–carcinoma sequence. In: Morson BC (ed) The pathogenesis of colorectal cancer. Saunders, Philadelphia (Major problems in pathology, vol 10)

Deschner EE, Lipkin M (1975) Proliferative patterns in colonic mucosa in familial polyposis. Cancer 35:413–418

Duke CL (1947) Explanation of differences between papilloma and adenoma of the rectum. Proc R Soc Med 40:829–830

Eide TJ (1986) Prevalence and morphological features of adenomas of the large intestine in individuals with and without colorectal carcinoma. Histopathology 10:111–118

Ekelund G (1963) On cancer and polyps of colon and rectum. Acta Pathol Microbiol Scand 59:165–170

Enterline H, Evans GW, Mercardo-Lugo R, Miller L, Fitts WT (1962) Malignant potential of adenomas of colon and rectum. JAMA 179:322–330

Falterman KW, Hill CB, Markey JC, Fox JW, Cohn I (1974) Cancer of the colon, rectum and anus: a review of 2313 cases. Cancer 34:951–959

Filipe MI (1975) Mucous secretion in rat colonic mucosa during carcinogenesis induced by dimethylhydrazine. A morphological and histochemical study. Br J Cancer 32:60–77

Filipe MI, Mughal S, Bussey HJ (1980) Patterns of mucous secretion in the colonic epithelium in familial polyposis. Invest Cell Pathol 3:329–335

Fitts WT (1961) Adenomas of the colon and rectum – their malignant potential. Am J Surg 101:87–90

Galandiuk S, Fazio VW, Jagelman DG, Lavery IC, Weakley FA, Petras RE, Badhwar K, McGonagle B, Eastin K, Sutton T (1987) Villous and tubulovillous adenomas of the colon and rectum. Am J Surg 153:41–47

Gebbers JO, Laissue JA (1986) Mixed hyperplastic and neoplastic polyp of the colon – an immunohistological study. Virchows Arch [A] 410:189–194

Goldman H, Si-Chun Ming, Hickok DF (1970) Nature and significance of hyperplastic polyps of the human colon. Arch Pathol 89:349–354

Greaves P, Filipe MI, Branfoot AC (1980) Transitional mucosa and survival in human colorectal cancer. Cancer 46:764–770

Haase P, Cowen DM, Knowles E, Cooper EH (1973) Evaluation of dimethylhydrasine induced tumours in mice as a model system for colorectal cancer. Br J Cancer 28:530–543

Heald RJ, Bussey HJR (1975) Clinical experiences at St. Mark's Hospital with multiple synchronous cancers of the colon and rectum. Dis Colon Rectum 18:6–10

Helwig EB (1959) Adenomas and the pathogenesis of cancer of the colon and rectum. Dis Colon Rectum 2:5–17

Horn RC (1971) Malignant potential of polypoid lesions of colon and rectum. Cancer 28:146–152

Konishi F, Morson BC (1982) Pathology of colorectal adenomas, a colonoscopic survey. J Clin Pathol 35:830–841

Lane N, Lev R (1963) Observations on the origin of adenomatous epithelium of the colon: serial section studies of minute polyps in familial polyposis. Cancer 16:751–764

Lanza G Jr, Altavilla G, Cavazzini L, Negrini R (1985) Colonic mucosa adjacent to adenomas and hyperplastic polyps – a morphological and histochemical study. Histopathology 9:857–873

Lipkin M (1974) Phase 1 and phase 2 proliferative lesions of colonic epithelial cells in disease leading to colonic cancer. Cancer 34:878–888

Mak KM, Slater CH, Hoff MB (1979) Inhibition of DNA synthesis by carcinogens in human colon mucosa in organ culture. JNCI 63:1305–1312

Maskens AP (1976) Histogenesis and growth pattern of 1,2-dimethylhydrasine induced rat colon adenocarcinoma. Cancer Res 36:1585–1593

Maskens AP (1979) Histogenesis of adenomatous polyps in the human large intestine. Gastroenterology 77:1245–1251

Morson BC (1966) Factors affecting the prognosis of early cancer of the rectum. Proc R Soc Med 59:607–608

Morson BC (1976) Genesis of colorectal cancer. In: Sherlak P, Zonchek N (eds) Clinics of gastroenterology, vol 5. Saunders, Philadelphia, pp 505–525

Morson BC (1978) The pathogenesis of colorectal cancer. Saunders, Philadelphia (Major problems in pathology, vol 10)

Morson BC, Bussey HJR, Day DW, Hill MJ (1983) Adenomas of large bowel. Cancer Surv 2:451–477

Muto T, Bussey HJR, Morson BC (1975) The evolution of cancer of the colon and rectum. Cancer 36:2251–2270

Muto T, Kamiya J, Sawada T, Konshi F, Sugihara K, Kubota Y, Adachi M, Agawa S, Saito Y, Morioka Y, Tanprayoon T (1985) Small 'flat adenoma' of the large bowel with special reference to its clinicopathologic features. Dis Colon Rectum 28:847–851

Nakamura SI, Kino I (1984) Morphogenesis of minute adenomas in familial polyposis coli. JNCI 73:41–49

Nakamura SI, Ohtawara Y, Naito Y, Kino I (1978) Cell kinetic of the mouse colonic epithelium after administration of N,N'-dimethylhydrasine dihydrochloride (in Japanese). In: Proceedings of 37th annual meeting of Japanese Cancer Assocation, p 204

Newberne PM, Rogers AE (1973) Animal model: DMH-induced adenocarcinoma of the colon in the rat. Am J Pathol 72:541–544

Ota DM, Drewinko B (1985) Growth kinetics of human colorectal carcinomas. Cancer Res 45:2128–2131

Potet F, Soullard J (1971) Polyps of the rectum and colon. Gut 12:468–482

Pozharisski KM (1975) Morphology and morphogenesis of experimental epithelial tumours of the intestine. JNCI 54:1115–1135

Pozharisski KM, Likhachev AJ, Klimashevski VF, Shaposhnikov JD (1979) Experimental intestinal cancer research with special reference to human pathology. Adv Cancer Res 30:165–237

Richards TC (1977) Early changes in the dynamics of crypt cell populations in mouse colon following administration of 1,2-dimethylhydrasine. Cancer Res 37:1680–1685

Spjut JJ (1972) Newer concepts of cancer of the colon and rectum: similarities between human and experimentally induced tumours of the large intestine. Dis Colon Rectum 15:94–99

Spratt JS, Ackerman LV, Moyer CA (1958) Relationship of polyps of colon to colonic cancer. Ann Surg 148:682–696

Stragand JJ, Bergerat JP, Allan White R, Robinson J, Drewinko B (1980) Biological and cell kinetic properties of a human colonic adenocarcinoma grown in athymia mice. Cancer Res 40:2846–2852

Sunter JP (1980) In: Appleton DR, Sunter JP, Watson AJ (eds) Cell proliferation in the gastrointestinal tract. Pitman Medical, London, p 255

Sunter JP, Appleton DR, Wright NA, Watson AJ (1978) Pathological features of the colonic tumours induced in rats by administration of 1,2-dimethylhydrasine. Virchows Arch [B] 29:211–223

Sunter JP, Appleton DR, Watson AJ (1981) Acute changes occurring in the intestinal mucosae of rats given a single injection of 1,2-dimethylhydrasine. Virchows Arch [B] 36:47–57

Terpstra OT, Blankenstein M, Dees J, Eilers GAM (1987) Abnormal pattern of cell proliferation in the entire colonic mucosa of patients with colon adenoma or cancer. Gastroenterology 92:704–708

Thurnherr N, Deschner EE, Stonehill EH, Lipkin M (1973) Induction of adenocarcinomas of the colon in mice by weekly injections of 1,2-dimethylhydrasine. Cancer Res 33:940–945

Urbanski SJ, Haber G, Hartwick W, Kortan P, Marcon N, Miceli P (1986) Mucosal changes associated with adenomatous colonic polyps. Am J Pathol 124:34–38

Valdes-Depera A, Beckfield WJ (1957) Adenomatous polyps of the large intestine; pathology and histogenesis. Gastroenterology 32:452–461

Ward JM (1974) Morphogenesis of chemically induced neoplasms of the large intestine in rats. Lab Invest 30:505–513

Welin S, Youker J, Spratt JS (1963) The rates and pattern of growth of 375 tumours of the large intestine and rectum observed serially by double contrast enema study (Malmo technique). Am J Roentgenol 90:673–687

Wiebecke B, Krey U, Lohrs U, Eder M (1973) Morphological and autoradiographical investigations on experimental carcinogenesis and polyp development in the intestinal tract of rats and mice. Virchows Arch [A] 360:179–193

Wiebecke B, Bradits A, Eder M (1974) Epithelial proliferation and morphogenesis of hyperplastic adenomatous and villous polyps of the human colon. Virchows Arch [A] 364:35–49

Wright NA (1984) Cell proliferation in gastrointestinal carcinogenesis. In: Wright NA, Alison M (eds) The biology of epithelial cell populations, vol 2. Clarendon, Oxford, pp 805–839

Cell Differentiation in Colorectal Carcinoma

S. C. Kirkland

Cancer Research Campaign, Cell Proliferation Unit, Department of Histopathology, Royal Postgraduate Medical School, Hammersmith Hospital, Ducane Road, London W12 0HS, UK

Contents

Introduction

Colorectal mucosa is composed of a flat surface epithelium and numerous invaginations or crypts, both lined by polarised columnar epithelial cells. The epithelium is composed of undifferentiated cells and several differentiated cell types including absorptive, mucous and enteroendocrine. It is a continually renewing epithelium, proliferation taking place in the crypt and differentiating cells migrating to the surface where they are eventually lost into the gut lumen. It has been proposed that multipotential stem cells located in the base of the crypt give rise to all cell types present in colorectal epithelium (the unitarian hypothesis). There are now several experiments which provide evidence supporting the unitarian hypothesis (Chang and Leblond 1971; Cheng and Leblond 1974; Ponder et al. 1985).

Differentiation can be assessed using morphological, biochemical and physiological criteria. Markers of differentiation in the colon and rectum include those associated with the transport function of the epithelium, as well as markers of mucous and enteroendocrine cells. The degree to which malignant cells express these differentiation markers should provide insight into the origin, development and behaviour of carcinomas. If the multipotential stem cells are the cells of origin of colorectal carcinoma the malignant cells might be expected to retain some ability to produce differentiated progeny.

This chapter will describe some of the differentiated features found in human colorectal carcinomas, experimental animal tumours and cell lines derived from human colorectal adenocarcinomas.

Differentiated Features of Normal Human Colorectal Mucosa

In the normal mucosa of the large intestine, a regular pattern of differentiation is observed as cells migrate from the crypt base to the surface epithelium. Four basic cell types are present; undifferentiated, columnar, mucous and enteroendocrine cells (Shamsuddin et al. 1982). Ultrastructurally a further three types of cells, intermediate, immature goblet and immature columnar cells can be identified (Kaye et al. 1973). In general, progressive maturation is observed from undifferentiated cells in the base of the crypt to immature goblet and absorptive cells in the mid-crypt and finally to fully mature goblet and absorptive cells in the upper one-third of the crypt and surface epithelium (Kaye et al. 1973). Unlike goblet and absorptive cells, mature entero-endocrine cells are generally located in the lower one-third of the crypt. Cell division is restricted to the lower two-thirds of the crypt (Lipkin et al. 1963). Although this is the basic pattern of cell differentiation, there are differences both in morphology and histochemical reaction between various segments of the large intestine (Shamsuddin et al. 1982). Differences are found both in the ratios of differentiated cells and in the ultrastructural characteristics of mucous and columnar cells.

All the differentiated cell types in colorectal epithelium are thought to be derived from multipotential stem cells (the unitarian hypothesis). The results of several investigations on cell renewal in normal rodent gastrointestinal tract provide evidence which supports the unitarian hypothesis. Cheng and Leblond exploited the radiosensitivity of the basal crypt columnar cells in mouse small intestine to kill them selectively with ^{3}H-thymidine: the surrounding cells phagocytosed the debris, and the fate of the remaining basal crypt cells containing labelled phagosomes was investigated. Labelled phagosomes were later observed in villous columnar, mucous and Paneth's cells, although only one enteroendocrine cell was shown to contain a phagosome (Cheng and Leblond 1974). Additional evidence in support of the unitarian hypothesis has been provided by studies using mouse embryo aggregation chimaeras. These experiments demonstrate that individual crypts of both small and large intestine are composed of epithelial cells of only one parental type (Ponder et al. 1985). Therefore it appears that the renewal of colorectal epithelium takes place by carefully balanced proliferation and differentiation of multipotential stem cells.

Differentiated Features of Human Adenocarcinomas

Studies of adenomatous epithelium have shown that it rarely differentiates past the partially differentiated cell stage observed in the lower one-third of the crypt. The majority of cells within the adenomatous epithelium retain both the morphological and proliferative characteristics of this immature cell type (Kaye et al. 1973). Cell division in adenomatous epithelium extends beyond the proliferative zone found in normal epithelium.

In adenocarcinoma, about 85% have a uniform tubular structure and secrete relatively small amounts of mucin (Morson and Dawson 1979). Malignant transformation is characterised by an increase in the proportion of undifferentiated and partially differentiated cells (Hickey and Seiler 1981). In a study of the differentiated features of adenocarcinomas, it was found that the degree of differentiation was related to the histological grading of the tumour (Seiler et al. 1984). Seven well-differentiated adenocarcinomas were all shown to contain immature mucous cells in varying proportions and cells with abundant microvilli. In this same study, only five of 29 moderately differentiated adenocarcinomas were shown to contain unequivocal intracytoplasmic mucin vacuoles (Seiler et al. 1984). Moderately well-differentiated tumours also contained absorptive cells with microvilli, but these had a less regular appearance than in the well-differentiated tumours. Poorly differentiated tumours were generally composed of sheets of undifferentiated cells; however, some remnants of intestinal differentiation, such as glycocalyceal bodies or dense core microvilli, could always be found on careful searching (Seiler et al. 1984).

Therefore the majority of colorectal adenocarcinomas are moderately differentiated histologically and contain a high proportion of immature absorptive cells and varying numbers of immature mucous cells. In addition to these two cell types, colorectal adenocarcinomas have also been shown to contain enteroendocrine cells (Ulich et al. 1983; Smith and Haggitt 1984). Endocrine cells were infrequently observed in poorly differentiated tumours but were found in 52% of other colonic adenocarcinomas (Smith and Haggitt 1984).

Although human colorectal carcinomas may often appear to be composed of a homogeneous population of cells, heterogeneity in the expression of membrane antigens can be demonstrated by immunostaining of sections with monoclonal antibodies (Daar and Fabre 1983). Cell populations can be isolated from single carcinomas which differ markedly in morphological and functional characteristics (Dexter et al. 1981; Brattain et al. 1981). At present the mechanisms which generate and maintain this heterogeneity are poorly understood.

In addition to functional and antigenic characteristics of normal adult colonocytes, human colorectal carcinoma cells can also express some antigens which are not usually present in normal adult colonic epithelium. Some colon carcinomas exhibit a pattern of enterocytic differentiation which is characteristic of the foetal colon. Such carcinoma cells express brush border hydrolases, such as sucrase-isomaltase, which are normally expressed in the foetal but not in the adult colon (Zweibaum et al. 1984). Carcinoembryonic antigen is another foetal antigen which is usually absent or present in traces in the adult colon but which is found in most colorectal carcinomas (Gold and Freedman 1965). In addition, HLA-DR can be demonstrated in histological sections of colonic adenocarcinomas, whereas normal colonocytes are HLA-DR negative except in certain pathological conditions (Daar et al. 1982; Rognum et al. 1983).

Human colorectal adenocarcinomas have been shown to contain cells with many of the characteristics of the three differentiated cell types present in normal colorectal epithelium. These observations support the concept of transformation of progenitor cells which retain varying degrees of ability to yield differentiated progeny. Although transformed cells retain some capacity to differentiate, their exact state of differentiation may differ from their normal counterparts as certain features of the transformed cell are not found within normal adult colorectal mucosa.

Experimental Carcinomas

Dimethylhydrazine (DMH) has been widely used to produce intestinal neoplasms in rodents (Druckrey 1970). Colonic carcinomas induced in rats by DMH are either moderately well or poorly differentiated adenocarcinomas with some benign adenomas (Sunter 1980). Using such experimental systems it has been possible to examine the differentiated features of cells within both carcinomas and early lesions.

DMH-induced adenocarcinomas in the rat have been shown to contain a predominance of cells morphologically resembling undifferentiated crypt cells of normal colonic epithelium. However, differentiated cell types including absorptive, mucous and endocrine cells, which were indistinguishable from their normal counterparts in normal epithelium are also present in small numbers (Barkla and Tutton 1978). In the mouse, early neoplastic lesions were identified as adenomatous structures lined with pseudostratified or stratified columnar epithelium without mucous cells. In the search for precursors of these early neoplastic lesions, hyperplastic abnormal crypts were noted. These crypts were composed of a homogeneous population of cuboidal or columnar cells without vacuoles or mucous droplets. Mucous cells were usually absent. Ultrastructurally, early neoplastic lesions were composed of cells with the features of the undifferentiated cells usually confined to the base of the crypt in normal colon. These results suggest a reduced ability of transformed cells to differentiate, as columnar, mucous and endocrine cells were usually absent from abnormal crypts in DMH-teated animals (Chang 1978).

In a detailed study of neuroendocrine cells within DMH-induced rat colorectal tumours, the tumours contained only types of endocrine cell which are normally found in colorectal epithelium. Glucagon, PYY and 5-hydroxytryptamine immunoreactive cells were frequently observed within well- or moderately well-differentiated tumours while poorly differentiated tumours were consistently negative (Johnston et al. 1986).

Endocrine cells have also been reported in another chemically induced rat colonic adenocarcinoma (Cox and Pierce 1982). This adenocarcinoma was shown to contain three recognisable cell lineages (columnar, mucous and endocrine) in addition to numerous undifferentiated cells. Single cell suspensions of this tumour gave rise to lung colonies which contained columnar, mucous, endocrine and undifferentiated cells. These experiments again support the concept that malignant cells have features in common with normal stem cells in that they are able to differentiate into mucous, columnar and endocrine cells. Therefore the undifferentiated cancer cell can be a multipotential stem cell closely resembling the undifferentiated stem cell of the colonic crypt. Indeed, ultrastructural comparison of undifferentiated cells within murine colonic carcinoma with normal undifferentiated cells showed that the normal stem cells are as undifferentiated as their malignant counterparts (Pierce et al. 1977). Such evidence suggests that carcinoma cells are derived from normal stem cells.

Human Colorectal Carcinoma Cell Lines

Although there are now a large number of cell lines derived from colorectal carcinomas (Fogh and Trempe 1975; Leibowitz et al. 1976; McBain et al. 1984), only a few of these exhibit differentiated features of normal colorectal epithelium. Some cell lines can be induced to differentiate by agents such as sodium butyrate (Chung et al. 1985; Morita et al. 1982; Augeron and Laboisse 1984) or by replacement of glucose in the culture medium with galactose (Pinto et al. 1982). These cell lines provide useful tools with which to study the functional and morphological characteristics of human carcinoma cells in the absence of contaminating normal cell types.

In general, the cells which "spontaneously" express differentiated features have the properties of absorptive or columnar epithelial cells. Some lines form polarised monolayers with a brush border (Namba et al. 1983; Pinto et al. 1983; Whitehead et al. 1985; Kirkland and Bailey 1986), while other lines are also able to demonstrate vectorial fluid transport (Dharmsathaphorn et al. 1984; Grasset et al. 1984; Kirkland 1985). In addition to a basal level of fluid transport, carcinoma cells have also been shown to respond to agents which act as secretagogues in normal epithelium, for example, vasoactive intestinal polypeptide (VIP) (Dharmsathaphorn et al. 1985; Grasset et al. 1985; Cuthbert et al. 1985). The short circuit current measured in these experiments is thought to be due to electrogenic chloride secretion (Grasset et al. 1984; Dharmsathaphorn et al. 1985; Cuthbert et al. 1987). In normal colorectal epithelium, crypts are the site of chloride secretion, and the surface epithelium is the site of sodium absorption (Welsh et al. 1986). Carcinoma cells maintained in vitro therefore show features of crypt cells as it has not yet been possible to demonstrate sodium absorption in colorectal cell lines (Cuthbert et al. 1987). Such results demonstrate that colorectal carcinoma cells can retain much of the structural and functional polarity characteristic of normal colorectal epithelial cells.

The presence of mucous cells has only been reported in three colorectal carcinoma cell lines in vitro. In the LIM 1215 cell line established from a patient with nonpolyposis colorectal cancer, mucous cells were demonstrated by electron microscopy, mucicarmine staining and staining with a monoclonal antibody to colonic mucous (Whitehead et al. 1985). Recently the same group (Whitehead et al. 1987) has described the establishment of a cell line, LIM 1863, which grows as organoids. These organoids contain both polarised columnar cells with a brush border and mucous cells which secrete mucous into the lumen of the organoids. Finally, colonies of mucous cells were reported in monolayer cultures of HT-29 following treatment with sodium butyrate (Augeron and Laboisse 1984).

Unlike primary colorectal carcinomas where endocrine cells are a common feature, only one human colorectal carcinoma cell line, HRA-19, has been shown to differentiate into endocrine cells. The HRA-19 cell line, established from a primary rectal adenocarcinoma, demonstrates some endocrine differentiation when grown as xenografts in nude mice (Kirkland 1986). Xenografts of a clone of this cell line have now been shown to contain endocrine, mucous and columnar cells. Therefore all epithelial lineages, at least in neoplastic epithelium, are of clonal origin (Kirkland 1988).

Studies on human colorectal carcinomas have confirmed the presence of heterogeneous cell populations. Subpopulations have been isolated from cultures of single carcinomas which differ in morphology, karyotype and cloning efficiency in soft agar (Dexter et al. 1981). Isolation of distinct subpopulations has been achieved from human colorectal carcinoma cell lines (Brattain et al. 1981; Dexter et al. 1981; Cuthbert et al. 1987) and primary cultures (Verstijnen et al. 1987). These subpopulations differ in their functional characteristics (Cuthbert et al. 1987), and there is also some evidence to suggest that they display differing differentiation features (Verstijnen et al. 1987).

The results obtained with the cell lines show that carcinoma cells in the absence of contaminating cell types can express many of the differentiated features of normal colonocytes. However, mucous and endocrine cell differentiation is rarely seen in these cell lines. This may be due to selection for less well-differentiated carcinoma cells when cell lines are established from primary tumours or to failure of the in vitro conditions to support differentiation. In addition, many workers have used tumours of high-grade malignancy to establish cell lines (McBain et al. 1984), and such tumours may provide a less well-differentiated starting material (Seiler et al. 1984).

Summary

Normal colorectal epithelium is composed of undifferentiated, absorptive, mucous and endocrine cells. There is now good evidence to support the unitarian hypothesis for cell renewal which proposes that multipotential stem cells give rise to all the differentiated cell types present in the epithelium. Observations on human and chemically induced rodent colorectal carcinomas show that they contain all the differentiated cell types found in normal mucosa. Experiments with colorectal carcinoma cell lines confirm that malignant cells can express differentiated features in the absence of contaminating normal cells. It has been shown that a single human rectal adenocarcinoma cell can differentiate into columnar, mucous and endocrine cells (Kirkland 1988). All these observations demonstrate similarity between malignant cells and undifferentiated stem cells and suggest that carcinomas arise from these stem cells. The differences observed in the differentiation potential of individual tumours may reflect either differences in the effect of transformation on cell function or may reflect similar effects on different target cells.

At present, little is known about the mechanisms controlling differentiation in normal colorectal epithelium. In other continually renewing systems such as the bone marrow, a range of growth and differentiation factors is known to influence the differentiation of the stem cell leading to different cell lineages. Factors controlling differentiation in colorectal epithelium have yet to be identified, but with the differentiating in vitro systems now available, the search for such factors is underway. The differentiation of human colorectal carcinoma cells can be modulated by changes in growth conditions (Kirkland 1986), therefore these cells retain some requirement for external stimuli for their differentiation. Considerable evidence exists which indicates that certain carcinoma cells can be induced to differentiate to mature end stage cells with no proliferative potential (Pierce and Wallace 1971; Sartorelli 1985). Thus it is conceivable that differentiation-inducing agents from colorectal epithelium could be used to induce malignant cells to differentiate into benign forms and therefore provide a new therapeutic approach to the treatment of colorectal cancer.

References

Augeron C, Laboisse CL (1984) Emergence of permanently differentiated cell clones in a human colonic cancer cell line after treatment with sodium butyrate. Cancer Res 44:3941–3969

Barkla DH, Tutton PJM (1978) Ultrastructure of 1,2-dimethylhydrazine-induced adenocarcinomas in the rat colon. JNCI 61:1291–1299

Brattain MG, Fine WD, Khaled FM, Thompson J, Brattain DE (1981) Heterogeneity of malignant cells from a human colonic carcinoma. Cancer Res 41:1751–1756

Chang WWL (1978) Histogenesis of symmetrical 1,2-dimethylhydrazine induced neoplasms of the colon in the mouse. JNCI 60:1405–1418

Chang WWL, Leblond CP (1971) Renewal of the epithelium in the descending colon of the mouse small intestine. I. Presence of three epithelial cell populations vacuolated, columnar, mucous and argentaffin. Am J Anat 131:73–100

Cheng H, Leblond CP (1974) Origin, differentiation and renewal of the four main epithelial cell types in the mouse small intestine. V. Unitarian theory of the origin of the four epithelial cell types. Am J Anat 141:537–567

Chung YS, Song IS, Erickson RH, Sleisenger MH, Kim YS (1985) Effect of growth and sodium butyrate on brush border membrane associated hydrolases in human colorectal cancer cell lines. Cancer Res 45:2976–2982

Cox WF, Pierce GB (1982) The endodermal origin of the endocrine cells of an adenocarcinoma of the colon of the rat. Cancer 50:1530–1538

Cuthbert AW, Kirkland SC, MacVinish LJ (1985) Kinin effects on ion transport in monolayers of HCA-7 cells, a line from a human colonic adenocarcinoma. Br J Pharmacol 86:3–5

Cuthbert AW, Egleme C, Greenwood H, Hickman ME, Kirkland SC, MacVinish LJ (1987) Calcium and cyclic AMP-dependent chloride secretion in human colonic epithelia. Br J Pharmacol 91:503–515

Daar AS, Fabre JW (1983) The membrane antigens of human colorectal cancer cells: demonstration with monoclonal antibodies of heterogeneity within and between tumours and anomalous expression of HLA-DR. Eur J Clin Cancer Clin Oncol 19(2):209–220

Daar AS, Fuggle SV, Ting A, Fabre JW (1982) Anomalous expression of HLA-DR antigens on human colorectal cancer cells. J Immunol 129:447–449

Dexter DL, Spremulli EN, Fligiel Z, Barbosa JA, Vogel R, VanVoorheees A, Calabresi P (1981) Heterogeneity of cancer cells from a single human colon carcinoma. Am J Med 71:949–956

Dharmasathaporn K, McRoberts JA, Mandel KG, Tisdale LD, Masui HA (1984) A human colonic tumor cell line that maintains vectorial electrolyte transport. Am J Physiol 246:G204–G208

Dharmasathaporn K, Mandel KG, Masui H, McRoberts JA (1985) Vasoactive intestinal polypeptide-induced chloride secretion by a colonic epithelial cell line. J Clin Invest 75:462–471

Druckrey H (1970) Production of colonic carcinomas by 1,2-dialkylhydrazines and azoxyalkanes. In: Burdette WJ (ed) Carcinoma of the colon and antecedent epithelium. Thomas, Springfield, IL, pp 267–279

Fogh J, Trempe G (1975) New human tumour cell lines. In: Fogh J (ed) Human tumour cells in vitro. Plenum, New York, pp 115–141

Gold P, Freedman SO (1965) Specific carcinoembryonic antigen of the human digestive system. J Exp Med 122:467–481

Grasset E, Pinto M, Dussaulx E, Zweibaum A, Desjeux JF (1984) Epithelial properties of human colonic carcinoma cell line Caco-2: electrical parameters. Am J Physiol 247:C260–C267

Grasset E, Bernabeu J, Pinto M (1985) Epithelial properties of human colonic carcinoma cell line Caco-2: effect of secretagogues. Am J Physiol 248:C410–C418

Hickey WF, Seiler MW (1981) Ultrastructural markers of colonic adenocarcinoma. Cancer 47:140–145

Johnston CF, O'Neill AB, O'Hare MMT, Buchanan KD (1986) Neuroendocrine cells within colorectal tumours induced by dimethylhydrazine. An immunocytochemical study. Cell Tissue Res 246:205–210

Kaye GI, Fenoglio CM, Pascal RR, Lane N (1973) Comparative electron microscopic features of normal, hyperplastic and adenomatous epithelium. Gastroenterology 64:926–945

Kirkland SC (1985) Dome formation by a human colonic adenocarcinoma cell line (HCA-7). Cancer Res 45:3790–3795

Kirkland SC (1986) Endocrine differentiation by a human rectal adenocarcinoma cell line (HRA-19). Differentiation 33:148–155

Kirkland SC (1988) Clonal origin of columnar, mucous and endocrine cell lineages in human colorectal epithelium. Cancer 61:1359–1363

Kirkland SC, Bailey IG (1986) Establishment and characterisation of six human colorectal adenocarcinoma cell lines. Br J Cancer 53:779-785

Leibovitz A, Stinson JC, McCombs WB, McCoy CE, Mazur KC, Mabry ND (1976) Classification of human colorectal adenocarcinoma cell lines. Cancer Res 36:4562-4569

Lipkin M, Bell B, Sherlock P (1963) Cell proliferation kinetics in the gastrointestinal tract of man. I. Cell renewal in the colon and rectum. J Clin Invest 42:767-776

McBain JA, Weese JL, Meisner LF, Wolberg WH, Willson JKV (1984) Establishment and characterisation of human colorectal cancer cell lines. Cancer Res 44:5813-5821

Morita A, Tsao D, Kim YS (1982) Effect of sodium butyrate on alkaline phosphatase in HRT-18, a human rectal cancer cell line. Cancer Res 42:4540-4545

Morson BC, Dawson IMP (1979) Gastrointestinal pathology. Blackwell Scientific, Oxford

Namba M, Miyamoto K, Hyodah F, Iwama T, Utsonomuja J, Fukushima F, Kimoto T (1983) Establishment and characterisation of a human colon carcinoma cell line (KMS-4) from a patient with hereditary adenomatosis of the colon and rectum. Int J Cancer 32:697-702

Pierce GB, Wallace C (1971) Differentiation of malignant to benign cells. Cancer Res 31:127-134

Pierce GB, Nakane PK, Martinez-Hernandez A, Ward JM (1977) Ultrastructural comparison of differentiation of stem cells of murine adenocarcinomas of colon and breast with their normal counterparts. JNCI 58:1329-1345

Pinto M, Appay MD, Simon-Assmann P, Chevalier G, Dracopoli N, Fogh J, Zweibaum A (1982) Enterocytic differentiation of cultured human colon cancer cells by replacement of glucose by galactose in the medium. Biol Cell 44:193-196

Pinto M, Robine-Leon S, Appay MD, Kedinger M, Triadou N, Dussaulx E, Lacroix B, Simon-Assman P, Haffen K, Fogh J, Zweibaum A (1983) Enterocyte-like differentiation and polarisation of the human colon carcinoma cell line Caco-2 in culture. Biol Cell 47:323-330

Ponder BAJ, Schmidt GH, Wilkinson MM, Wood MJ, Monk M, Reid A (1985) Derivation of mouse intestinal crypts from single progenitor cells. Nature 313:689-691

Rognum TO, Brandtzaeg P, Thorud E (1983) Is the heterogeneous expression of HLA-DR antigens and CEA along with DNA profile variations evidence of phenotypic instability and clonal proliferation in human large bowel carcinomas? Br J Cancer 48:543-557

Sartorelli AC (1985) Malignant cell differentiation as a potential therapeutic approach. Br J Cancer 52:293-302

Seiler MW, Reilova-Velez J, Hickey W, Bono L (1984) Ultrastructural markers of large bowel cancer. In: Wolman SR, Mastromarino AJ (eds) Progress in cancer research and therapy, vol 29. Raven, NY, pp 51-65

Shamsuddin AM, Phelps PC, Trump BF (1982) Human large intestinal epithelium: light microscopy, histochemistry and ultrastructure. Hum Pathol 13:790-803

Smith DM, Haggitt RC (1984) The prevalence and prognostic significance of argyrophil cells in colorectal carcinomas. Am J Surg Pathol 8(2):123-128

Sunter JP (1980) Experimental carcinogenesis and cancer in the rodent gut. In: Appleton DR, Sunter JP, Watson AJ (eds) Cell proliferation in the gastrointestinal tract. Pitman Medical, Tunbridge Wells, Kent, pp 254-276

Ulich TR, Cheng L, Glover H, Yang K, Lewin KJ (1983) A colonic adenocarcinoma with argentaffin cells: an immunoperoxidase study demonstrating the presence of numerous neuroendocrine products. Cancer 51:1483-1489

Verstijnen CPHJ, Arends JW, Moerkerk PTM, Geraedts JPM, Sekikawa K, Uttendaal MP, Bosman FT (1987) The establishment and characterisation of two new cell lines derived from a single human colonic adenocarcinoma. Virchows Arch [B] 53:191-197

Welsh MJ, Smith PL, Fromm M, Frizzell RA (1982) Crypts are the site of intestinal fluid and electrolyte secretion. Science 218:1219-1221

Whitehead RH, Macrae FA, James D, St John B, Ma JA (1985) A colon cancer cell line (LIM1215) derived from a patient with inherited nonpolyposis colorectal cancer. JNCI 74:759-765

Whitehead RH, Jones JK, Gabriel A, Lukies RE (1987) A new colon carcinoma cell line (LIM1863) that grows as organoids with spontaneous differentiation into crypt-like structures in vitro. Cancer Res 47:2683-2689

Zweibaum A, Hauri HP, Sterchi E, Chantret I, Haffen K, Bamat J, Sordat B (1984) Immunohistological evidence, obtained with monoclonal antibodies, of small intestinal brush border hydrolases in human colon cancers and foetal colons. Int J Cancer 34:591-598

Attempts for Diagnostic
and Therapeutic Approaches

Immunoassay for Fecal Occult Blood and Early Detection of Colorectal Cancer

H. Schmidt-Gayk*

Chirurgische Klinik der Universität Heidelberg, Abt. 2.1.1

Contents

Haemoccult Testing – Chemical Detection of Fecal Occult Blood

"Fecal occult bleeding", i.e., macroscopically undetectable bleeding, is generally defined as a blood loss of less than 50 ml/d (Songster 1980). The detection of colorectal
carcinoma by testing for occult blood in feces is possible, but it is questionable

* The author wishes to thank H. G. Bischoff (Heidelberg), D. Theuer (Heilbronn), L.-M. Mao,
E. Wieland, H. M. Thon, T. Vogel, P. Schorb, A. Quentmeier, and C. Herfarth (Heidelberg) for
their cooperation.

whether this method permits early recognition in the majority of colorectal cancer patients because the sensitivity of many tests for occult blood is fairly low.

The Haemoccult Test, a Chemical Assay for Occult Bleeding
(for review see Köbberling and Windeler 1985)

In 1901, Boas started the search for occult blood to diagnose gastric bleeding. He used the gum guaiac method developed by van Deen in 1864. Initially, guaiac solutions and tablets were used. For these tests, the stool specimens had to be collected and tested in the laboratory, a fairly unpleasant procedure. In 1967, Greegor reported his experiences with a new test principle, which was an easy procedure and convenient for the laboratory staff. This test (Haemoccult) was introduced in the Federal Republic of Germany in 1972 when promising reports had been received from the United States. In 1979 it was incorporated into the German program for early cancer recognition.

Test Principle

The test is based on guaiac-impregnated filter paper to which a small stool sample is added. For evaluation, an H_2O_2-containing solution is applied to the reverse side of the filter paper. A complete test contains six samples; duplicate samples of three successive stools are usually collected.

If at least one sample is positive (bluish discoloration), the test series is considered positive. By its pseudo-peroxidase activity, hemoglobin oxidizes the colorless guaiac to the blue color. H_2O_2 in the developer solution acts as oxygen donor. For this reaction, only heme is responsible, and the hemoglobin protein chains are not necessary.

For this reason, the test yields false-positive results if animal hemoglobin and myoglobin are present. In addition, peroxidases from food or vegetables may also lead to the bluish discoloration. *False-positive* reactions are induced by black pudding, red meat, liver, horseradish, radishes, bananas, tomatoes, cherries, iodine in polyvidon, iodine as disinfectant, iron. *False-negative* results are produced by vitamin C in fruit juices or drugs.

Most authors recommend a diet rich in fiber for some days before and during the test. This diet increases the stool volume, and peristaltic waves and reduced passage time may provoke bleeding of the tumor by mechanical alteration. The test results are interpreted differently by different authors; some speak of false-positive results if other causes of bleeding such as polyps, diverticulosis, or colitis are found in addition to colorectal cancer. Other authors consider the results as false-positive, if no bleeding source can be detected despite intensive follow-up. Kruis et al. (1979) failed to reveal any pathological findings in 17.2% of their Haemoccult-positive patients. Ribet et al. (1980) reported 81% false-positive Haemoccult tests. False-positive guaiac tests entail high costs during follow-up investigation and are a considerable burden for the patient.

Determining the in vivo sensitivity of guaiac tests, several authors have found that in patients with colorectal cancer or adenoma, some of the tests remained negative (Anderson 1981; Griffith et al. 1981; Schewe et al. 1979). The rate of false-negative

Table 1. Rate of false-negative results in negative guaiac testing

Reference	Cancer	False-negative		Adenoma	False-negative	
	(n)	(n)	(%)	(n)	(n)	(%)
Deyhle[a]	23	3	13	17	7	41
Warm and Bloch[a]	12	7	58	84	55	65
Schewe et al. (1979)	84	30	35.7	53	31	58.5
Gnauck (1984)	176	25	14	451	191	42
Schüler (1984)	150	50	33 (HemoFEC)			

[a] Cited in Frühmorgen (1984).

results was endoscopically confirmed by different investigators in negative guaiac testing. Some of these investigations are listed in Table 1.

False-negative results have fatal consequences. Colorectal cancers or adenomas in a still operable condition remain undiscovered, and a real chance for cure is lost. Frühmorgen (1984) states that a single undetected cancer – mainly in the early stage – is undoubtedly of more importance than some false-positive results.

Immunological Detection of Fecal Occult Blood

Double Diffusion

The double diffusion method was described by Ouchterlony in 1947 (for review see Ouchterlony and Nilsson, 1978). It may be used as a qualitative test for occult bleeding. For diffusion, agar gel is poured onto a plastic or glass plate, and holes are punched into the gel. In the one-dimensional procedure, antigen (fecal extract) is pipetted into one hole, and antibody (for example, against human hemoglobin) into another one. Antigen (human hemoglobin) and antibody (against hemoglobin) diffuse against each other and form a precipitation line. The relative position of this precipitation line depends on the local concentration of antigen antibody. If the blood loss is high, the precipitation line is found near the antibody-containing well; if the blood loss is low, the line is near the antigen-containing well.

Latex Test

By agglutination of latex particles, a simple and rapid qualitative assay for fecal occult blood was developed by Heinrich (1984). This assay is extremely sensitive, and in a tube test procedure 200 nl blood per 100 g feces is detected. In a filter paper procedure, the in vitro sensitivity limit is approximately 2 µl/100 g feces.

In a comparative study with three chemical occult blood tests, Heinrich and Benn reported the following results in 1982: in 11 patients with histologically confirmed colorectal cancer, the tube version of the latex agglutination test was positive in all patients (100%), and the filter method in 82%. With the Fecatest, positive results were obtained in 36%, with the Feca-Nostic in 55%, and with the Haemoccult test in 18%. Seven patients with colorectal adenoma were all positive in the tube version of the latex agglutination test, and only one single patient had a positive Feca-Nostic test, whereas the Fecatest and Haemoccult were negative in all patients.

The in vitro sensitivity of the latex agglutination test is approximately 1000-fold higher than the guaiac test. Whereas a high sensitivity latex test detects a blood loss of more than 2 µl/day, the guaiac test will detect a blood loss of more than 2 ml/day.

Immunofluorescence Test for Fecal Occult Blood

This method was developed by Vellacott et al. (1981). After centrifugation of a mixture of feces in water, fluorescent anti-human hemoglobin was added to the supernatant. The nonbound antibody was separated after 10 min by a filter membrane coated with human hemoglobin. By comparing the fluorescence detection of this antibody with the hemoglobin standard, the hemoglobin concentration of the fecal samples was determined. Vellacott et al. (1981) reported a sensitivity limit of 100 mg hemoglobin per 100 g feces. The usefulness of this procedure remains to be demonstrated.

Radial Immunodiffusion

Immunochemical quantitation of antigens by single radial diffusion has been described by Mancini et al. (1965). This simple technique requires neither high-titer nor strictly monospecific antiserum. A gel film (thickness approximately 2 mm) composed of 1% agarose in phosphate buffer at pH 7.4 is cast into a supporting plate. Holes are punched into the gel as shown in Fig. 1. The antigen diffuses radially from the starting hole into the gel containing the antibody. The diameter of the precipitation ring is proportional to the amount of antigen, e.g., hemoglobin, in a feces sample.

Development of a New Test Tube for Collection of More Representative Fecal Samples and Combined Use of Immunological Hemoglobin and Albumin Determination in Feces

New Test Tube

A new test tube was developed as shown in Fig. 2. Two samples of one stool specimen were taken up at different positions to obtain a fairly representative amount of feces. The tubes were labeled with the patient's surname, first name, and date of birth and stored frozen at −18°C. An information sheet was given to the patient for instruction and to facilitate feces collection for the hospital staff. The patient received this instruction sheet together with six tubes for feces collection and six small plastic spades.

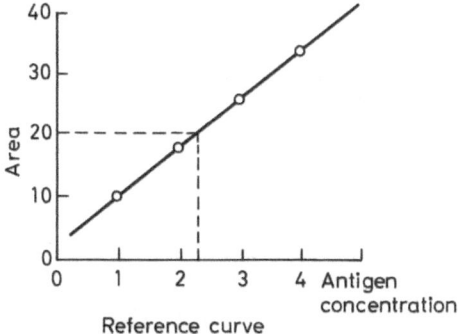

Reference curve

Fig. 1. Reference curve for the radial immunodiffusion method. On the *x-axis* the antigen concentration and on the *y-axis* the area of the precipitation ring are depicted

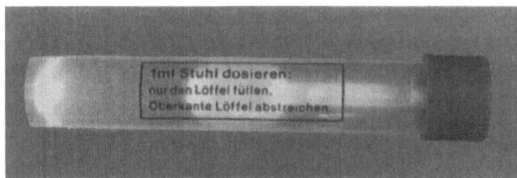

Fig. 2. Test tube for the collection of 1 ml (approximately 1 g) of feces. The spoon is firmly connected to the cap of the tube. With the spoon, 1 ml of feces is collected, the spoon is introduced into the tube, and the tube is closed firmly

Instruction Sheet

With this test, occult blood can be detected in feces. For investigation, two samples from three successive stools must be collected. No pain relieving drugs or drugs against rheumatic diseases should be taken during the collection of the stool samples. Females should not perform this test during menstruation. Since samples from three successive stools are used, please start with sample collection early enough before your next visit to your physician.

Instructions for Use (Read Carefully)

1. Use the spoon at the cap of the tube to collect one sample of feces.
2. Use the additional spade to wipe feces from above the upper edge of the spoon. The spoon should be entirely filled with feces (do not fill the whole tube with feces!!).
3. Screw the cap carefully.
4. Use a second tube to collect feces from another site of the same stool sample.
5. After the spoons have been filled and the tubes closed they must be kept frozen (for example in the freezing compartment of your refrigerator). The tubes are air- and water-tight so that no bacteria or fumes can leave the tube. There is no risk of contaminating the freezing compartment of your refrigerator.
6. At the next and after the following bowel movement follow the identical procedure outlined in points 1–5 of this instruction sheet. Again, use two tubes for the next and two tubes for the last collection.

7. Immediately before the next visit to your physician, take the six tubes from the freezing compartment of your refrigerator, add the labels containing your surname, first name, and date of birth, and give the tubes to your physician.

Aim of the Study

1. In animal experiments with carcinogen-induced colorectal cancer, the sensitivity of this immunological technique according to Mancini et al. (1965), which allows identification of occult blood loss, was compared with the guaiac test.
2. In healthy controls and endoscopically confirmed colorectal carcinoma and adenoma patients, the sensitivity and specificity of the methods were determined.
3. Finally, this method was used in screening for colorectal carcinoma and adenoma.

Materials and Methods

Preparation of the Immunodiffusion Plate

– Prepare a 1% agarose solution. Take 1 g of Difco Bacto-Agar (Difco, Detroit, Michigan, USA) in 100 ml phosphate buffer pH 7.4 with 0.2 g gelatine, 0.1 g sodium azide, 0.04 g ethylenediaminetetra-acetic acid (EDTA), and 3 g polyethylene glycol 6000 (PEG). The phosphate buffer has to be heated with the gelatine up to 50°C until the latter has dissolved. After cooling, sodium azide, EDTA, and PEG are added.
– Addition of PEG makes the precipitation rings more distinct, and the diameter may be determined with better precision.
– The agarose solution with PEG is heated on a magnetic stirrer up to a temperature of 95°C. Cooling down to 56°C is monitored with a thermometer. This temperature is kept constant in a heated water bath.
– At this temperature, 250 µl anti-albumin (or 2.5 ml anti-hemoglobin) are added for every 25 ml of agarose solution and mixed. This amount is sufficient for four plates (Immunodiffusion Plates, calibrated, unfilled, Code No. 42-150-1, Miles Laboratories Inc., Elkart, IN 46515, USA). This antibody-agarose solution is poured onto an immunodiffusion plate, 6 ml/plate.
– Within approximately 8 min, the solution transforms into a gel, and with a Cutter & Template Kit, three parallel lines with six holes each, a total fo 18 holes per plate, are cut. The cutter has a diameter of 3 mm and is connected by a tube to a vacuum pump.
– The immunodiffusion plate is covered with a cap and may be stored for up to 4 weeks in a moist chamber in a refrigerator at 4°–8°C.

Preparation of the Fecal Samples

– The frozen fecal samples are thawed and centrifuged briefly (approximately 30 s) at 3800 rpm (approximately 3000 × g) to remove fecal contamination at the upper rim of the tube.

- Two milliliters of the phosphate buffer with gelatine, sodium azide, EDTA, and polyethylene glycol are pipetted into each tube, and the sample at the bottom of the tube is mixed with the phosphate buffer with a Whirlmixer. After 15 min, the samples are mixed again.
- Thereafter the tubes are centrifuged for 15 min at 3800 rpm (approximately $3000 \times g$).
- One milliliter of the supernatant is transferred to an Eppendorf reaction vial (1.3-ml test tubes, Item No. 72690, Sarstedt, 5223 Nümbrecht-Rommelsdorf, FRG) and centrifuged for 15 min in an Eppendorf centrifuge (Eppendorf-Gerätebau, Netheler and Hintz GmbH, 2000 Hamburg, FRG) at 13000 rpm (approximately $12000 \times g$).
- Thereafter the supernatant is transferred to new Eppendorf reaction vials. The tubes are numbered, and 10 µl supernatant from each is transferred to the Mancini immunodiffusion plate. One drop may be added to a Haemoccult slide and used for guaiac testing. The Eppendorf reaction vial containing the clean fecal supernatant may be stored frozen again and re-used for control studies.
- In addition to the transfer of 10 µl of the buffered fecal supernatant from this Eppendorf reaction vial to one immuno-diffusion plate for human hemoglobin, 10 µl are transferred to a second immunodiffusion plate impregnated with an antibody against human albumin. This means that human hemoglobin and human albumin are determined in each sample.
- The immunodiffusion plate is covered, and the date, number, and antibody are stated on an adhesive label. The immunodiffusion plate is incubated at room temperature for 24 h in a humid chamber.
- For Haemoccult testing, the fecal slide of Haemoccult is opened, and 25 µl of the supernatant is applied to the filter paper. The Haemoccult slide is then closed again. The reverse side of the Haemoccult slide is opened, and two drops of a developer solution are added. A positive outcome of the test is indicated by a bluish discoloration. If the bluish coloration does not occur within 30 s, the test is considered negative. The Haemoccult must be viewed after 30 s because the bluish discoloration slowly fades.

Evaluation of the Immunodiffusion Plate

After 24 h, the cover is removed from the immunodiffusion plate, and the plate is viewed under a Behring Viewer (Meßprojektor, Behringwerke AG, 6000 Frankfurt/Main 80, FRG). An example of an immunodiffusion plate is shown in Fig. 3.

Results

Animal Experiments

We compared a commercially available test based on guaiac with an immunological assay for fecal occult blood. The latter method was based on antibodies against rat hemoglobin (Bischoff 1987).

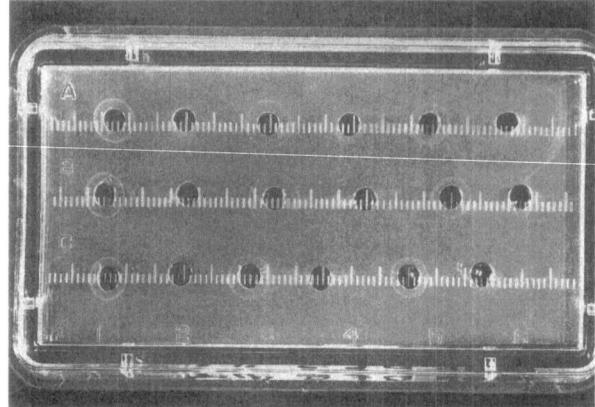

Fig. 3. Immunodiffusion
plate against human
albumin. The holes *A1*, *B1*,
and *C1* are positive, whereas
A2, *B2*, and *C2* are negative

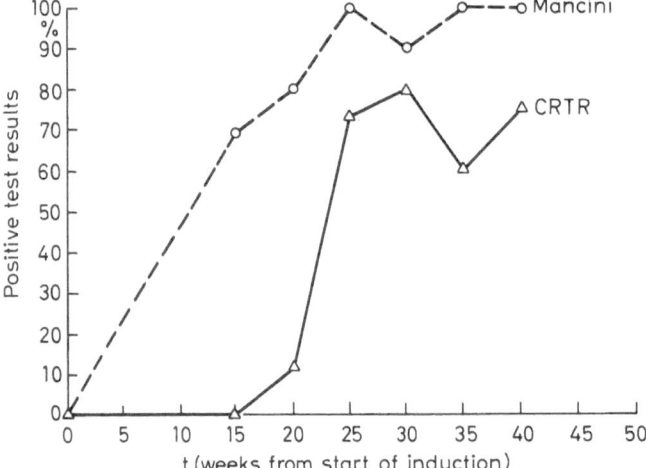

Fig. 4. Comparison of both testing methods at different times. Test results obtained by radial immunodiffusion for rat hemoglobin (*MANCINI*) and Colo-rectal-test-Roche (*CRTR*) are shown

As a tumor model, the acetoxymethyl-methyl-nitrosamine-induced (AMMN) colon tumor of the rat was chosen because of its many parallels to human colorectal carcinoma. By weekly intrarectal application of 2 mg/kg AMMN[1] for 10 weeks, colorectal tumors were induced in male Sprague-Dawley (SD) rats (WIGA, Sulzfeld, FRG). The initial weight of the rats was 200 g. The animals were kept under standard laboratory conditions and received altromin pellets and water ad libitum. Fecal samples were collected initially and at weeks 15, 20, 25, 30, 35, and 40. As a commercially available guaiac-based test the colo-rectal-test-Roche[2] (CRTR) was used. The immunoassay was performed by radial immunodiffusion according to Mancini et al. (1965).

_____

[1] Synthesized by P.D.M. Wiessler, DKFZ, Heidelberg, FRG.
[2] Hoffmann-La Roche, Basel, Switzerland.

Antibodies were raised in rabbits against rat hemoglobin by i.m. injection of 1 ml (3.5 mg hemoglobin) of an emulsion of rat hemoglobin with incomplete Freund's adjuvant. Injections were performed at monthly intervals for a total of four injections. Four weeks after the final booster injection, blood was collected and serum separated by centrifugation.

Preparation of the feces was done as described under Materials and Methods. In these experiments, the precipitation ring diameter was measured after 48 h of incubation. The standard curve was measured with samples of known hemoglobin concentration. AMMN induced colorectoral tumors in 100% of the animals between the 15th and the 25th weeks. The tumors were mainly adenocarcinomas. As shown in Fig. 4, fecal occult bleeding was confirmed by both methods. However, radial immunodiffusion detected occult bleeding 5–10 weeks earlier. All samples that were negative by radial immunodiffusion were also negative by guaiac testing. All guaiac-positive samples were also positive by radial immunodiffusion.

Healthy Controls and Patients with Endoscopically Confirmed Colorectal Carcinoma and Adenoma

One hundred and four healthy subjects served as a control group. Their ages ranged from 19 to 73 years; 59 were males and 55 were females. Seventy-four were 19–40 years, 30 were 41–60, and 10 were 60–73 years of age. There was no suggestion of gastrointestinal disease in any of the control subjects at the time of investigation, and none of them had symptoms of gastrointestinal or other acute diseases. Six stool samples were collected on three different days and investigated. Two of the 104 controls showed more albumin than a 1:1000 serum dilution in buffer, equal to 0.1 ml/100 ml of feces. One of these two also had detectable levels of hemoglobin in feces. Endoscopy revealed multiple polyps, and polyposis coli was diagnosed. For the other control subject with increased albumin concentration (more albumin than a 1:1000 human serum dilution in buffer) endoscopy revealed mild ulcerative colitis. After 6 months, the disease became symptomatic. In 53 patients with colorectal cancer who were sent to a gastroenterologist (D. Theuer) for endoscopy, fecal samples were collected before a biopsy had been performed. The age of these patients was 32–85 years. In two patients all tests were negative in all samples. Twenty-six of the 53 patients were positive in the Haemoccult test, 47 in the radial immunodiffusion for hemoglobin, and 35 in the radial immunodiffusion for albumin. By combined use of the radial immunodiffusion for hemoglobin and albumin, 51 of the 53 patients with colorectal cancer were positive in one or both of the radial immunodiffusion methods. Sensitivity was 96% for colorectal cancer by radial immunodiffusion and 49% by the Haemoccult test. Specificity was 98% for healthy controls (2/104 positive) by radial immunodiffusion and 100% by the Haemoccult test (104/104 negative). The shortcomings of this investigation will be discussed later.

Screening of Patients

A total of 2011 patients of internal wards at two hospitals in Heidelberg (Krankenhaus Salem and Speyererhof) were screened for occult blood by the Haemoccult test

Table 2. Screening of 2011 patients for colorectal cancer by immunological detection of occult blood

Group number	Patient group – final diagnosis	Patients (n)
1	Negative, no intestinal disease	1378
2	Adenomas (polyps), newly detected	69
3	Colorectal cancer, newly detected	24
4	Colorectal cancer, previously known	17
5	Other cancers, known	23
6	Inflammatory intestinal disease	76
7	Diverticulosis, diverticulitis	74
8	No cause detected (false-positive)	27
9	No diagnostic evaluation permitted	295
10	Other causes, partly questionable	28
		2011

Table 3. Test results ($n = 2011$)

Group number	Hb HSA HO	Hb HO	HSA HO	Hb HSA	HSA	Hb	HO	All tests negative
1								1378
2	5	5	1	26	21	11	–	–
3	4	4	1	7	5	3	–	–
4	4	–	1	5	1	3	–	3
5	4	2	3	3	5	–	1	5
6	5	2	1	13	7	8	1	39
7	2	4	1	11	16	2	1	37
8	–	1	2	4	16	1	3	–
9	25	2	2	74	148	29	15	–
10	5	2	–	6	13	–	2	–
	54	22	12	149	232	57	23	1462

Hb, hemoglobin; HSA, human serum albumin; HO, Haemoccult.

as well as by radial immunodiffusion for albumin and hemoglobin. Of these, 1378 showed negative results in all tests. Sixty-nine patients with colorectal adenomas or polyps and 24 patients with colorectal cancer were newly discovered by positive test results followed by endoscopy or radiography of the colon and rectum. The results are given in detail in Tables 2–4.

Table 4. Details of groups in Tables 2 and 3

Group 1	All tests negative, no symptoms of intestinal disease, negative Hemoccult tests, no precipitation ring in the hemoglobin radial immunodiffusion test, a diameter of albumin precipitation ring less than 5.5 mm (5.5-mm diameters are obtained with a serum dilution in buffer of 1:1000)
Group 2	Villous and tubular adenomas, hyperplastic polyps
Group 3	Twelve colon carcinomas, five sigma carcinomas, six rectal carcinomas, one patient with colon and simultaneous rectal carcinoma; eleven patients had metastases
Group 4	Colorectal cancer, previously known: three were negative in all tests
Group 5	Other cancer cases: eight gastric, eight pancreatic, two gallblader, two ovarian, one Vater's papilla, one esophageal, and one prostatic
Group 6	Twelve cases of ulcerative colitis, six of M. Crohn, 42 of gastritis, 16 cases with other inflammatory intestinal diseases
Group 7	Of the 74 patients, 64 were diagnosed as having diverticulosis
Group 8	No cause detected, false-positives: radiography or endoscopy of colon and rectum revealed no abnormalities; gastroscopy was not performed
Group 9	No diagnostic evaluation permitted: this group consisted of 295 patients; evaluation was refused by either patient or physician
Group 10	Other causes, partly questionable; some subjects were taking antirheumatic drugs, some had had surgery for gastric, colonic, or prostatic cancer months or years before

Discussion

Animal Experiments

The results from the animal experiments show that the immunological occult blood test for hemoglobin is more sensitive than the chemical test based on guaic. Furthermore, there were no false-positives. AMMN-induced cancer was detected earlier by the immunological method.

Healthy Controls and Patients with Colorectal Carcinoma

Several tests for the detection of fecal occult blood have been developed in recent years. The chemical test has been improved by the introduction of Haemoccult-II (Kornborg et al. 1986). Vellacot et al. (1981) have described an immunological test for fecal occult blood with fluorescein-labeled anti-human hemoglobin, but to our knowledge this has not been used for mass screening. Schwartz et al. (1983) have developed a sensitive test (HemoQuant) based on the conversion of nonfluorescent heme to fluorescent porphyrin. However, the disadvantage of using an heme-based test is that heme is equal in different species.

Various immunological tests have been described in recent years: Kim et al. (1985) developed an immunoprecipitation test and showed that this test has a higher sensitivity than the guaiac-based Haemoccult-II. However, the numbers of patients and specimens were fairly small (24 specimens). Turunen et al. (1984) described a two-phase kit for fecal occult blood combining a sensitive guaiac test [Fecatwin(S)ensitive] with an immunological test for human hemoglobin (FECA-EIA). They compared this procedure with three current guaiac tests (Fecatest, Fecatwin, Haemoccult) in 19 colorectal cancer patients and 11 controls on a restricted diet. The FECA-EIA was the most sensitive test, giving one (3%) false-negative result in the 30 tests performed on colorectal cancer patients, and no false-positives in the control subjects. It was also the only test that detected low-degree tumor bleeding. They suggested that for screening purposes only the positive results of the very sensitive guaiac test (Fecatwin S) should be tested with the FECA-EIA to eliminate false-positive results. With this approach the diagnostic accuracy of the two-phase test would be approximately twice as good as that of the Haemoccult test.

In 1985 Kapparis and Frommer published their results of immunological detection of occult blood in bowel cancer patients with an agarose gel immunodiffusion technique. They used a very similar radial immunodiffusion assay with the same antisera we use (Dakopatts, Denmark, rabbit antiserum to human hemoglobin). However, they used small paper discs 3 mm in diameter, to which smears of feces were applied. These discs were added to each well in the radial immunodiffusion plate. In our procedure, a much greater amount of feces is tested (1 g). Kapparis and Frommer obtained 3.3% positive results in 1200 samples from 200 control subjects by the immunological technique, 5.0% by Haemoccult-II with rehydration, and 2.3% without rehydration, representing 7.5%, 10.5% and 5.0% of the subjects, respectively. A total of two carcinomas and six polyps were detected in the 27 positive subjects. False-positive results were 4.5% for the immunological technique, 7.5%, and 3.0% for Haemoccult-II with and without rehydration.

All 40 patients with colorectal carcinoma had at least one of six samples positive on immunological testing, and 79.2% of all samples were positive. By the Haemoccult-II test without rehydration, 52.1% of the samples and 71.8% of the patients were positive. These values increased to 66.3% and 87.5% with rehydration. The authors conclude that the proportion of false-positive results on immunological testing is low enough to allow the screening of populations for colorectal carcinoma by using this technique. However, Kapparis and Frommer did not perform screening. Using six fecal samples from six bowel movements, this technique detected bleeding in 100% of colorectal carcinoma patients. The results of these authors were very similar to those we obtained in our patients with colorectal cancer and which we used to determine the sensitivity of the procedure, and they were also very similar to our control group with regard to specificity. Preliminary data on sensitivity and specificity have been presented by our group in 1986 (Wieland et al.).

From our results in 53 endoscopically confirmed cases of colorectal carcinoma (see p. 341) and from the results of our screening group 4 (colorectal cancer previously known, 17 cases), five cases of this total of 70 ($=7\%$) were missed by the immunological technique (sensitivity$=93\%$). If the 24 newly detected colorectal cancer cases are added, five of 94 cases of colorectal cancer would have been missed ($=5.3\%$) by the immunological technique.

This is similar to the calculation of Kapparis and Frommer; they detected in 100% of the patients ($n=40$) occult bleeding when six fecal samples (from six bowel movements, one sample per movement) were tested; they would have missed 5.6% of the patients if feces from only three bowel movements had been tested. The 93% sensitivity of our combined procedure would drop to 87% (12 cases from 94 were missed) if only the hemoglobin assay had been employed. The specificity of the combined procedure was 98% in healthy controls (two of 104 were "false" positive, however; one had polyposis, and the other developed ulcerative colitis 6 months later). Therefore, specificity in this group can be regarded to be 100%.

Screening of Patients

In the screening program, 27 of 2011 subjects were "false" positive (1.3%); no cause was found by barium enema or endoscopy of the colon and rectum. However, upper gastrointestinal disease was not excluded. Specificity was 98.7% by the combined procedure of hemoglobin and albumin determination. This specificity would have increased to 99.5% if the albumin determination had been omitted. On the other hand, 21 adenomas and five colorectal cancers would not have been detected. Therefore we prefer to continue the combined procedure of hemoglobin and albumin determination.

The screening of "in house" patients resulted in a fairly high detection rate: 24 cases of colorectal carcinoma among 2011 screened patients. The detection rate of 12/1000 is higher than the rate obtained in screening programs of the standard risk group (Winawer, 1980). The standard risk group includes men and women above the age of 40 who have no underlying disease and no past history or family history that would place them at higher risk for colorectal cancer. In the standard risk group a detection rate of 3–4/1000 is normally expected (Gnauck, 1984). We suggest that the high detection rate in our patients was caused by the fairly high mean age of about 70 years.

High sensitivity and specificity of immunological detection of human blood in stool have been previously described by Barrows et al. (1978) and Songster et al. (1980). The sensitivity of their radial immunodiffusion assay was approximately ten-fold higher than the Haemoccult test and gave complete specificity. However, Songster et al. (1980) found only 65% of the patients (97 of 150 consecutive colorectal carcinomas) positive in their test. We suggest that our sensitivity of 93% was mainly achieved by combining the radial immunodiffusion test with the advantage of the new test tube, by which a more representative amount of feces could be tested (1 g) in comparison to a feces sample on filter paper which was punched out in their procedure (punch-disk test system). Songster et al. (1980) reported a 40% sensitivity for the Haemoccult fecal smear (60 of 150 patients with colorectal carcinoma were positive), which is similar to our 42.5% sensitivity (40 of 94 patients with colorectal carcinoma were positive in the Haemoccult).

As described by Barrows et al. (1978), foods, drugs, or chemicals do not interfere with the immunological test. Cross-reactivity with animal hemoglobin and myoglobin contained in the diet was absent. The same specificity for other animal species has been described by Kim et al. (1985). We tested the specificity of both radial immunodiffusion tests, hemoglobin and albumin, and observed no cross-reactivity at concentrations that might occur in feces (blood diluted 1:100, 1:1000, and 1:10000).

The sensitivity of our radial immunodiffusion method gives visible precipitation rings at human blood dilutions in distilled water of 1:100 and 1:1000, and negative results at 1:10000. Whereas in the hemoglobin assay every precipitation ring was regarded as positive, only precipitation rings with a diameter of >5.5 mm (a 1:1000 blood dilution results in a precipitation ring of 5.5 mm diameter) were regarded as positive in the albumin assay. Small amounts of albumin are found in the feces of some healthy persons, and therefore this "cut-off" had to be introduced.

Summary

An immunochemical test for fecal occult blood by radial immunodiffusion for rat hemoglobin, human hemoglobin, and human albumin was developed. The assays employ antisera against rat hemoglobin, human hemoglobin, and human albumin, obtained from rabbits. In rats, colonic tumors were induced by AMMN, and the feces were collected and tested for occult blood by the radial immunodiffusion test and by the guaiac method (Colo-Rect). The immunological technique was more sensitive than the guaiac method.

To estimate the amount of human albumin and hemoglobin in feces, a new 10-ml centrifuge tube equipped with a spoon for 1 ml of feces was developed, as well as a buffer for the solubilization of feces. The buffer used for solubilization delays the degradation of albumin and hemoglobin in feces. The minimal quantity of detectable hemoglobin and albumin is equivalent to 0.1 ml blood in 100 g feces. One hundred and four healthy controls (age 19–73 years) were investigated, of whom 103 were hemoglobin negative in the immunodiffusion. One subject was positive for hemoglobin immunodiffusion and albumin (albumin cut-off: diameter of precipitation ring more than 5.5 mm), and another one was positive for albumin only. In these two positive controls, polyposis and ulcerative colitis were detected by follow-up investigation. Specificity in this group was considered to be 100%. Immunodiffusion showed small amounts of albumin in some healthy persons (diameter of precipitation ring less than 5.5 mm).

The sensitivity of the immunochemical tests was determined in 53 patients with colorectal cancer detected by endoscopy, the ages of the patients ranging from 32 to 85 years. Six stool samples were collected, and a minimum of four samples was required for evaluation. Of the 53 colorectal cancer patients, 51 were positive in the radial immunodiffusion test for hemoglobin or albumin (sensitivity 96.2%), 47 were positive in hemoglobin and 35 in albumin radial immunodiffusion. The Haemoccult determination was positive in 26 of the 53 colorectal cancer patients.

After the determination of sensitivity and specificity, 2011 patients who had been admitted to internal wards were screened. From these, six stool samples were likewise collected on three different days. Twenty-four colorectal cancers were newly detected by immunological screening and only nine patients by Haemoccult testing. Twenty-seven of the 2011 patients were regarded as false-positives in the screening program (specificity 98.7%). These results suggest that immunological screening for occult blood loss combined with the new test tube will permit a high detection rate of colorectal cancer.

The manufacturers of test systems and equipments described in this paper will be provided on request by the author (Laboratorium Dr. H. J. Limbach, Prof. Dr. H. Schmidt-Gayk und Kollegen, Im Breitspiel 15, D-6900 Heidelberg, FRG).

References

Anderson JM (1981) False-negative results of Haemoccult-test in colorectal cancer. Br Med J 283:1123–1124

Barrows GH, Burton RM, Jarret DD, Russell GG, Alford MD, Songster CL (1978) Immuno-chemical detection of human blood in feces. Am J Clin Pathol 69:342–346

Bischoff HG (1987) Scientific Proceedings, Fourth Symposium of the Section of Experimental Cancer Research (SEK) of the German Cancer Society, Heidelberg, FRG, March 18–21, 1987 (Abstr S 12)

Boas I (1901) Über okkulte Magenblutungen. Dtsch Med Wochenschr 27:315–321

Frühmorgen P (1984) Prävention und Früherkennung des kolorektalen Karzinoms. Springer, Berlin Heidelberg New York, pp 125–192

Gnauck R (1984) Übersicht und Beweiskraft europäischer und amerikanischer Haemoccult-Studien. In: Frühmorgen P (1984) Prävention und Früherkennung des kolorektalen Karzinoms. Springer, Berlin Heidelberg New York, pp 99–109

Greegor DH (1967) Diagnosis of large-bowel cancer in the asymptomatic patient. J Am Med Ass 201:943–945

Griffith CDM, Turner DJ, Saunders JH (1981) False-negative results of Haemoccult test in colorectal cancer. Br Med J 283:472

Heinrich HC (1984) Ultrasensitiver immunochemischer Okkultblutnachweis im Stuhl. In: Frühmorgen P (ed) Prävention und Früherkennung des kolorektalen Karzinoms, 1st edn. Springer, Berlin Heidelberg New York, pp 59–82

Heinrich HC, Benn HP (1982) Chemischer oder immunologischer Okkultblut-Nachweis im Stuhl bei der Frühdiagnostik des kolorektalen Karzinoms? Dtsch Med Wochenschr 107:307–310

Kapparis A, Frommer D (1985) Immunological detection of occult blood in bowel cancer patients. Br J Cancer 52:857–861

Kim YD, Nolan JM, Malkin A, Barch D, Tomita JT (1985) A qualitative agar gel immunopre-cipitin (IP) test for detection of fecal occult human hemoglobin. Clin Chim Acta 152:175–184

Köbberling J, Windeler J (eds) (1985) Der Test auf okkultes Blut im Stuhl: Studie zum Aussage-wert für die Früherkennung kolorektaler Karzinome. Thieme, Stuttgart

Kronborg O, Fenger C, Olsen J, Pedersen KM (1986) A randomized trial of screening for colorectal cancer with Haemoccult-II. In: Transactions of XX Nordic Congress in Clinical Chemistry, Odense, Denmark, Ann Clin Biochem 23 (1986) Suppl

Kruis W, Weinzierl M, Eisenberg J (1979) Endoskopische Diagnosen bei positivem und negati-vem Haemoccult-Test. Med Klin 74:1641–1644

Mancini G, Carbenara AO, Heremans JF (1965) Immunochemical quantitation of antigens by single radial diffusion. Immunochemistry 2:235–254

Ouchterlony O, Nilsson LA (1978) Immunodiffusion and immunoelectrophoresis, 19.1–19.44. In: Weir DM (ed) Handbook of experimental immunology, vol 1 Immunochemistry, 3rd edn. Blackwell Scientific, Oxford

Ribet A, Frexinos J, Escourrou J, Delpu J (1980) Occult-blood test and colorectal tumors. Lancet 1:417

Schewe S, Feifel G, Heldwein W, Weinzierl W, Wolf W, Bolte HD, Konrad E (1979) Sensitivität des Haemoccult-Tests bei kolorektalen Tumoren. Dtsch Med Wochenschr 104:253–256

Schüler H (1984) Okkultbluttestung in der Praxis. In: Frühmorgen P (ed) Prävention und Früherkennung des kolorektalen Karzinoms. Springer, Berlin Heidelberg New York, pp 209–211

Schwartz S, Dahl J, Ellefson M, Ahlquist D (1983) The "HemoQuant" test: a specific and quantitative determination of heme (hemoglobin) in feces and other materials. Clin Chem 29:2061–2067

Songster CL, Barrows GH, Jarrett DD (1980) Immunochemical detection of fecal occult blood. The fecal smear punch-disk-test: a new non-invasive screening test for colorectal cancer. Cancer 45:1099–1102

Turunen MJ, Liewendahl K, Partanen P, Adlercreutz H (1984) Immunological detection of faecal occult blood in colorectal cancer. Br J Cancer 49:141–148

Van Deen J (1864) Tincture guaijaci, und ein Ozonträger, als Reagens auf sehr geringe Blut-
   mengen, namentlich in medicoforensischen Fällen. Arch Holländ Beitr Natura Heilk
   3:228–231
Vellacott KD, Baldwin RW, Hardcastle JD (1981) An immunofluorescent test for faecal occult
   blood. Lancet 1:3
Wieland E, Thon M, Theuer D, Quentmeier A, Schmidt-Gayk H (1986) Immunoassay of fecal
   albumin and hemoglobin in colorectal carcinoma. 18. Deutscher Krebskongreß, Deutsche
   Krebsgesellschaft e.V., München
Winawer SJ (1980) Screening for colorectal cancer: An overview. Cancer 45:1093–1098

Experimental Models to Study New Chemotherapeutic Agents in Colorectal Cancer

F. T. Garzon, M. R. Berger, and D. Schmähl

Institute of Toxicology and Chemotherapy, German Cancer Research Center,
Im Neuenheimer Feld 280, 6900 Heidelberg, FRG

Contents

Introduction

Clinical Situation of Colorectal Cancer

Colorectal cancer is one of the most frequent malignancies in the Western world, with rising incidence and mortality rates (Silberg and Lubera 1986). Prognosis appears to be related to the stage of the disease at the time of diagnosis. Patients with colorectal cancer whose primary lesions are confined to the bowel wall have a higher cure rate after surgical excision than those in whom the tumor has spread regionally through the serosa to the pericolic fat or to adjacent lymph nodes.

Despite complete surgical resection of all evidence of malignant disease, the rate of recurrence is greater than 50%, thus implying the presence of clinically undetectable micrometastases, whose elimination through the use of adjuvant chemotherapy might lead to an improved survival time for these patients. The role for radiation therapy on advanced disease seems to be limited to palliation of symptoms, although there might be some minimal benefit for those patients with rectal cancer.

More than 40 chemotherapeutic agents have been evaluated in the treatment of colorectal cancer. However, only three classes of drugs have been shown to exert limited activity: the fluoropyrimidines, the nitrosoureas, and mitomycin-C. Since the introduction of 5-fluorouracil (5-FU) 30 years ago, this drug has remained a classical agent in the treatment of colorectal cancer, with an overall response rate of 21%.

No great progress has been achieved lately regarding new effective chemotherapeutic agents against colorectal cancer. The results of adjuvant chemotherapy on this
tumor still remain controversial and disappointing (Gastrointestinal Tumor Study
Group 1984). New effective chemotherapy against solid, slowly growing tumors,
especially against the most frequent, e.g., colorectal tumors, is urgently needed.

Screening Systems

In order to select new effective chemotherapeutic agents, several screening systems
have been developed. One of the most common and simple screening systems is the
in vitro assay with cells of human or murine origin as a first screen (Salmon and von
Hoff 1981; Weisenthal 1981). So far, no compound derived from this system has
proven its efficacy in human beings. This lack of predictivity due to the obvious
limitations of this system could be explained by the following characteristics: (a) lack
of mechanisms of metabolic activation other than those exhibited by the tumor cells;
(b) lack of pharmacokinetic influences or pharmacodynamic processes; (c) limited
accuracy in predicting response (true positive); (d) established cell lines are highly
selected clones from originally multiclonal tumors; (e) changing characteristics of
tumor cells under in vitro conditions; and (f) lack of cell cycle heterogenicity in tumor
cell culture.

In recent years the former National Cancer Institute (NCI) system, which was
based on transplanted mouse tumors, has been supplemented by tumors of human
origin inoculated into nude mice. It was hoped at the time of the introduction, that
xenografts derived from a certain type of human cancer, e.g., colonic cancer, would
help in selecting active compounds against this tumor in human beings. Once again
this system showed its limitations and failed to predict or select active compounds
against tumors of the gastrointestinal tract (Atassi 1984).

A major difficulty in the evaluation of most anticancer agents is the lack of correlation of the animal tumor model with the drug response obtained in the respective
types of human cancer (Venditti 1981). In addition, the conventionally used, rapidly
proliferating rodent tumors have failed to identify new agents with marked activity
in the treatment of large bowel cancer (Goldin et al. 1981). This situation challenges
the development of new models and/or the use of rational combinations of preclinical
systems which permit a more reliable selection of new compounds (Kraemer and
Sedlacek 1984; Fiebig et al. 1986).

Acetoxymethyl-Methylnitrosamine-Induced Colorectal Cancer

Special attention is merited by chemically induced colorectal cancer in rodents, in
which the tumors grow autochthonously in the bowel of the animals. They mimic the
human situation more closely than transplanted tumors (Zeller and Berger 1984).
Among these models we have chosen and developed further the acetoxymethyl-
methylnitrosamine (AMMN)-induced colorectal cancer in male Sprague-Dawley
rats. This model offers similarity to the human situation with respect to the origin of
neoplasms, the growth of tumors, histology, and chemosensitivity (Berger et al. 1986;

Bischoff 1986; Garzon 1986). Intrarectal administration of AMMN was chosen for induction, because this method yields higher incidence with a shorter tumor manifestation time than does intrarectal instillation of N-methyl-N-nitrosourea or N-methyl-N'-nitro-N-nitrosoguanidine. In addition, AMMN-induced tumors present unilocular growth as compared with systemic induction by dimethylhydrazine (DMH).

The increased effort required for induction, diagnosis, and subsequent therapy of these tumors are all properties which limit the use of this model as compared with transplanted tumor systems. Thus, a few compounds of specific interest were selected following stringent preevaluation. They included: flavone acetic acid (Fig. 1), 4-amino-N-(2'-aminophenyl)benzamide (Fig. 2), inorganic metal complexes derived from either titanium (Fig. 3) or ruthenium (Fig. 4), a pyrimidine derivative, 5'-deoxy-5-fluorouridine (5'dFUR; Fig. 5), and a biological response modifier, interleukin-2 (IL-2). They were evaluated in terms of tumor growth inhibition.

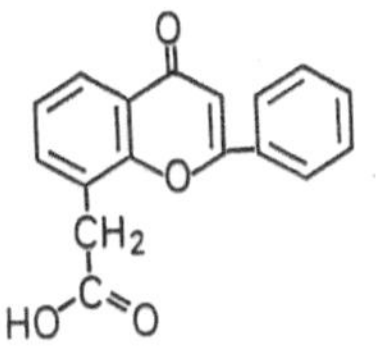

Fig. 1

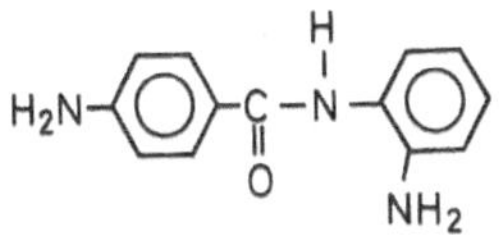

Fig. 2

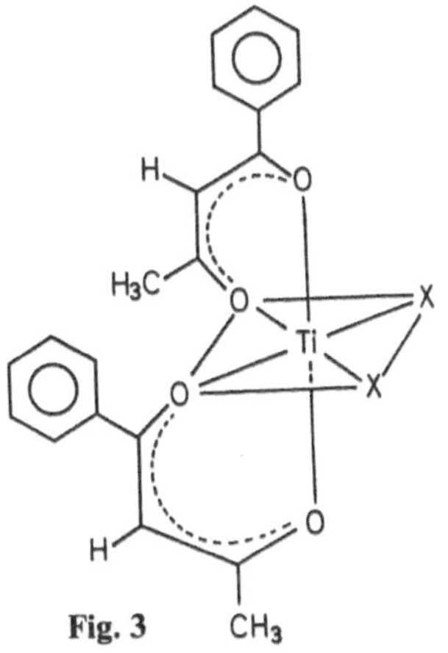

Fig. 3

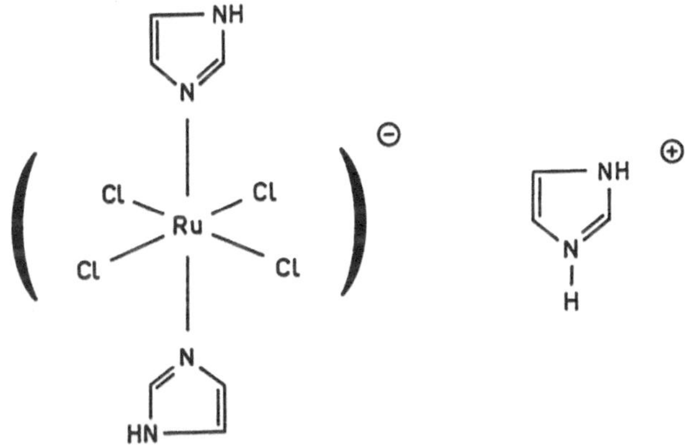

Fig. 4

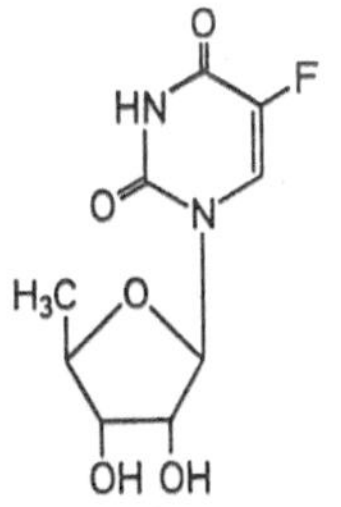

Fig. 5

Fig. 1. Structure of 4-oxo-2-phenyl-4H-1-benzopyran-8-acetic acid (LM975, flavone acetic acid)

Fig. 2. Structure of 4-amino-N-(2'-aminophenyl)benzamide (GOE1734)

Fig. 3. Structure of diethoxybis(1-phenylbutane-1,3-dionato)titanium (IV), (Ti(bzac)$_2$ (OEt)$_2$)

Fig. 4. Structure of imidazolium-bis(imidazole)tetrachlororuthenate (III), (ImH(RuIm$_2$Cl$_4$))

Fig. 5. Structure of 5'-deoxy-5-flurouridine (5'dFUR)

Methodology

Animals and Tumor Induction

Male Sprague-Dawley rats (Charles River Breeding, Sulzfeld, FRG) were purchased at a weight of 140–160 g and thereafter kept under conventional conditions (two rats per Macrolon III cage, temperature $22° \pm 2°$ C, relative air humidity $55\% \pm 10\%$, dark-light cycle of 12 h). Altromin 1320 laboratory chow and tap water were given ad lib. The induction of colorectal carcinomas was performed using fresh 0.2% solutions of AMMN (Rice et al. 1975; Wiessler 1975) in physiological saline; 2 mg/kg was administered intrarectally at weekly intervals for 10 weeks through a rectal tube, the tip of which reached the colonic flexure of rats when fully inserted.

According to the time between the end of the induction period and the diagnosis of the tumors, this animal model can be used in two modes (Fig. 6): (a) treatment starting immediately after the end of the induction period, normally for 10 weeks, represents the concept of treating nonestablished tumors – this setting was also used to evaluate immunologic approaches; (b) treatment starting after the endoscopic diagnosis of the tumors (which was performed in the 5th, 7th, and 9th weeks after the end of the induction period) represents the concept of treating established tumors.

A double control group, one sacrificed before and the second sacrificed after the treatment, serves to evaluate tumor regression in this model. In all cases the animals were randomized before the experiment into treatment and control groups.

Antineoplastic Agents

4-Amino-N-(2′aminophenyl)benzamide (GOE 1734; Fig. 2; Gödecke AG, Freiburg, FRG) was suspended in 0.8% methocel (Nordmann-Rasman, Hamburg, FRG) at a concentration of 0.6%. 5′dFUR (Fig. 5; Hoffmann-La Roche, Grenzach-Whylen, FRG) was dissolved in distilled water at a concentration of 10%. 4-Oxo-2-phenyl-4H-1-benzopyran-8-acetic acid (LM 975; flavone acetic acid, Fig. 1; LIPHA,

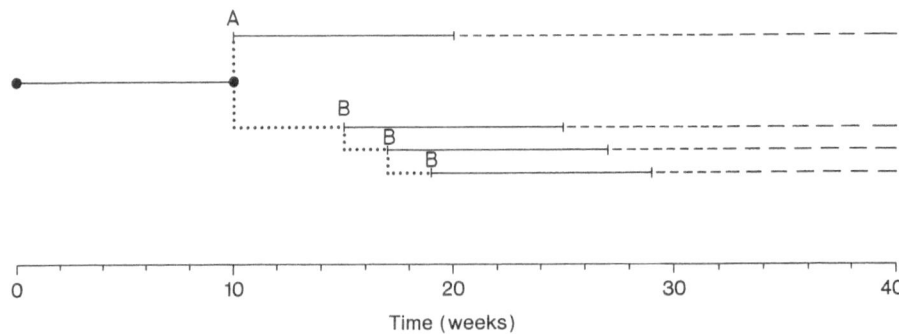

Fig. 6. Sequence of the induction of colorectal cancer in Sprague-Dawley rats with acetoxy-methyl-methylnitrosamine and subsequent treatment; *A*, treatment starts before the manifestation of tumors; *B*, treatment starts following endoscopical diagnosis of tumors.
Black circles, induction period; *solid line,* treatment; *dotted line,* time to tumor occurrence; *broken line,* termination of experiment or follow-up

Lyon, France) was dissolved (2.5%) in distilled water. Diethoxybis(1-phenyl-butane-1,3-dionato)titanium (IV), ([Ti(bzac)$_2$(OEt$_2$)]; Fig. 3) and imidazolium-bis(imidazole)tetrachlororuthenate (III) ([ImH(RuIm$_2$Cl$_4$)]; Fig. 4) were kindly supplied by Dr. B. Keppler (Department of Inorganic Chemistry, University of Heidelberg, FRG). Ti(bzac)$_2$OEt$_2$ was dissolved in a coprecipitate containing drug/cremophor EL/propylene glycol in the ratio 1/9/1, which was diluted with 0.9% NaCl to a concentration of 1%. ImH(RuLm$_2$Cl$_4$) was diluted in 0.9% NaCl solution at a concentration of 0.4%. IL-2 was administered by daily s. c. injection or by means of osmotic minipumps (Alzet, Palo Alto, USA; 0.2 cc = 20 000 U IL-2 recombinant, Bio-test Laboratory, Frankfurt, FRG) which were implanted subcutaneously under ether narcosis in the dorsal region of the animals and renewed every 15 days. Mafosfamide (Asta Werke, Bielefeld, FRG) was diluted in 0.9% NaCl at a concentration of 2%.

Diagnosis and Evaluation of the Treatment

For endoscopic examination the animals were anesthesized with intraperitoneal administration of chloral hydrate (3 g/kg diluted in physiological saline), followed by inspection of the colon (Narisawa et al. 1975; Merz et al. 1981) using a children's bronchoscope (Olympus BF, Type 4C2, Olympus Optical Co., Tokyo, Japan). All animals were inspected twice daily and weighed once weekly during induction and treatment periods. Moribund rats were inspected separately and killed shortly before their natural death. The rest of the animals were sacrificed after 5 or 10 weeks of treatment. They were dissected and the last 20 cm of the gut were removed, opened, and weighed. The number of tumors was recorded, and the volume of each lesion was estimated by measuring three diameters according to the formula a × b × c/2. Macroscopically changed organs and tumors were fixed in a 7% formalin solution and processed for histological evaluation. Tumor volumes of the experimental groups were compared for significant differences using the multiple rank sum test (Dunn 1964). In addition, the percentage tumor to control ratio (T/C% < 42) was used to estimate significance.

Results and Discussion

The titanium complex was found to be remarkably nontoxic in preceding experiments on transplanted tumors (Keller et al. 1982, 1983; Keppler 1985) thus making it suitable for prolonged therapy. Administration of this compound starting immediately after the end of the induction period showed a dose dependent tumor growth inhibition of 77% and 55%, respectively, and the observed toxicity was also dose related (Table 1; Bischoff 1986).

Preliminary experiments on ruthenium derivatives have shown promising results on transplanted tumor systems (Keppler and Rupp 1986) and also on this animal model (Garzon et al. 1987). The growth of colorectal tumor was inhibited by more than 80% in comparison with untreated controls, and a dose-related toxicity was observed (Table 2). Since this compound is easier to solubilize than the titanium complex, it might have some advantages in routine practice. Further experiments on this derivative and on structurally related congeners are currently being performed.

Table 1. Therapy of AMMN-induced colorectal rat adenocarcinoma with diethoxy-bis(1-phenylbutane-1,3-dionato)titanium(IV) [Ti(bzac)$_2$(OEt)$_2$]

Animals (n)	Treatment schedule[a]	Median tumor volume (mm^3) per rat (95% confidence limits)	T/C × 100	Median tumor number per rat (95% confidence limits)	Mortality (n)(%)	
25	Control	60 (26–102)	100	4 (2–6)	0	0
30	2 × 10 mg/kg Ti(bzac)$_2$(OEt)$_2$ i.v.	14 (6–27)	23[b]	2 (2–3)	6	20
30	Control	123 (86–164)	100	6 (5–6)	0	0
30	2 × 6,3 mg/kg Ti(bzac)$_2$(OEt)$_2$ i.v.	56 (33–88)	45	4 (3–5)	0	0

[a] Treatment was applied twice a week for 10 weeks and started immediately after the end of the induction period (week 11).
[b] $P < 0.05$.

Table 2. Therapy of AMMN-induced colorectal rat adenocarcinoma with imidazolium-bis(imidazol)tetrachlororuthenate(III) [ImH(RuIm$_2$Cl$_4$)]

Animals (n)	Treatment schedule[a]	Median tumor volume (mm^3) per rat (95% confidence limits)	T/C × 100	Median tumor number per rat (95% confidence limits)	Mortality (n)(%)	
20	Control	386 (120–683)	100	4 (2–5)	0	0
20	2 × 14 mg/kg ImH(RuIm$_2$Cl$_4$) i.v.	80 (14–315)	21	3 (2–4)	9	45
12	2 × 12 mg/kg ImH(RuIm$_2$Cl$_4$) i.v.	78 (4–506)	20	2 (1–3)	1	8
10	2 × 7 mg/kg ImH(RuIm$_2$Cl$_4$) i.v.	69 (24–401)	18	4 (3–5)	0	0

[a] Treatment was applied twice a week for 10 weeks and started after endoscopical diagnosis of the tumors (week 15).

Flavone acetic acid (LM975) is a compound without activity in leukemia P388; however, this compound had a remarkably high anticancer efficacy in nine transplanted solid tumors (Corbett et al. 1986). Seven of these tumors were derived from the gastrointestinal tract, including pancreatic tissue. LM975 showed the following interesting properties: it had anticancer activity in vitro, it displayed a narrow range of active doses in vivo, split doses were no better than one full dose, and its half-life was relatively long (about 7 h).

Our results in AMMN-induced colorectal carcinomas obtained after 10 weeks of treatment immediately following the end of the induction period confirm this activity: there was a remarkable antitumoral effect (Table 3) at a marginal toxic dose as measured by tumor growth inhibition. A similar activity was displayed by 5'dFUR. Interestingly, the combination of both drugs showed an synergistic effect at a nontoxic dose level. Therefore, this compound could easily be combined with established cystostatic therapy in the treatment of human colorectal cancer.

Table 3. Treatment of AMMN-induced colorectal carcinomas with flavone acetic acid (LM975), 5′-deoxy-5-fluorouridine (5′dFUR) and the combination of both agents

Treatment schedule[a] LM975 (mg/kg)	5′dFUR (mg/kg)	Animals (n)	Median tumor volume (95% confidence limits)	T/C ×100	Median tumor number (95% confidence limits)	Mortality (n)(%)	
Control		30	123 (86–169)	–	6 (5–6)	0	0
100	–	20	135 (81–172)	110	5.5 (3–6)	0	0
200	–	20	53 (26–82)	43	4 (3–4)	2	10
–	300	20	85 (58–108)	69	5 (4–6)	0	0
–	600	20	58 (19–77)	47	3 (2–5)	2	10
Control		20	167 (48–589)	–	3 (2–3)	0	0
100	300	20	14 (3–60)	8[b]	2 (1–3)	0	0

[a] Two interperitoneal administrations per week for 10 weeks started immediately after the end of the induction period (week 11)
[b] $P < 0.05$.

Table 4. Treatment of established AMMN-induced colorectal carcinomas with 4-amino-N(2′-aminophenyl)benzamide (GOE1734)

Dosage/week (mg/kg)	Animals (n)	Median tumor volume (95% confidence limits)	T/C ×100	Median tumor number (95% confidence limits)	Rats without tumors (n)(%)		Mortality (n)(%)	
Control I[a]	20	36.5 (24–74)	–	2 (1–3)	0	0	0	0
Control II[b]	20	389 (264–1046)	100	4 (3–7)	0	0	1	5
7.9; days 1–5	20	28 (12–68)	7.2[c]	3 (2–4)	1	5	6	30
6.3; days 1–5	20	53 (19–101)	13.6[c]	3 (2–4)	0	0	2	10
12.6; days 1, 3, 5	20	126 (33–180)	32.4[c]	4 (3–4)	0	0	3	15

[a] Animals sacrificed at diagnosis to establish tumor size before treatment.
[b] Controls parallel to treated groups.
[c] $P < 0.05$.

GOE1734 shares similar characteristics with flavone acetic acid regarding its inactivity toward quickly growing leukemias (Berger et al. 1985). There was, however, high antineoplastic effectiveness in AMMN-induced colorectal rat adenocarcinoma when the animals were treated before or after the endoscopic diagnosis of tumors. The appearance of tumors was protracted, and their growth was inhibited in a dose-related manner. Moreover, a tumor growth inhibition of 95% was observed when compared with the control groups before or after the treatment. Together with the antineoplastic efficacy the toxicity was dose dependent (Table 4).

Compared to these new cytostatic agents, the anticancer activity of the biological response modifier was modest when administered before the manifestation of tumors in order to influence the immunologic state of the animals (Garzon et al. 1986). This situation mimics patients with minimal residual disease (Duncan 1982). In fact, a somewhat lower tumor volume and tumor number were observed following daily subcutaneous applications over a 5-week period (Table 5). Subsequent experiments

Table 5. Therapy of AMMN-induced colorectal rat adenocarcinoma with IL-2

Animals (n)	Treatment schedule	Median tumor volume (mm³) per rat (95% confidence limits)	Median tumor number per rat (95% confidence limits)	Median weight difference (week 5–week 1) (%)	Mortality (n)(%)
10	Controls	25 (3–129)	4 (3–4)	+9	1 10
12	10 000 units/kg IL-2 [a]	9 (4–27)	3 (1–5)	+4	0 0

[a] Daily s.c. administration for 5 weeks

Table 6. Treatment of AMMN-induced colorectal rat adenocarcinoma with interleukin 2 (IL-2) and low-dose mafosfamide

Experiment no.	Animals (n)	Treatment schedule	Median tumor volume (mm³) per rat (95% confidence limits)	T/C × 100	Median tumor number per rat (95% confidence limits)	Mortality (n)(%)
1	20	Control	68 (32–152)	100	2.5 (2–3)	0 0
1	20	1200 units IL-2 [a]	13 (5–17)	20 [b]	2 (1–2)	0 0
1	20	1200 units IL-2 [a] × 10 mg/kg mafosfamide i.p.	6 (1–12)	9 [b]	2 (1–3)	1 5
2	20	Control	62 (28–78)	100	3 (3–4)	1 5
2	15	1200 units IL-2 [a]	12 (4.5–69)	19	2 (2–3)	0 0
2	15	1200 units IL-2 [a] + 10 mg/kg mafosfamide i.p.	20 (8–72)	32	2 (2–3)	1 5

Experiment 1: treatment before the manifestation of the tumors.
Experiment 2: treatment started following endoscopical diagnosis of the tumors.
[a] Continuous subcutaneous administration by osmotic minipumps.
[b] $P < 0.05$.

with this agent alone and in combination with an oxazaphosphorine-derivative (mafosfamide) confirmed these results (Table 6).

Conclusions

A careful selection of suitable preclinical models should result in the more effective finding of new drugs which are active against slowly growing solid tumors, especially those derived from the gastrointestinal tract, e.g., colorectal cancer. A couple of promising new compounds with an effect against autochthonous colorectal rat adenocarcinoma have been found and preclinically characterized; however, they still await clinical evaluation.

References

Atassi G (1984) Do we need new chemosensitive experimental models? Eur J Cancer Clin Oncol 20:1217–1220

Berger MR, Bischoff H, Fritschi E, Henne T, Herrmann M, Pool B, Satzinger G, Schmähl D, Weiershausen U (1985) Synthesis, toxicity and therapeutic efficacy of 4-amino-*N*-(2'-aminophenyl) benzamide: a new compound active in slowly growing tumours. Cancer Treat Rep 69:1415–1424

Berger MR, Bischoff H, Garzon FT, Schmähl D (1986) Autochthonous, acetoxymethyl-methylnitrosamine-induced colorectal cancer in rats: A useful tool in selecting new active antineoplastic compounds? Hepato-gastroenterol. 33:227–234

Bischoff H (1986) Chemotherapie eines Nitrosamin-induzierten autochthonen Colontumors bei SD-Ratten mit *β*-Diketonato-Verbindungen von Titan, Zirkonium und Hafnium, im Vergleich mit *cis*-Platin, Cyclophosphamid, 5-Fluorouracil und 5'-Deoxy-5-Fluorouridin. Thesis, Heidelberg University, Heidelberg

Corbett T, Bissery M, Wosniak A, Plowman J, Polin L, Tapazoglou E, Dieckman J, Valeriote F (1986) Solid tumor activity of flavone acetic acid (FAA). Proc Am Assoc Cancer Res 27:281

Duncan W (1982) Prospects in management. In: Duncan W (ed) Colorectal cancer. Springer, Berlin Heidelberg New York, pp 135–149 (Recent results in cancer research, vol 83)

Dunn OJ (1964) Multiple comparisons using ranks suns. Technometrics 6:241–252

Fiebig HH, Schmid JR, Henss H, Dentler V, Schildge J, Löhr GW (1986) Bedeutung des Kolonie-Assays als In-vitro-Verfahren zur Tumorsensibilitätstestung und für die Zytostatikaentwicklung. In: Drings P, Schmähl D, Vogt-Moykopf I (eds) Bronchialkarzinom. Zuckschwerdt, Bern, pp 132–161 (Aktuelle Onkologie vol 26)

Garzon FT (1986) Versuche zur Evaluation neuer antineoplastisch wirksamer Verbindungen an autochthonen Acetoxymethyl-methylnitrosamin-induzierten kolorektalen Tumoren der SD-Ratte. Thesis, Heidelberg University, Heidelberg

Garzon FT, Salas M, Berger MR, Kirchner H (1986) Effect of interleukin-2 on the manifestation and growth of acetoxymethyl-methylnitrosamine induced colorectal rat adenocarcinoma. J Cancer Res Clin Oncol 111:79–81

Garzon FT, Berger MR, Keppler BK, Schmähl D (1987) Comparative antitumor activity of ruthenium derivatives with 5'-deoxy-5-fluorouridine in chemically induced colorectal tumors in SD rats. Cancer Chemother Pharmacol 19:347–349

Gastrointestinal Tumor Study Group (1984) Adjuvant therapy of colon cancer – results of a prospectively randomized trial. N Engl J Med 310:737–743

Goldin A, Venditti JM, MacDonald JS, Muggia FM, Henney JE, Devita VT (1981) Current results of the screening program at the division of cancer treatment. National Cancer Institute. Eur J Cancer 17:129–142

Keller HJ, Keppler B, Schmähl D (1982) Antitumor activity of *cis*-dihalogenobis(1-phenyl-1,3-butanedionato)titanium(IV) compounds against Walker 256 carcinosarcoma. Drug Res 32:806–807

Keller HJ, Keppler B, Schmähl D (1983) Antitumor activity of *cis*-dihalogenobis(1-phenyl-1,3-butanedionato)titanium(IV) compounds. J Cancer Res Clin Oncol 105:109–110

Keppler B (1985) Synthesis and preclinical evaluation of bis-*β*-diketonatotitanium(IV) complexes as a new class of antitumor agents. J Cancer Res Clin Oncol 109:A43

Keppler B, Rupp W (1986) Antitumor activity of imidazolium-bisimidazole-tetrachlororuthenate(III). J Cancer Res Clin Oncol 111:166–168

Kraemer HP, Sedlacek HH (1984) A modified screening system to select new cytostatic drugs. Behring Inst Mitt 74:301–328

Merz R, Wagner I, Habs M, Schmähl D, Amberger H, Bachmann U (1981) Endoscopic diagnosis of chemically induced autochthonous colonic tumors in rats. Hepato-gastroenterol 28:53–57

Narisawa T, Ching-Quo Wong DS, Weisburger JH (1975) Evaluation of endoscopic examination of colon tumors in rats. Am J Dig Dis 20:928–934

Rice JM, Joshi SR, Roller PP (1975) Methyl(acetoxymethyl)-nitrosamine. A new carcinogen highly specific for colon and rectum. Proc Am Assoc Cancer Res 16:32

Salmon SE, Von Hoff DD (1981) In vitro evaluation of anticancer drugs with the human tumor stem cell assay. Semin Oncol 8 (4):377–385

Silberg E, Lubera J (1986) Cancer statistics, 1986. CA 36:9–25

Venditti JM (1981) Preclinical drug development: rationale and methods. Semin Oncol 8 (4):349–361

Weisenthal LM (1981) In vitro assays in preclinical antineoplastic drug screening. Semin Oncol 8 (4):362–376

Wiessler M (1975) Chemie der Nitrosamine, II. Synthese α-funktioneller Dimethylnitrosamine. Tetrahedron Lett 30:2575–2578

Zeller J, Berger MR (1984) Chemically induced autochthonous tumor models in experimental chemotherapy. Behring Inst Mitt 74:201–208

Recommendation

Dietary Prevention of Colorectal Cancer

J. H. Weisburger

American Health Foundation, Dana Road, Valhalla, New York 10595-1599, USA

Contents

Introduction

In the general field of intestinal diseases, cancer in the intestinal tract is often referred to as "large bowel cancer" or "colorectal cancer". From the perspective of elucidating the complex etiologic factors for these types of neoplastic disease, however, this term, referring to the entire intestinal tract, from the ileocecal junction to the anus, is incorrect, for it does not properly reflect what has been learned so far about etiologic factors. Through the techniques of geographic pathology and observations of time trends in the occurrence of cancer in the intestinal tract, international incidence data have been carefully reviewed, and it has become clear that distinction needs to be made between cancer in the ascending colon (proximal colon cancer), descending and sigmoid colon (distal colon cancer), and rectal cancer, the latter being designated as being 8 cm from the anal verge. The rationale for this distinction has been discussed in this volume and previously by a number of reviewers (Morson et al. 1983; Netscher and Larson 1983; Jensen 1984; Butcher et al. 1985; Howson et al. 1985; Tajima et al. 1985; Devesa et al. 1987; LaVecchia et al. 1987; Thomas and Karagas 1987; Weisburger and Wynder 1987).

The international classification of diseases (ICD) provides the basis for a standard categorization of malignancies in the intestinal tract. Thus, from the perspective of etiologic factors, the ICD classification 153.0 (proximal colon cancer) needs careful discrimination from 153.2 and 153.3 (distal and sigmoid colon cancer). It is not yet clear how to classify the relatively infrequent lesions found in the transverse colon (153.1) as regards etiologic factors. Clearly, however, 154.0 and 154.1 (rectal cancer) are distinct again. Death certificates should present mortality data according to the ICD classification.

Time trends as a function of area of residence display distinct incidence and mortality rates (see Frentzel-Beyme, this volume; Weisburger and Wynder 1987). In the United States, for example, the main type of intestinal neoplasm, that in the descending or sigmoid colon, has had a slightly increasing incidence in the last 40 years with a barely rising mortality rate in males and a modestly declining mortality rate in females. In contrast, rectal cancer has been decreasing in the United States in men and women. In countries with a formerly low incidence and mortality of distal colon cancer, a continuing increase, recently at a somewhat accelerated rate as in Japan, has been observed (Tajima et al. 1985). Interpretation of these combined data reporting incidence and time trends suggests that proximal colon, distal colon, and rectal cancer have distinct etiologic factors, which occur to different extents at different times as a function of area of residence. In some instances these factors have decreased in importance in one area but have increased in another. Examination of incidence rates of large bowel cancer for each segment in migrants from regions of low rates to those of high rates supports the view that current residence and related life styles play a key role in the development of these diseases.

Mechanisms of Carcinogenesis

In view of the complex nature of the etiologic factors bearing on "colorectal" cancer, it may be useful to outline what is known about causative factors in relation to probable mechanisms of action that, in turn, may provide an excellent basis for recommendations on the prevention of one or the other type of intestinal cancer.

A variety of approaches has expanded our knowledge as to the mechanisms of carcinogenesis. Historically, experimenters have demonstrated on the skin of mice that polycyclic aromatic hydrocarbons (PAHs) could act as initiators when administered as relatively small single doses, but that other agents such as croton oil, an irritant natural oil from the eucalyptus family which was used initially as the test agent, can act as powerful promoters although by themselves they are not significantly carcinogenic (Berenblum 1974). These pioneering experiments, reproduced many times, were extended to other organs, such as liver, bladder, breast, and colon, by utilizing distinct, organ-specific initiating carcinogens, followed by distinct promoting elements (Slaga and Montesano 1983; Appel and Hildebrandt 1985; Butterworth and Slaga 1987).

In relation to the specific mode of action, initiators can be construed to be genotoxic, that is, they can interact through specific biochemical and metabolic reactions with DNA and the genetic material of the cell. Duplication of cells bearing such a carcinogen-modified genetic material, as a result of oncogene codon transfer and amplification, results in cells with an abnormal DNA typical of that of the neoplastic cell. Any agent that increases cell duplication rates in the presence of a genotoxic carcinogen can augment the effectiveness of the genotoxic carcinogen by increasing

Table 1. Mechanisms postulated for etiologic factors bearing on segments of large bowel cancer

Disease	Carcinogen	Promoting elements	Protective elements	Suggested mechanisms
Hereditary adenomatosis Familial polyposis Gardner's syndrome	Cellular Genome	?	Vitamin C?	Genetically mediated program towards neoplasia
Ulcerative colitis	?	Refined carbohydrates	Cereal fiber, calcium salts, low-fat diets	Higher cell turnover rates favor carcinogenesis
Crohn's disease	?	Refined carbohydrates, smoking	Cereal fiber, calcium salts, low-fat diets	
High-risk nonpolyposis	Fried food?	Dietary fat (bile and fatty acids)	Cereal fiber, calcium salts, yellow-green vegetables, low-fat diets	Higher cell turnover; other mechanisms may be similar to those for distal colon cancer
Proximal colon neoplasms	?	Dietary fat (bile and fatty acids)? Estrogen? Obesity? Cholecystectomy?	Cereal fiber, calcium salts, yellow-green vegetables?	?
Distal colon neoplasms	Fried food	Dietary fat (bile and fatty acids)	Cereal fiber, calcium salts, yellow-green vegetables, olive oil, fish oils	Initiation by carcinogens produced during cooking; also postulated are mutagens stemming from specific bacterial cell membranes. Enhancement (promotion) by bile and fatty acids related to total fat intake (except olive and fish oils). Protection by stool bulk (cereal fiber), calcium binding of bile or fatty acids, or unknown mechanisms through yellow-green vegetables, control of cell proliferation by calcium or suitable lower pH.
Rectal neoplasms	?	Dietary fat? Alcohol?	Cereal fiber? Calcium salts?	Some data show parallel, but not identical, factors as for distal colon cancer. However, there are also sharply distinct elements. Basically unknown mechanisms although effects on cell duplication rates are relevant

the chances for a modification of the genetic apparatus. Such agents, not carcinogenic by themselves, are called "cocarcinogens". Other types of chemicals, promoters, practically control the development of early neoplastic cells and thus give rise to the overt neoplasms. Promoting agents may operate by a variety of mechanisms, including the inhibition of transfer of growth control elements between normal and neoplastic cells by breaking gap junctions, effects on the differentiation of cell systems, and the like.

In exploring the complex environment leading to any specific kind of cancer, it is important to obtain information on the genotoxic causative elements as well as any cocarcinogens or promoting factors (Table 1). If such factors with multiple modes of action have been outlined, it will be possible to make recommendations for preventive maneuvers based on the elimination or reduction of any of the elements playing a role in causation or development, without necessarily being in a position to reduce all of them. In the overall process of cancer causation, predictions can be made as to the probable effectiveness of a given inhibiting procedure that would depend on the mechanism of action of the factor, that is, the target of the planned decreased effect.

Causes of Proximal Colon Cancer

Proximal colon cancer has a moderate incidence around the world. In Western countries the incidence is somewhat higher than in Asia, but the data base is not robust since many registries merge proximal and distal colon cancer into one category (see Boyle et al. 1985; Faivre et al. 1985). At this time virtually no hypotheses exist as to possible genotoxic carcinogens or promoting agents. In view of our ignorance in this area, it is not possible to make any sound, fact-based recommendations on preventive approaches for proximal colon cancer.

Causes of Distal Colon Cancer

Distal colon cancer is a major type in the Western world, with a high incidence in men and women. It displays an increasing tendency in some formerly low-incidence regions such as Japan and eastern Europe. Migrants from a low-risk region to a high-risk region acquire the higher incidence of the host population. Thus, the high-risk region offers an environment propitious for the induction of this neoplasm.

Genotoxic Carcinogens

The laboratory of Bruce (1987) discovered relatively powerful direct-acting mutagens in the stools of some individuals on a Western diet. Supplementation of the diet with fiber and both vitamins C and E lowered activity, as did a vegetarian diet. The mutagenic activity was identified as belonging to a class of fecapentaenes, a novel polyunsaturated, reactive chemical structure (Wilkins et al. 1981; Hirai et al. 1982; Gupta et al. 1983, 1984). We are investigating the carcinogenic activity to the intestinal tract. Pure fecapentaene in contact with the intestinal epithelium failed to induce micronuclei (Bruce 1987), a characteristic shown by specific intestinal carcinogens, although they can damage intestinal DNA (Curren et al. 1987; Hinzman et al. 1987). Thus, at this time it is not possible to relate the presence of this type of chemical in the intestinal tract to potential cancer risk.

Sugimura (1985) discovered 10 years ago that powerful mutagens were formed during cooking of fish or meat. These mutagens are heterocyclic amines, typified by 2-amino-3-methylimidazoquinolines or quinoxalines. They display potent activity in a battery of in vitro tests, which permits classification of these agents as genotoxic (see Knudsen 1986). Bioassays for carcinogenicity have demonstrated that several of these chemicals can induce cancer at specific sites including the breast, and proximal and distal colon. The amounts present in fried foods are relatively small, and for this reason it has not yet been fully established that these food-borne intestinal carcinogens are actually causative in intestinal carcinogenesis. However, while the amount consumed at any one time is relatively small, in most instances the intake begins in childhood and occurs on an almost daily basis. Furthermore, as will be noted below, intestinal carcinogenesis and cancer induction in breast and pancreas, all target organs for this class of novel carcinogen, are highly susceptible to cocarcinogenesis and promotion (Slaga and Montesano 1983; Weisburger 1987). Thus, it is at least plausible that the mode of cooking can generate specific carcinogens for the colon. We have developed a number of modalities such as dilution of ground beef by soy protein or addition of antioxidants, or of indole-containing amino acids such as L-tryptophan or L-proline to abolish carcinogen formation during cooking (Vuolo and Schuessler 1985; Jones and Weisburger 1988).

Cocarcinogenesis and Promoting Factors

Deschner et al. (1984) and Lipkin (1988) have contributed a number of studies demonstrating the probable relationship between the rate of cell cycling, the movement of cells in the intestinal crypt up to the point of shedding, and intestinal cancer risk. Higher-risk individuals had a faster rate, as did animals with increased sensitivity to carcinogenesis. Based on current knowledge of the mechanisms of carcinogenesis, genetically mediated or environmentally controlled rates of synthesis and mitosis appear to translate into a specific risk of cancer. Thus, any element increasing the rate of cell cycling would be construed to have cocarcinogenic activity, and any element lowering cell cycling would be interpreted to have an inhibitory effect. Bile acids, especially secondary bile acids increase cell cycling, whereas calcium salts have the opposite effect (Bird et al. 1985; Lipkin and Newmark 1985; Buset et al. 1986; Stadler et al. 1988; Ponz de Leon et al. 1988).

Diet, Nutritional Traditions and Distal Colon Cancer

International epidemiologic studies and geographic pathology relate the customary intake of certain foods traditionally consumed to risk for distal colon cancer. In the Western world the typical diet includes 40% – 45% of calories as total fat. In recent years, as a result of recommendations by governmental agencies and voluntary associations on the prevention of heart disease, a lower intake of total fats and redistribution between polyunsaturated and saturated fats has taken place (Consensus Conference 1985; Joossens and Geboers 1985; Ip et al. 1986; Wynder et al. 1986; Simopoulos 1987). These changes have occurred in the United States to a certain extent, in part accounting for a lower mortality rate from heart disease. Introduction of these changes in other parts of the Anglo-Saxon community have been less successful. In Japan and other parts of the Orient, the food intake traditionally included only 10% – 15% of calories as fat, and a good part of this lipid spectrum included oils from fish. In the Mediterranean countries the total fat intake is also lower, approximately 30% – 35% of total calories, and the main lipid is olive oil consisting principally of monounsaturated oleic acid (Simopoulos 1987). In animal models, Reddy (1986) has observed that the type of fat as well as the amount of fat is important in colon carcinogenesis. A diet fed to rodents at the Western level of fat, 40% of calories, led to a higher colon cancer incidence when the fat component was corn or safflower oil, which contains appreciable amounts of omega-6 polyunsaturated fatty acids, compared to a diet of 10% fat calories mimicking a low-risk situation. However, certain fats (olive oil, coconut oil, fish oils) given at the higher level, 40% of calories, yielded approximately the same tumor incidence as when fed at 10% of calories. This finding compares with the epidemiologic findings that populations consuming fat as fish oils or olive oil have a lower incidence of colon cancer compared with other countries. One underlying, mechanistic element in each instance is the production of bile acids, although a possible additional parameter of action at the cellular or intracellular level, mediating the production and metabolism of specific prostaglandins, needs to be considered as well (Weisburger 1987). Also, fat is a high energy component of food and thus may play a nonspecific enhancing action (Garfinkel 1986; Graham 1986; Lyon et al. 1987; Simopoulos 1987). However, it is a fact derived from human studies and animal models that different types of fat have distinct effects in colon carcinogenesis, even though their caloric content is identical.

One key element relevant to the etiology of distal colon cancer is the underlying mechanism, namely a given amount and type of fat control cholesterol and, thence, bile acid biosynthesis. In turn, bile acids have demonstrated promoting effects in animal models as well as in in vitro bioassay systems designed to demonstrate a promoting effect via breakage of gap junctions. Bile acids are not genotoxic or carcinogenic. A 50-year-old proposal that bile acids were converted to 3-methylcholanthrene, a PAH carcinogenic to mouse skin and select other target organs, has never been realized experimentally and certainly does not arise under in vivo conditions, despite continuing mention of this particular hypothesis even in the current literature. In fact, except for a special model of inbred hamster where high dosages of 3-methylcholanthrene administered or applied directly and repeatedly to the colon mucosa led to a small incidence of colon cancer (see Wang et al. 1985), no one has observed any sensitivity of the colon mucosa of other rodents to PAHs. Intake of PAH through eating fried meat has not led to PAH excretion in stools, and thus such carcinogens are probably absent in the human distal colon (Hecht and LaVoie 1981).

Bile acids play a key role in enhancing the development of colon cancer by promoting mechanisms. Some fatty acids possibly present in the intestinal tract of individuals on a high fat intake may have similar properties (Bird et al. 1985).

In certain animal models for colon cancer, the simultaneous administration of selenium salt has lowered the incidence of induced colon cancer. Claims have been made about the occurrence of higher rates of colon cancer in regions displaying a deficiency of selenium in the soil (Levander 1987). Considering the diversity of food consumed by man, it is not clear how local prevailing geographic soil properties would explain this kind of association. For the same reason, the claimed inhibiting effect of potassium in colon cancer requires clarification and detailed documentation (Jansson 1985).

Role of Cereal Fiber, Yellow-Green Vegetables, and Calcium

International epidemiologic studies have discovered an unusually low incidence of distal colon cancer in Finland, especially rural Finland, compared with neighboring Denmark or other parts of the Western world including the United States and Great Britain. Investigation by two groups (Reddy et al. 1980; Jensen et al. 1982) has demonstrated that the people in rural Finland normally consume sizable amounts of cereal fiber leading to a large stool bulk. Intermediary findings were made in comparisons between northern Sweden and southern Sweden (Reddy 1986), or rural and urban Finland or Denmark (Jensen 1985). These findings have clearly indicated that an absence of constipation and sizeable stool bulks of the order of 200 g per day may be protective. One explanation is that bile acids and fatty acids are diluted through bulk, although there may be additional protective mechanisms with wheat bran (Calvert et al. 1987). In individuals studied in the New York area, the average bile acid concentration in the stool was 12 mg/g, but in rural Finland it was 3 or 4 mg/g. The type and amount of fiber, and degree of milling may affect colon carcinogenesis through diverse, specific mechanisms (Block and Lanza 1987; Weisburger 1987; Wilpart and Roberfroid 1987). Incidentally, the same low bile acid concentration in stools was found in people in Japan where it is derived from a low fat intake and not a high fiber intake. An additional parameter typical of the Finnish diet is a high intake of dairy products, excellent sources of calcium. Several approaches have suggested that calcium may confer a protective effect in colon cancer development (see Lipkin 1988; Pence and Buddingh 1988). Studies by Byers and Graham (1984) in western New York have found a somewhat protective effect by yellow-green vegetables. The active protective elements in vegetables have not yet been elucidated. No studies have been performed as to a potential effect on stool bulk. Wattenberg (1985) has performed basic biochemical studies demonstrating that certain vegetables modify the biochemical properties and especially the levels of certain enzymes in the intestinal tract. However, intake of yellow-green vegetables has not yet been shown to inhibit colon carcinogenesis in animal models, nor have specific mechanisms been proposed. Hirayama (1985) observed that regular intake of such vegetables had a protective effect for several types of cancer.

Role of Exercise

Several reports have described a lower incidence of colon or colorectal cancer in individuals who were said to have some form of regular physical activity compared with controls who were sedentary (see Weisburger and Wynder 1987). The underlying mechanism has not been explored but may rest on physiologic stimulation of intestinal motility.

Rectal Cancer

The incidence and mortality data for rectal cancer need to be reviewed critically on a worldwide basis. Indeed, it is only in the last 10–15 years that there has been general agreement on specifically delineating the rectum as constituting the tissue 8 cm from the anal verge, in contrast to the rectosigmoid area. If an area of the world has a high incidence of cancer in the rectosigmoid, it is possible that this particular lesion might have been classified with rectal cancer, which might then have an erroneously high rate. Other situations can be postulated where the reverse may have occurred, and rectal cancer was described with an incidence lower than actual. This situation is apt to occur if the disease was discovered clinically only when it had attained an appreciable size and the exact site of origin could not be outlined (Devesa et al. 1987).

Little information exists on etiologic factors for rectal cancer. Virtually nothing is known about any genotoxic carcinogens specifically affecting the rectum. Epidemiologic studies show some parallelism between the occurrence of rectal cancer and distal colon cancer. Reasonably firm data show that in the United States the male:female ratio for rectal cancer is 1.4:1, but for colon cancer is about 1:1. Rectal cancer also displays a declining trend in the United States, but distal colon cancer does not (in males). However, a weak association is noted in international data between distal colon and rectal cancer, perhaps accounted for by a possible promoting element common to both distal colon and rectal cancer, such as bile acids (Stadler et al. 1988). Clearly, this may be spurious, since the rectum is usually not bathed continuously by intestinal contents as is the distal colon. Some epidemiologic studies, but not others, have related the customary intake of alcoholic beverages, especially beer, to a finding of rectal cancer (Kabat et al. 1986; Seitz and Simanowski 1987; Wu et al. 1987; Weisburger and Wynder 1987). Laboratory studies attempting to explore a role for alcohol in rectal cancer have for the most part been fruitless, but Seitz's group have found that alcohol stimulates cell cycling in the rectum of rats (Simanowski et al. 1986; Seitz and Simanowski 1987). By the definition given previously, alcohol would therefore be classified as a cocarcinogen.

Recommendations for Prevention

Subsequent to the discussion of colorectal cancer as three distinct diseases with different causative and developmental factors, we will develop recommendations based on this concept.

Since the etiologic factors for *proximal colon cancer* are not known, we are not in a position to make any recommendations to lower the risk for this neoplasm except to state that greater research efforts need to be exerted to discover genotoxic carcinogens and promoters as well as inhibitors for this neoplasm.

For *distal colon cancer*, the major neoplasm in the Western world and one of growing importance in Japan, the following elements can be considered:

The Type and Amount of Fat. We are inclined to recommend that the individual diet contain no more than 20%–25% total fat intake, unless the major part of the fat intake is in the form of lipids that have no enhancing qualities such as fish oils, olive oil, and perhaps palm or coconut oil. A high level of palm or coconut oil, with fairly high proportions of saturated fatty acids, is undesirable because these oils have a demonstrated action in raising serum cholesterol levels and, thence, risk of coronary heart disease. There is little information about the effect of a mixed intake of various fats. In breast cancer research, however, it has been demonstrated that total fat calories are important, provided that a minimum of essential fatty acids from polyunsaturated omega-6 fatty acids (4.5%) was available (Ip et al. 1986).

Type and Amount of Fiber. A regular intake of cereal fiber or bran obtained from whole grains – wheat, corn, rye, or oats is recommended. The key element to consider is the effect of this type of fiber on stool bulk. Bran from different grains may have distinct biochemical effects (Jenkins et al. 1987). Wheat bran displays little effect in controlling serum cholesterol levels, but oat bran definitely lowers serum cholesterol, possibly by interfering with the enterohepatic cycling of bile acids. Pectin has little effect in modifying stool bulk but apparently has an effect on biochemical functions of the liver and perhaps of the intestinal tract. Pectin appreciably lowered the effect of azoxymethane in colon carcinogenesis but had no action when *N*-methyl-*N*-nitrosourea was used as the carcinogen. The first chemical requires metabolism by the liver and the second is direct acting. Thus, the interpretation of these distinct findings is that pectin affects the metabolism of azoxymethane (Reddy 1986).

The mode of action of most fibers is not well known as regards effects on the intestinal tract, except for those fibers such as wheat bran that increase stool bulk. The example of rural Finland suggests that adequate intake of cereal bran fiber in people on an otherwise well-balanced, mixed diet can be instrumental in lowering the risk for colon cancer development without any obvious adverse effects. Some have expressed fears that the phytic acid content of bran fiber might lead to mineral imbalances that may have potential adverse effects on human physiology. Such effects, however, were demonstrated only in populations on a uniformly poor diet, as in Iran. Such a situation is not relevant in most countries where the people of various socioeconomic groups consume a diet containing more than adequate amounts of micronutrients, including minerals.

Micronutrients. A number of vitamins, especially carotene and retinoids generally, have been studied, and no discernible effects on colon cancer were noted. Likewise, where studied, no real effect of the water-soluble vitamins, especially vitamin C, has been observed. Several reports have alluded to a favorable effect of calcium, including adequate amounts of vitamin D to control the biochemical effects of calcium (Garland et al. 1985). Based on several lines of investigation, an adequate intake of calcium from certain vegetables and low-fat or skimmed milk is desirable, even though not all of the mechanisms underlying calcium action have been fully elucidated (Bruce 1987; Lipkin 1988).

Physical Activity or Exercise. Physical activity has also been noted to lower colon cancer risk, possibly by favorably affecting intestinal motility and the passage of intestinal content. Any additional specific biochemical and physical effects of exercise have not received adequate study.

Conclusion

The above recommendations mainly address effects that at the cellular and tissue level reflect promoting actions. Research has demonstrated the production of genotoxic carcinogens specific for the colon by frying or broiling meats and fish, and means of inhibiting their formation have been developed. More research is necessary, however, to outline the role of carcinogens formed during cooking in the overall scheme leading to colon cancer.

On the basis of reasonably secure present knowledge, the risk for distal colon cancer could be reduced by a fat intake of no more than 25% of calories; by selecting fats such as olive or fish oils that present lower risk; by the intake of adequate amounts of bran fiber in whole grain breads and cereals to secure a stool bulk of about 200 g; by the regular intake of low-fat milk or yogurt as a source of calcium ions; by the consistent consumption of fruits and vegetables, including complex carbohydrates, and by regular exercise to assist in intestinal motility and weight control (Tables 2 and 3).

Table 2. Recommendations for probable lower risk life styles for colon and rectal cancer

Action	Mechanisms
1. Regular exercise	Increased intestinal motility
2. Lower total fat intake (20%–25% of calories)	Lower total bile acid and fatty acid flux with promoting and cytotoxic actions
3. Increase proportion of monounsaturated fats (olive oil, special rapeseed oils)	Lower total bile acid flux
4. Increase intake of fish and fish oils	Protective effect of omega-3 fatty acids (prostaglandin synthetases and metabolism)
5. Have optimal intake of bran cereals, whole grain bread, unrefined rice	Avoids constipation, nonneoplastic intestinal diseases antecedent to neoplasia. Optimal amount gives daily stool of about 200 g
6. Have optimal intake of yellow-green and brassica vegetables (cauliflower, Brussels sprouts, broccoli)	Specific mechanisms not clear, provides micronutrients and bulk, replacing harmful, more energy-dense foods
7. Have optimal intake of calcium-rich foods (some vegetables, but especially low- or no-fat yogurt or milk)	Controls intestinal cell duplication rates
8. Avoid excessive intake of alcoholic beverages	Lower cell turnover rates in rectum
9. Lower intake of highly fried or broiled, browned foods	Possible lower intake of intestine-specific carcinogens

Table 3. Some practical life style and dietary recommendations

Avoid	Use
White bread	Whole grain bread
Baked goods with refined flour	Baked goods made with whole grains
Low-fiber cereals	Bran breakfast cereals; wheat, oat, corn bran cooked cereals
White rice	Brown, unrefined rice
Peeled fruits	Fruits with peels
French fried potatoes	Baked potatoes with skin
Vegetables with butter or fatty sauces	Steamed or microwaved vegetables
Whole milk or cream	Low-fat or skimmed milk
Ice cream	Ice milk or frozen low-fat yogurt
Sour cream	Low-fat yogurt
Most cheeses	Low-fat, low-salt cheeses
Oil, mayonnaise or fatty dressings	Tomato sauce, lemon juice, low-fat yogurt, herbs
Fatty meats and poultry, frankfurters, most sausages	Lean cuts of beef, pork, lamb, veal; chicken or turkey without skin; fish (broiled, baked, or microwaved)
Most cakes, pastries, pies	Fresh fruits

The United States National Cancer Institute program in cancer prevention and control has summarized certain of these recommendations (Greenwald et al. 1987). Other countries with a high incidence of colon cancer may benefit from a systematic, deliberate application of such recommendations not only to their healthy population beginning at young ages as a means of primary prevention but also to "cured" patients as a possible scheme to prevent recurrences.

Acknowledgement. Research by the author is supported by USPHS grants CA-24217, CA-42381, and CA-45720 from the National Cancer Institute.

References

Appel KE, Hildebrandt AG (eds) Tumorpromotoren. Iga Schriften 6. MMV Medizin, München

Berenblum I (1974) Carcinogenesis as a biological problem. Frontiers of biology, vol 34. North-Holland, Amsterdam

Bird RP, Medline A, Furrer R, Bruce WR (1985) Toxicity of orally administered fat to the colonic epithelium of mice. Carcinogenesis 6:1063–1066

Block G, Lanza E (1987) Dietary fiber sources in the United States by demographic group. JNCI 79:83–91

Boyle P, Zaridze DG, Smans M (1985) Descriptive epidemiology of colorectal cancer. Int J Cancer 36:9–18

Bruce WR (1987) Recent hypotheses for the origin of colon cancer. Cancer Res 47:4237–4242

Buset M, Lipkin M, Winawer S, Swaroop S, Friedman E (1986) Inhibition of human colonic epithelia cell proliferation in vivo and in vitro by calcium. Cancer Res 46:5426–5430

Butcher D, Hassanein K, Dudgeon M, Rhodes J, Holmes FF (1985) Female gender is a major determinant of changing subsite distribution of colorectal cancer with age. Cancer 56:714–716

Butterworth BE, Slaga TJ (eds) (1987) Nongenotoxic mechanisms in carcinogenesis. Banbury Report No. 25 Cold Spring Harbor, NY

Byers T, Graham S (1984) The epidemiology of diet and cancer. Adv Cancer Res 41:1–69

Calvert RJ, Klurfeld DM, Subramanian S, Vahouny GV, Kritchevsky D (1987) Reduction of colonic carcinogenesis by wheat bran independent of fecal bile acid concentration. J Natl Cancer Inst 79:875–880

Consensus Conference (1985) Lowering blood cholesterol to prevent heart disease. JAMA 253:2080–2086

Curren RD, Putman DL, Yang LL, Haworth SR, Lawlor TE, Plummer SM, Harris CC (1987) Genotoxicity of fecapentaene-12 in bacterial and mammalian cell assay systems. Carcinogenesis 8:349–352

Deschner EE, Long FC, Hakissian M, Cupo SH (1984) Differential susceptibility of inbred mouse strains forecast by acute colonic proliferative response to methylazoxymethanol. J Natl Cancer Inst 72:195–198

Devesa SS, Silverman DT, Young JL, Pollack ES, Brown CC, Horm JW, Percy CL, Myers MH, McKay FW, Fraumeni JF (1987) Cancer incidence and mortality trends among whites in the United States. JNCI 79:701–770

Faivre J, Boutron MC, Hillon P, Bedenne L, Klepping C (1985) Epidemiology of colorectal cancer. In: Joossens JV, Hill MJ, Geboers J (eds) Diet and human carcinogenesis. Excerpta Medica, Amsterdam, p 123

Garfinkel L (1986) Overweight and mortality. Cancer 58:1826–1829

Garland C, Shekelle RB, Barrett-Connor E, Criqui MH, Rossof AH, Paul O (1985) Dietary vitamin D and calcium and risk of colorectal cancer: a 19-year prospective study in men. Lancet 1:307–309

Graham S (1986) Hypotheses regarding caloric intake in cancer development. Cancer 58:1814–1817

Greenwald P, Cullen JW, McKenna JW (1987) Cancer prevention and control: from research through applications. JNCI 79:389–400

Gupta I, Baptista J, Bruce WR, Che CT, Furrer R, Gingerich JS, Grey AA, Marai L, Yates P, Krepinsky JJ (1983) Structures of fecapentaenes, the mutagens of bacterial origin isolated from human feces. Biochemistry 22:241–245

Gupta I, Suzuki K, Bruce WR, Krepinsky JJ, Yates P (1984) A model study of fecapentaene: mutagens of bacterial origin with alkylating properties. Science 225:521–523

Hecht SS, LaVoie EJ (1981) Analysis of feces for benz(a)pyrene after consumption of charcoal-broiled beef. In: Bruce WR, Correa P, Lipkin M, Tannenbaum SR, Wilkins TO (eds) Gastrointestinal cancer: endogenous factors. Banbury report, no 7. Cold Spring Harbor, NY, pp 381–391

Hinzman MJ, Novotny C, Ullah A, Shamsuddin AM (1987) Fecal mutagen fecapentaene-12 damages mammalian colon epithelial DNA. Carcinogenesis 8:1475–1479

Hirai N, Kingston DGI, Van Tassell RL, Wilkins TD (1982) Structure elucidation of a potent mutagen from human feces. J Am Chem Soc 104:6149–6150

Hirayama T (1985) Diet and cancer: feasibility and importance of prospective cohort study. In: Joosens JV, Hill MJ, Geboers J (eds) Diet and human carcinogenesis. Excerpta Medica, Amsterdam, pp 191–198

Howson CP, Hiyama T, Wynder EL (1985) Is the shift towards right-sided colon cancer in the United States abating? Prev Med 15:192–194

Ip C, Birt DF, Rogers AE, Mettlin C (eds) (1986) Dietary fat and cancer. Progress in clinical and biological research, vol 222. Liss, New York

Jansson B (1985) Geographic mappings of colorectal cancer rates: a retrospect of studies, 1974–1984. Cancer Detect Prev 8:341–348

Jenkins DJA, Jenkins AL, Rao AV, Thompson LU (1987) Starchy foods, type of fiber, and cancer risk. Prev Med 16:545–553

Jensen OM (1984) Different age and sex relationship for cancer of subsites of the large bowel. Br J Cancer 50:825–829

Jensen OM (1985) The role of diet in colorectal cancer. In: Joossens JV, Hill MJ, Geboers J (eds) Diet and human carcinogenesis. Excerpta Medica, Amsterdam, p 137

Jensen OM, MacLennan R, Wahrendorf J (1982) Diet, bowel function, fecal characteristics, and large bowel cancer in Denmark and Finland. Nutr Cancer 4:5–19

Jones RC, Weisburger JH (1988) L-Tryptophan inhibits formation of mutagens during cooking of meat and in laboratory models. Mutat Res 206:343–349

Joossens JV, Geboers J (1985) Diet, cancer, and other diseases. In: Joossens JV, Hill MJ, Geboers J (eds) Diet and human carcinogenesis. Excerpta Medica, Amsterdam, p 277

Kabat GC, Howson CP, Wynder EL (1986) Beer consumption and rectal cancer. Int J Epidemiol 15:494–501

Knudson I (ed) (1986) Genetic toxicology of the diet. Progress in clinical and biological research, vol 206. Liss, New York

Levander OA (1987) A global view of human selenium nutrition. Ann Rev Nutr 7:227–250

LaVecchia C, Negri E, DeCarli A, D'Avanzo B, Gentile A, Franceschi S (1988) A case-control study of diet and colo-rectal cancer in northern Italy. Int J Cancer 41:492–498

Lipkin M (1988) Biomarkers of increased susceptibility to gatrointestinal cancer: new application to studies of cancer prevention in human subjects. Cancer Res 48:235–245

Lipkin M, Uehara K, Winawer S, Sanchez A, Bauer C, Phillips R, Lynch HT, Blattner WA, Fraumeni JF (1985) Seventh-Day Adventist vegetarians have a quiescent proliferative activity in colonic mucosa. Cancer Lett 26:139–144

Lyon JL, Mahoney AW, West DW, Gardner JW, Smith KR, Sorenson AW, Stanish W (1987) Energy intake: its relationship to colon cancer risk. J Natl Cancer Inst 78:853–861

Morson BC, Bussey HJR, Day DW, Hill MJ (1983) Adenomas of large bowel. Cancer Surv 2:451–477

Netscher DT, Larson GM (1983) Colon cancer: the left to right shift and its implications. Surg Gastroenterol 2:13–18

Pence BC, Buddingh F (1988) Inhibition of dietary fat-promoted colon carcinogenesis in rats by supplemental calcium or vitamin D. Carcinogenesis 9:187–190

Ponz de Leon M, Roncucci L, DiDonato P, Tassi L, Smerieri O, Amorico MG, Malagoli G, DeMaria D, Antonioli A, Chahin NJ, Perini M, Rigo G, Barberini G, Manenti A, Biasco G, Barbara L (1988) Pattern of epithelial cell proliferation in colorectal mucosa of normal subjects and of patients with adenomatous polyps or cancer of the large bowel. Cancer Res 48:4121–4126

Reddy BS (1986) Diet and colon cancer: evidence from human and animal model studies. In: Reddy BS, Cohen LA (eds) Diet, nutrition, and cancer: a critical evaluation, vol I. CRC, Boca Raton, pp 47–65

Reddy BS, Cohen LA, McCoy D, Hill P, Weisburger JH, Wynder EL (1980) Nutrition and its relationship to cancer. Adv Cancer Res 32:237–245

Seitz HK, Simanowski UA (1987) Metabolic and nutritional effects of ethanol. In: Hathcock JN (ed) Nutritional toxicology, vol II. Academic, New York

Simanowski UA, Seitz HK, Baier B, Kommerell B, Schmidt-Gayk H, Wright NA (1986) Chronic ethanol consumption selectively stimulates rectal cell proliferation in the rat. Gut 27:278–282

Simopoulos A (ed) (1987) Diet and health: scientific concepts and principles. Am J Clin Nutr 45 (suppl):1015–1410

Slaga TJ, Montesano R (eds) (1983) Tumour promotion and human cancer. Cancer Surv 2:519–621

Stadler J, Yeung KS, Furrer R, Marcon N, Himal HS, Bruce WR (1988) Proliferative activity of rectal mucosa and soluble fecal bile acids in patients with normal colons and in patients with colonic polyps or cancer. Cancer Lett 38:315–320

Sugimura T (1985) Carcinogenicity of mutagenic heterocyclic amines formed during the cooking process. Mutat Res 15:33–41

Tajima K, Hirose K, Nakagawa N, Kuroshishi T, Tominaga S (1985) Urban-rural differences in the trend of colo-rectal cancer mortality with special reference to the subsites of colon cancer in Japan. Jpn J Cancer Res (Gann) 76:717–728

Thomas DB, Karagas MR (1987) Cancer in first and second generation Americans. Cancer Res 47:5771–5776

Vuolo LL, Schuessler GJ (1985) Review: putative mutagens and carcinogens in foods. VI. Protein pyrolysate products. Environ Mutagen 7:577–598

Wang CX, Watanabe K, Weisburger JH, Williams GM (1985) Induction of colon cancer in inbred Syrian hamsters by intrarectal administration of benzo[a]pyrene, 3-methylcholanthrene and N-methyl-N-nitrosourea. Cancer Lett 27:309–314

Wattenberg LW (1985) Inhibitors of carcinogenesis and their implication for cancer prevention in humans. In: Joosseens JV, Hill MJ, Geboers J (eds) Diet and human carcinogenesis. Excerpta Medica, Amsterdam, p 49

Weisburger JH (1987) On the mechanisms relevant to nutritional carcinogenesis. Prev Med 16:586–591

Weisburger JH, Wynder EL (1987) Etiology of colorectal cancer with emphasis on mechanism of action. In: DeVita VT, Hellman S, Rosenberg SA (eds) Important advances in oncology. Lippincott, Philadelphia, p 197

Wilkins TD, Lederman M, Van Tassell RL (1981) Isolation of a mutagen produced in the human colon by bacterial action. In: Bruce WR, Lipkin M, Tannenbaum SR, Wilkins TO (eds) Gastrointestinal cancer endogenous factors. Banbury report no 7. Cold Spring Harbor, NY, pp 205–214

Wilpart M, Roberfroid M (1987) Intestinal carcinogenesis and dietary fibers: the influence of cellulose, or fybagel chronically given after exposure to DMH. Nutr Cancer 10:39–51

Wu AH, Paganini-Hill A, Ross RK, Henderson BE (1987) Alcohol, physical activity and other risk factors for colorectal cancer: a prospective study. Br J Cancer 55:687–694

Wynder EL, Field F, Haley NJ (1986) Population screening for cholesterol determination; a pilot study. JAMA 256:2839–2842

Subject Index

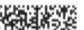